MAINE'S PREMIER MEDICAL COMMUNITY

Physician Inspired Stories of Innovation and Excellence

Created and Produced by
Stuart G. Gilbert MD

Editors
Stuart G. Gilbert MD
Stephen R. Blattner MD MBA
Roger T. Pezzuti MD
Tracey F. Weisberg MD

Dedication

To the founding physicians of our medical community who recruited us, inspired us, and by their example, established a culture of excellence in patient care. Their vision, hard work, and high standards established the foundation for the present day success of Portland's physicians and medical center.

TABLE OF CONTENTS

Organizations

Foreign Medical Missions

PROLOGUE

Beginning in about 1950 a remarkable transition in the medical community of Portland, Maine began to take place. What started out as a private practice based medical community comprised primarily of general practitioners, internists, and general surgeons had evolved by the turn of millennium to become a world class professional community with primary care specialists as well as a level of subspecialist depth matching or exceeding that of most academic medical centers.

What makes this transition truly noteworthy is that it occurred in a small northern New England city lacking a large population or extensive wealth and resources. Portland's major hospital had not even been constituted into its modern form until the mid 1950's when Maine General Hospital, Portland Children's Hospital and the Maine Eye and Ear Infirmary came together to form the Maine Medical Center (MMC).

This book was conceived to document the critical role played by physicians, largely as owners of their own small businesses, in the creation of the sophisticated and highly functional medical community we know today and to ensure the story of this now aging generation is not overlooked. Although the role of the hospital in supporting the aspirations of its primarily voluntary medical staff during this period should be noted, it was primarily the creativity and entrepreneurial spirit of the physicians that spearheaded this remarkable transition. Indeed progress was at times made despite budgetary or other barriers imposed by the hospital and the state. In the end, with support from hospital administrations, Boards, and a generous community, both a vibrant medical community and an outstanding medical center resulted.

From the late 1970's through the 1990's the medical staff at MMC doubled in size as many well trained subspecialists came to Portland with the training, experience, energy, work ethic, and business sense to transform the medical community into the clinical powerhouse that currently exists. The initial investment, risk, and personal effort required to recruit the best available subspecialists from academic centers to Portland and the responsibility to support their salaries during their early years was borne almost exclusively by the physicians and their private practices.

This book is a compilation of 36 chapters that represent individual narratives told through the eyes of the participants in each story. The chapters trace the development of many of Portland's medical specialties, group practices, departments and other entities that together make this an outstanding medical community that also forms the medical staff of MMC. Each chapter is authored by one or more key physicians who played a role in this evolution. We have imposed relatively little editorial discipline, respecting the principle of letting each spokesperson tell the story through his or her eyes. As a result, the chapters vary considerably in style, yet each documents the spirit, energy, collegiality, and generosity of practicing physicians as key elements in the successful creation of this unique medical community.

Since the year 2000, physicians coming to this and most other communities have increasingly been recruited into large corporate or hospital owned practices. This is because health care has become a far more complex industry, with success requiring larger than ever capital outlays for facilities, equipment, information systems and support personnel. We believe that physicians, who are centered on caring for patients, should continue to have a significant role in management decisions in the future. Our book documents what physicians can and have accomplished. We hope that the awareness of these contributions will influence administrators and physicians to coordinate their efforts and responsibilities for the good of our patients, the community, and the medical system as a whole.

Editors' Note

The editors wish to acknowledge at the outset that this book does not include the story of every physician or organization that has been important to the medical community in Portland Maine. Many highly respected individuals, specialties and entities have made significant contributions but have not, for varying reasons, been included. This is not intended to diminish the significance of their work in any way. It simply reflects the realities the editors faced in gathering a sufficient number of authors able to create chapters in representative clinical and service areas. In the end, we wanted to tell the overall story in a meaningful way while at the same time keeping the book manageable in length.

DEPARTMENT OF ANESTHESIOLOGY AND PERIOPERATIVE MEDICINE

By Thomas VerLee MD, Norman Wilson MD and Richard Flowerdew MD

Introduction

In 1948, following the lead of nearby Boston hospitals, Maine Medical Center hired its first fulltime Board Certified Anesthesiologist,[1] John Lincoln MD who trained at Yale University. He was soon joined by Elio Baldini MD and Howard Sawyer MD[2]. These three anesthesiologists formed the core of the newly established MMC Department of Anesthesiology. They assumed supervision of Nurse Anesthetists and in the 1950's established an Anesthesiology Residency to train physicians in this evolving specialty.

Nidus for Growth

Proverbs 13:20 says: "Walk with the wise, and you will become wise…". A corollary to this sage advice has been extrapolated and exported to academic medicine: "Quality physicians attract quality physicians". Over the course of the next several decades, the complexity and sophistication of surgical services demanded parallel growth in the skills of anesthesia administration. It was easy to attract quality physicians to MMC because of the excellence of its staff and the progressive attitude of the institution. It didn't hurt that the community of Portland was at the same time becoming an attractive place to raise a family. In 1974 Kate Sewall MD[3] became the first fellowship-trained anesthesiologist at MMC, with specialized skills in pediatric anesthesiology. The cardiac surgery program initiated by Chris Lutes MD and Richard White MD in 1969[4] experienced exponential growth. In response, several fellowship-trained cardiac anesthesiologists joined the staff. Increased surgical volumes in orthopedics and neurosurgery, a budding transplant program, as well as changes in the delivery of obstetrical care, demanded fellowship-trained quality in anesthesiology as well. Skilled graduates from highly respected universities were attracted to MMC's Department of Anesthesiology because they wanted to work in a climate of medical excellence that also offered a community of educational and cultural distinction. Resident graduates who desired to continue their careers at MMC were required to complete a year or more of fellowship training at a major university before applying for a staff position.

Anesthesiology

The Department of Anesthesiology at MMC was also distinguished from other departments at institutions around the country because of its operating principles. Each member of the Department, regardless of academic credentials, was equal to the others. Compensation, call responsibilities, and benefits were always shared among the physician staff, including the Chief. When a person brought new skills to the Department, it was expected that he/she would share and teach those skills, raising the level of excellence of the entire group. At meetings, everyone had an equal voice.

The Chief of the Department of Anesthesiology fulfilled several roles within the group. He/she was:

- The director for the delivery of anesthesia services throughout the hospital;

- The face and spokesperson for the Department at medical staff meetings, with Chiefs of other departments, planning boards, and with the Chief CRNA;

- The Department's chief administrator, tracking clinical statistics, documentation, reporting requirements, safety practices, privileging, etc.; and

- The convener of group staff meetings.

At the same time, the Chief was expected to carry a proportionate share of the clinical care and call responsibilities. The Department of Anesthesiology has been fortunate to have strong, visionary Chiefs throughout its history.

Chief	Year
John Lincoln MD	1948-1971
Howard Sawyer MD	1971-75
Philip Villandry MD	1975-1979
Donald Klopp MD	1979-1988
Norman Wilson MD	1989
Theodor Rintel MD	1989-91
Kenneth Raessler MD	1991-2003
John Allyn MD	2003-2017
R. David Waters MD	2017-

Anesthesiology and Patient Safety

Before the 1980's undergoing anesthesia for surgery presented several significant risks to the patient.[5] Common risks at that time included airway difficulties, undiagnosed hypoxia with resultant brain damage, unanticipated hypotension with resultant organ failure, and equipment failure. The incidence of significant problems at that time was about 2 in 10,000 cases. Tolerable if you needed the surgery, perhaps not so much if the surgery was elective.

Anesthesiologists have a long history of interest in improving patient safety. From the early days of the specialty, they have faithfully documented patient care management in the form of a real-time patient record. Retrospective analysis of this data has long been used as a tool (the weekly case conference) to learn from historical problems and situations.

Three key developments in the 1980's led to dramatic, effective, and indisputable improvement in patient safety when undergoing anesthesia.

I. Pulse Oximetry

The Pulse Oximeter was introduced clinically in 1985. It offered real-time beat-to-beat determination of a patient's hemoglobin oxygen saturation, far more quickly and reliably than a visual assessment, all with a simple non-invasive clip on the fingertip. Anesthesiologists quickly found the instrument to be exceptionally valuable in avoiding hypoxic episodes. Oximetry was also helpful as a heart rate monitor. No other technology has moved so quickly from introduction to being a standard of care.[6]

II. Standards for Basic Patient Monitoring Under Anesthesia (Harvard)

In the mid-80's a Harvard committee[7] studied the causes of anesthesia accidents. This analysis led to the first standards of practice for minimum intraoperative monitoring, a strategy for preventing anesthesia accidents. In 1986, the American Society of Anesthesiologists adopted these in an expanded form as a national standard. This was a landmark step for a medical professional society which epitomized the lead role taken by anesthesiology in the nascent patient safety movement.

III. The American Society of Anesthesiologists (ASA) Closed Claims Project:

Analysis of Poor Outcomes

In 1984, there was little comprehensive information on the scope and cause of anesthetic injury in the United States. Because significant anesthesia injury is a relatively rare occurrence, it is difficult to study prospectively or by retrospective medical record review, even from multiple institutions.

The study of insurance company closed claims provided a cost-effective approach to data collection. Extensive data on injuries that occurred in many different institutions were collected in a centralized location. Typically, a closed claim file consisted of the hospital record, the anesthesia record, narrative statements of the involved healthcare personnel, expert and peer reviews, deposition summaries, outcome reports, and the cost of settlement or jury awards. These files provided a concentrated collection of information on the relatively rare events leading to anesthesia-related injury.

The ASA Closed Claims Project identified several major areas of anesthesia-related patient injury. These data were used to design strategies to improve patient safety[8] .

With technology, standardization of monitoring, and analysis of accident causes, the frequency of death or serious injury from anesthesia steadily, and dramatically, declined from 1:5000 in 1970 to 1:200,000-300,000 in 1995.

Demand for Anesthesia Services Outside the OR

As the delivery of anesthesia care became safer and more acceptable to patients, demand for services expanded outside the operating room. Certain radiologic procedures were best done with patients anesthetized or heavily sedated. Urologic procedures like lithotripsy required anesthesia to be administered in a semi-trailer in the hospital parking lot. Children needing diagnostic MRI required anesthesia in a high-intensity magnetic field. Sophisticated endoscopic procedures required anesthesia in a dark room. Many heart catheterization and ablation procedures required the patient to be motionless for hours. MMC anesthesiologists soon found themselves deployed through all levels of the hospital to provide anesthesia care.

Free-Standing Day Surgery Centers and Peripheral Hospitals

The first private free-standing surgery center in Maine was established by plastic surgeon Jean Labelle MD and colleagues in1987. Ophthalmology groups soon followed. In 1989 Orthopedic Associates opened a multi-OR complex primarily for arthroscopic surgery. These early centers were initially single-specialty clinics. MMC anesthesiologists were invited to provide care at all these centers. A few years later MMC merged with the Brighton Medical Center and made it a multi-specialty surgical center. In 2010 MMC opened the ten OR Scarborough Surgery Center.

Because of clinical excellence and administrative expertise, other hospitals around Maine looked to MMC and its private practice group of Spectrum anesthesiologists to provide coverage and care to their patients. Stephens Memorial Hospital in Norway in 1997, then SMMC in Biddeford in 1999, were added to the practice roster. In the 21st century similar requests came from MidCoast Hospital in Brunswick, Miles Hospital in Damariscotta, and in 2008, the Mercy Hospital in Portland.

To meet the demand for this kind of growth, the Department grew from 13 anesthesiologists in 1982, to 55 in 2015.

Critical Care Medicine and Anesthesiology

Anesthesiologists were among the first critical care medicine (CCM) specialists. It was a logical path, as their experience in the anesthesia recovery room (now called PACU, for Post-Anesthesia-Care-Unit) could easily be translated into longer term critical care. Critical care units at university hospitals in the US, especially those emphasizing post-surgical care and trauma, were usually staffed by anesthesiologists.

Historically MMC was not a university hospital, but a community/regional hospital, and adopted a different model. Critical care staffing was primarily provided by pulmonologists, with anesthesiologists acting as consultants for airway management and certain procedures.

Nevertheless, anesthesiologist-CCM physicians frequently brought a different perspective to critical care. Their participation was seen as valuable and important. In 1988 Carol Dean MD was the first anesthesiologist-trained and Board Certified in CCM physician to join the MMC staff. She allocated 12 weeks annually to CCM, with the remainder dedicated to OR responsibilities. Dr. Dean was later joined by Kolleen Dougherty MD, and William Swartz MD. With the development of a new Trauma-Surgical ICU, three additional anesthesiologist-CCM physicians joined the staff for a total of six by 2017. Although part of their role was to satisfy training requirements for resident anesthesiologists, these anesthesiologist-CCM physicians viewed themselves as being multi-disciplinary, and integral to the teaching of residents of all specialties who rotated through these units.

In addition W. Daniel Kovarik MD, Division Director of Pediatric Anesthesiology, was also a Board Certified pediatric intensivist who provided staff coverage in the Neonatal and Pediatric Intensive Care Units.

Obstetrical Analgesia, Post-Op Pain Management and the Anesthesia Pain Management Service (APMS)

The administration of local anesthesia via an epidural catheter in the lumbar spine was infrequently used as early as 1940 to provide analgesia for labor and delivery. In the 1970's, the introduction of new and safer local anesthetics, better understanding of side effects, and improved monitoring, led to a dramatic increase in the use of epidural analgesia for labor. Childbirth moved from a "natural" process to a highly managed one. Intermittent boluses of a local anesthetic were administered during the first and second stages of labor. By the 1980's, the use of continuous infusions of dilute local anesthetics became common practice for labor analgesia. After delivery, the epidural catheter was removed. It was rare to leave an epidural in place longer than 18-24 hours.

On July 13, 1985, President Ronald Reagan underwent a right hemicolectomy for colon cancer at Bethesda Naval Hospital. Henry F. Nicodemus MD,[9] then Chief of Anesthesiology, placed an epidural catheter preoperatively, and infused morphine and a local anesthetic to provide post-surgical analgesia. The goal was to reduce or eliminate the need for a parenteral narcotic with its potential for sedation and confusion. Just three hours after surgery, in the Recovery Room, President Reagan declared he felt "fit as a fiddle" and promptly resumed his role as President under the 25th Amendment. He was discharged home six days later.

That news spread quickly. Anesthesiologists around the country, including those at MMC, promptly extended the epidural concept into the surgical world. The epidural catheter could remain in place not for just hours, but days, with medication delivered continuously by a small pump. Post-op pain was better controlled, without side effects like sedation. Patients were pleased, and surgeons were impressed.

Initially these epidural patients at MMC remained in PACU for several days for management. They were transferred to special rooms on R3 or SCU.

At about this same time the concept of patient-controlled analgesia (PCA) was introduced. Using a special electronic pump with programmed lockouts to prevent overdose, patients could self-administer potent analgesics on their own schedule, without waiting for a nurse. This was a radical concept for many floor nurses at the time, initially meeting significant resistance.

Anesthesiologist Norman Wilson MD recognized the importance of these new modalities of pain management and the potential they had to dramatically improve patient comfort after surgery. He also realized that education of medical staff, physicians, nurses, and pharmacists was critical to the success of these programs. In 1990, Dr. Wilson recruited Robyn Dixon RN, an experienced and respected PACU nurse with outstanding relational and problem-solving skills. Together they developed the MMC Anesthesia Pain Management Service (APMS).

To quote Robyn Dixon:[10]

> *"We spent the majority of our time developing the infrastructure of the service, writing policies and vetting them through the seemingly endless approval committees and creating order sets. Many hours were spent in outreach and establishing relationships with other departments and their leadership and with educating the medical, nursing and pharmacy staff. This resulted in an improved understanding and trust on the part of those outside the department. Gradually the acceptance of these techniques, the twenty four hour support of the anesthesia staff via the APMS pager, and the recognition of the benefit the APMS provided patients led to a loosening of nursing department restrictions. PCAs and epidural catheters became widely accepted across all units including Pediatrics/NICU.*

> *With eventual universal acceptance by patients and medical staff, the APMS steadily grew to become a busy service providing acute pain management and consultative services to a wide variety of patients. The involvement of the service in the management of malignant pain and the use of tunneled intrathecal (IT) catheters for end stage oncology patients was one of the most personally rewarding developments during my time with the service. We were able to extend our care into the home as these patients were able to achieve adequate analgesia allowing them to be discharged with the IT catheter and spend their last days at home, in comfort, with their families."*

Due in part to this expanding expertise in management of both acute and chronic pain, in the mid 90's the Department was renamed the Maine Medical Center Department of Anesthesiology and Pain Management.

Growth of Regional Anesthesia and Integration into Practice

Local anesthetic drugs have a long history of clinical use by anesthesiologists, surgeons, and dentists.[11] Anesthesiologists trained in the 20th century generally received training in basic peripheral nerve blocks. However, peripheral nerve blocks were not widely utilized for a number of reasons:

- Short duration of action;

- Side effects of the drugs;

- Difficulty in placement, nerve injury, and incomplete results;

- Poor patient acceptance; and

- Extra time required for placement.

Nevertheless, some anesthesiologists maintained a keen interest in developing and perfecting clinical expertise with regional anesthesia techniques.

The advances in postoperative pain management initiated by epidural analgesia (cited above) were recognized and soon extended to peripheral nerve blocks. Charles Higgins MD was an early advocate and leader in this field. When portable ultrasonography was introduced around 2001 many of the objections to peripheral nerve block placement were minimized. With direct visualization of anatomic structures success rates dramatically improved with a concurrent reduction in complications and placement time. Patients awakened from anesthesia with minimal pain and lack of sedation.

Dr. Higgins was eager to teach these techniques to anesthesiology residents, and to provide this service on a broad scale to patients. In 2002 he established the Regional Block Program to provide this service perioperatively to MMC surgical patients. Today over 30% of all surgical patients receive a local anesthetic drug and technique as part of their care.

Documentation and Analysis of Patient Outcomes

Anesthesiologists have always carefully maintained a real-time record of intraoperative management of each patient – charting monitors and vital signs, drug administration, airway management, and a host of other parameters. Until recently, these records were handwritten which made it difficult to group and analyze them collectively.

As early as 1986 the MMC Anesthesiology Department began collecting general patient case data which was manually entered for subsequent computer tabulation.[13] Compliance and consistency with data entry was significantly improved in 1998 when computerized scanning and collation were adopted. At about the same time data collection was extended to the PACU. For the first time it became possible to accurately track the incidence of common events related to anesthesia. Coupled with intraoperative data, this has become a powerful tool to help document the incidence of problems like postoperative nausea and vomiting, residual neuromuscular blockade, post-dural puncture headache, hypothermia, and sentinel events. Craig Curry MD was an early leader and persistent champion of this new technology, using this data and analysis to help shape Departmental protocols and practices. Dr. Curry and the Spectrum Medical Group were pioneers in this quality assurance process. Together they developed and refined these methods to the point of successfully marketing their product to other anesthesia practices around the nation.[14]

Standardization of Care and Protocols

In the past, success or difficulty in management of a particular anesthetic procedure was easily shared with what was a small number of anesthesia colleagues. A notebook of guidelines for anesthesia management of particular types of cases was kept in each operating room. These guidelines served as reminders to ensure that particular steps occurred in conformity with Departmental standards and practice. Drugs were administered at certain times, specific monitors were placed, and surgeon preferences were acknowledged.

As the Department grew, and the number of anesthetizing locations multiplied, tools like notebooks (above) became more difficult to maintain and update. Changes did not always get communicated. At the same time, surgeons expected consistency in management of their patients. They assumed that any change in their preferences would automatically be shared with all other anesthesiologists.

In the mid-90's, handheld electronic pocket organizers like the Palm Pilot[15] became available. These devices were quickly adopted by many anesthesiologists. For the first time notes on case management could not only be quickly and legibly updated, but shared almost instantly with colleagues. Groups of anesthesiologists could often be seen in hallways, "beaming" information back and forth between themselves.

Later in the 90's, use of the internet grew from simple emails to something we now know as the internet, or world wide web. With a little technical knowledge a web site could be established where information could easily be accessed from any computer, anywhere in the world. This was clearly a major step forward as just one copy of a document or note was necessary. It was easily updated, searched for, and shared quickly by anyone with computer access. Thomas VerLee MD was quick to realize this. In 1998 he established a clinical anesthesia web site for the Department. This practical database organized and made available all Departmental guidelines and patient protocols. Providers could access this information before a case, at home the night before, and even in the operating room. In 1999, Maine Medical Center, University of North Carolina, and Stanford had the only three anesthesiology departments in the nation using this technology[16]. Other centers nationwide soon appreciated its value and developed web sites of their own, modeled after MMC.

Medical Simulation in Teaching and in Practice

As the practice of anesthesiology became progressively and steadily safer, the incidence and frequency of adverse intraoperative events dramatically diminished.

From the patient's perspective, this decrease in adverse events was a positive and important trend in improved outcomes.

From a teaching and experiential viewpoint, however, how doctors responded to a sudden, unexpected, or unplanned intraoperative event had always been used secondarily as a teaching tool. We always asked:

- What happened?

- What was the differential diagnosis?

- How should we have responded?

- What can we do better to predict or avoid this the next time?

Decreased frequency of adverse events meant a corresponding decreased opportunity to learn, albeit on real patients. Such was the conundrum of learning how to handle what were becoming low frequency, high-risk events.

Before beginning his anesthesiology residency at MMC in 1989, J. Randy Darby MD was Chief of Flight Medicine at Reese Air Force Base, Texas. During his tenure there he flew T-37 and T-38 aircraft as part of his joint clinical/operational role. The USAF incorporated flight simulation into the curriculum using state of the art aircraft simulation technology. Part of Dr. Darby's experience was recognizing the strong emphasis by the military aviation community on the use of simulation to train both novice and experienced pilots over the course of their careers. Simulation allowed pilots to repetitively practice the response to in-flight emergencies in a safe, virtual environment.

Dr. Darby saw direct parallels and recognized the possibilities during his anesthesia training at MMC. During subsequent fellowship training in Boston he developed a close liaison with the newly built Boston Anesthesia Simulation Center.[17] The Center supported the consortium of Harvard Anesthesia Programs under the leadership of Jeffery Cooper PhD.[18] On return to MMC as a staff anesthesiologist in 1993, Dr. Darby started taking MMC anesthesiology residents to the Harvard Simulation Center on Saturdays – first in his car and subsequently by van – once every three months. MMC was thus the first non-Harvard hospital in New England to gain access to high fidelity medical simulation and use it on a regular basis. Dr. Darby led this program on behalf of the MMC Anesthesiology Department through 2005.

In 2006, the MMC Department of Medical Education recognized the growing importance of medical simulation. Michael Gibbs MD, Chief of the Department of Emergency Medicine, worked diligently at the Chiefs' level to drive the inclusion of medical simulation in Maine Medical Center's future educational goals. Dr. Darby was enlisted to help lead a team of facility planners, architects, finance and IS/IT staff pulled together inside of MMC to drive the design and development of the project. Funding was approved in 2008 by the Board of Trustees and augmented by a gift from the Hannaford Foundation. In 2010, a new 18,000 sq. ft. state of the art simulation center was completed in the old surgical and recovery room spaces on the Brighton Campus. Dr. Darby was appointed the first Medical Director of the Hannaford Center for Safety, Innovation and Simulation.

As of this writing in 2017, simulation is a core element used during the education of residents in all of MMC's GME programs. New anesthesiology residents undergo two weeks of "Boot Camp" before ever touching a real patient or setting foot in the

OR. By 2017 the anesthesiology residency includes over 140 hours of dedicated practice in the simulation spaces, incorporating a mixture of procedural skills labs, high fidelity OR cases and standardized (actor) patient encounters. Surgeons practice new techniques in the virtual world of the simulation lab before transitioning to the OR. Emergency Medicine and Surgical residents learn trauma skills within a robust ER-centric simulation curriculum working as a team. All of this is done in a safe, state of the art facility. In the near future facilities like the Hannaford Center will be used to train and evaluate the proficiency of all physicians throughout their careers.

Continued Growth and Excellence

As the Maine Medical Center moves into the coming decades, demand for anesthesia and pain management services continues to grow. National healthcare design and policy changes demand new paradigms for patient management of surgery, diagnostic, and therapeutic procedures. Under the leadership of Allen Hayman MD, Maine Medical Center is taking the steps to establish a Perioperative Surgical Home, a patient-centered system that seamlessly guides the continuity of care, from the moment the decision to have surgery is made, all the way through recovery, discharge and beyond. The central idea is not to "clear the patient for surgery" but rather to optimize the patient for surgery based on risk factors and evidence-based protocols. Under this model, each patient will receive the right care, at the right place and the right time.

Standardization of anesthetic/nursing/surgical protocols is a critical component of this concept, with all protocols determined in advance. Similarly, nutrition management, a recovery plan, rescue from medical complications and smooth transition of care are all part of this pathway. The goal is to proactively pursue care redesign strategies and enhance the surgical patient's experience, improve quality and outcomes and reduce costs.

This component of the practice of Anesthesiology has become so central and important to the overall specialty that the Department has again been renamed the MMC Department of Anesthesiology and Perioperative Medicine. The Department, and Spectrum Medical Group, its parent and private practice partner, are committed to the common goal of the best possible patient care in New England.

[1] *Hartford Courant*, 22 August 1988

[2] *Portland Press-Herald*, 10 October 2010

[3] Norman Wilson MD, Personal Communication

[4] *Portland Press-Herald*, 13 June 2007

[5] Institute of Medicine. *To Err Is Human: Building a Safer Health System*. Washington, DC: National Academies Press; 2000:144–145.

[6] *J Anesth Hist*. 2017 Jan;3(1):24-26. doi: 10.1016/j.janh.2016.12.003.

Epub 2016 Dec 21.

[7] *Standards for Basic Anesthesia Monitoring*, American Society of Anesthesiologists, 21 October 1986

[8] Cheney FW . *The American Society of Anesthesiologists Closed Claims Project: what have we learned, how has it affected practice, and how will it affect practice*

in the future? Anesthesiology. 1999; 91(2):552–556

[9] *Newsweek Magazine*, "Doctors You Can't See", 18 November 1985, pp104-106.

[10] Dixon RN Robyn, Personal Communication

[11] Eger II MD, Edmond I, Saidman MD, Lawrence J., Editors, "A History of Regional Anesthesia", *The Wondrous Story of Anesthesia; Springer NY*; pp 859-870

[12] Internal Review Document, MMC Department of Anesthesiology

and Pain Management, July 2003

[13] VerLee MD, Thomas, Personal Communication

[14] Fides Website: http://www.fidesqa.com/

[15] https://en.wikipedia.org/wiki/PalmPilot

[16] Society for Technology in Anesthesia Annual Meeting 2000

[17] https://harvardmedsim.org/

[18] http://www.massgeneral.org/anesthesia/research/researchlab.aspx?id=1537

CARDIAC SURGERY

By Jeremy R. Morton MD

Early Days of Cardiac Surgery at MMC

The modern approach to cardiac disease began in Portland with the establishment of the Surgical Cardiac Diagnostic Clinic in 1951. The Clinic met monthly, staffed by members of cardiology, surgery, pediatrics and radiology, with cardiology consultants visiting from Boston. A cardiac catheterization facility was created shortly thereafter in the old Maine General Building with an image intensifier. In 1953, the first open heart operation in this country using a mechanical heart lung machine, was performed by Dr. John Gibbon in Pennsylvania. Over the next several years, several of the leading academic centers began performing these procedures using one of several improved versions of Dr. Gibbon's device. The early cardiac operations involved correction of relatively simple congenital abnormalities including atrial septal defect and aortic and pulmonic valve stenosis. As techniques improved, ventricular septal defects, pulmonary vein anomalies and Tetralogy of Fallot repairs were included. Patients from Maine were worked up in the Portland Clinic and sent to Boston for surgery. In late 1957, the staff at Maine Medical Center (MMC) decided to establish an open heart surgery program here. Those primarily involved were Dr. Edward Matthews, pediatric cardiologist; Dr. Emerson Drake, surgeon; Drs. Peter Rand and William Austin, both postdoctoral fellows on NIH grants; and Dr. Manu Chatterjee, research associate at MMC. Of the four modifications of the heart lung machine then in use, the team selected the membrane oxygenator model developed by Clowes. (see photograph of HL Machine below). After the machine arrived a team of volunteers spent 15 months experimenting

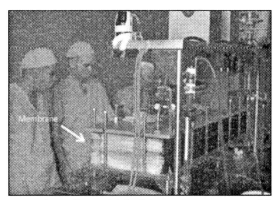

From Archives of Maine Medical Center: Permission granted for use

with, adjusting, and practicing with the system before they were ready to use it on a human. The first patient was operated on in May of 1959. Over the next year, 18 patients underwent open heart surgery without a mortality. Of these, 16 had atrial septal defects, some with associated anomalous pulmonary veins, and 2 had pulmonic stenosis (Rand, et al., JMMA, August, 1961).

The Mark-Clowes heart lung machine with a membrane oxygenator was in use at Maine Medical Center in 1959. Sixteen units of donor blood were needed to prime this heart-lung circuit.

Dr. Drake was the consummate surgeon - energetic, gifted and curious. After he began the cardiac surgery program with these outstanding results, other surgeons were attracted to practice cardiovascular and thoracic surgery in Portland. Drs. Hiebert, Lutes, White, and Morton continued to build the program in the late 1960's and through the 1970's.

Clement A. Hiebert MD grew up in Lewiston, Maine. He completed his medical and surgical training at Harvard followed by a thoracic surgery fellowship in England before returning to Maine and establishing a practice in general and thoracic surgery in 1959. He had a keen mind and boundless energy. He spent much of his free time, when not skiing, inventing better ways of doing things in and out of the operating room. Later in his career, he served as a Director of the American Board of Surgery, as Chief of Staff and then Chief of Surgery at the Maine Medical Center. In 1962, the first aortic valve replacement was performed by Dr. Albert Starr in Portland, Oregon, using a ball-and-cage prosthesis. Dr. Hiebert performed the same operation at MMC later the same year. Dr. Drake was the Chief of Surgery at MMC at the time and had made it clear that no heart surgery would be done by anyone without his permission. As Dr. Hiebert felt that this permission was not likely to be forthcoming, he scheduled the first case when Dr. Drake was on vacation and arranged for Dr. George Sager, a general surgeon, to be his assistant. Fortunately, the surgery went very well and a new hurdle was surmounted.

Chris Lutes MD went to Brown, a year ahead of Dr. Walter Goldfarb, and then to Tufts Medical School. He completed his general surgery residency at Maine Medical Center, then spent two years at Michigan in thoracic and cardiac surgery. He returned to Portland in 1965 to join Drs. Phillip Lape and Ferris Ray in surgical practice. For the first two years in practice he did primarily general and pulmonary surgery as he made preparations to join the cardiac surgery program. In 1966, with updated equipment and techniques, Dr. Lutes brought in a new surgeon Dr. Richard White, to be his assistant. The two began preforming open heart procedures, which were primarily uncomplicated atrial septal defects and aortic and pulmonic valvotomies at first, followed by more complex congenital repairs and adult valve replacements the following year. By 1971, over 100 open heart cases were being done each year with outcomes similar to those of other major cardiac programs

Dr. Jeremy Morton came to MMC in 1971, through a chance encounter with Dr. Hiebert at a surgery meeting in Chicago in 1970. It was his final year of surgical training in Houston and he was looking for a place to practice. Dr. Morton went to medical school at Johns Hopkins and interned there in internal medicine. After a year of surgery training at Hartford Hospital, in 1963, he decided to focus more on the developing field of vascular surgery and moved to Houston to train with Drs. DeBakey and Cooley. He spent the next four years in a rigorous and exciting residency program involving heavy exposure to vascular and trauma surgery. Dr. DeBakey did not believe in limited duty hours, and residents worked every other night usually spending most of each duty night in the operating room. They loved it. Each resident, during his (no women) second year, completed a three-month rotation on Dr. DeBakey's service, managing the surgical intensive care unit, a relatively new concept at the time, and caring for the 8-10 major vascular cases operated upon each day. In order to maximize continuity of care, Dr. DeBakey insisted that the resident on his service remain in the hospital for the entire three months. Dr. Morton's wife and two kids would come each Sunday for lunch and a visit. It was a little harsh but a remarkable learning experience. Dr. Morton's original plan was to extend his residency for another year to include thoracic surgery training, but the year was 1967, the Vietnam war was in full swing, and the army had other plans for him. He spent the next two years as a military surgeon, much of it in a MASH hospital where his trauma surgery training was fully utilized.

While Dr. Morton was in Vietnam, cardiac surgery, which was in its infancy when he left, advanced significantly. He returned to Houston for two more years for thoracic and cardiac training. At this time Dr. Favoloro at the Cleveland Clinic was demonstrating that obstructed coronary arteries could be effectively bypassed with saphenous veins. DeBakey and his associates had been working on the idea of coronary bypass surgery and had done one successful vein bypass procedure in 1965, but did not consider it a feasible procedure at the time. With Favoloro's success, it was immediately apparent that this would launch a major, and much anticipated, advance in cardiac surgery, and Dr. Morton was in the right place at the right time and was trained to do this new procedure, coronary artery bypass grafting, "CABG" surgery.

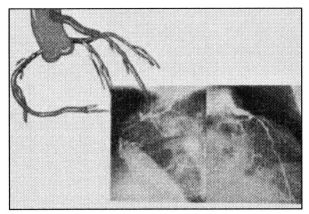

*Images of first coronary artery bypass performed by Doctors Ed Garrett
and Jimmy Howell.
From Methodist Debakey Cardiovasc J. 2015 Jul-Sep; 11(3 Suppl): 5–17.*

Dr. Morton grew up in Massachusetts, spent summers in Maine, and had a strong desire to return to New England and practice vascular and cardiac surgery in a modest-sized, medically active community. When he wrote to Dr. Drake he was assured that there was no room for another cardiovascular surgeon in Portland. He discovered, however, at the meeting in Chicago, that Dr. Hiebert had an interest in having a partner with cardiac surgery training and the following year Dr. Morton arrived in Portland for interviews with Dr. George Maltby, chairman of the Credentials Committee, who mumbled his approval; Douglas Pennoyer, who thought everyone was great; Walter Goldfarb who examined and approved of his sense of humor; and finally, as the ultimate test, he was taken to dinner with Marilyn VanSaun, Dr. Hiebert's private scrub nurse, for her analysis and approval, which he received.

Two years later, in 1971, when he arrived in Portland, he found a young, energetic and forward-thinking group of surgeons, internists and cardiologists who were enthusiastically embracing the latest advances in medicine and surgery. Drs. Lape and Ray and Dillihunt were doing vascular surgery, Drs. Lutes and Hiebert were doing pediatric and adult cardiac surgery, and two nephrologists, Drs. Drewry and Leeber, were to arrive within the year to begin a dialysis, and later, a renal transplant program. Everything seemed to be in motion for him to play his special card and do a CABG operation. The significant obstacle was the lack of a cath lab and cardiology expertise capable of accomplishing the necessary coronary angiograms required to visualize the obstructed arteries.

Eight months later, in March, 1972, Dr. Morton received a referral from a doctor in New Hampshire of a patient with severe angina and a tightly narrowed LAD coronary artery. The patient came with a 35 mm angiogram movie film showing the narrowed coronary artery, but MMC had no projector to observe the films. Dr. Hiebert made an arrangement with the projectionist of a local movie theater in town, open in the middle of the day, to project the films. This was the State Theater which at the time was a local pornography theater. The MMC surgeons and cardiologists sat in the audience amongst the other surprised and perhaps disappointed spectators to prepare themselves for the first coronary bypass operation performed at MMC and in Maine.

Subsequently, a new cath lab was completed and Dr. Cathel McLeod, a cardiologist from Cleveland, joined the medical staff to manage the cath lab and introduce us to the latest techniques in coronary arteriography. Within a few months, the other three thoracic surgeons - Drs. Lutes, White, and Hiebert - had mastered the technique and all were available to absorb the rapidly growing influx of new coronary patients.

Initially, the patients with coronary disease were relatively young and healthy with one or two obstructed arteries and limited diffuse disease. The operations were uncomplicated and the results were excellent. As expected, over time, the patients increased in number and were older, sicker and had more advanced coronary disease requiring more complicated procedures and more advanced post-operative care. The introduction of various methods of arresting, cooling and preserving the heart during the operation, and advances in the technology of the heart-lung machine, made longer and more complicated procedures possible with fewer complications and better results. This wave of new patients and surgical procedures required a significant reallocation and increase in resources, which was met with some resistance from the hospital administration and other specialties at first, but over time, the numbers and potential economic benefit to the hospital justified the cause, and the hospital responded with construction of new operating rooms and intensive care units.

Second Generation MMC Cardiac Surgeons

During this transition, three new cardiac surgeons joined the MMC staff, Edward Nowicki and Joan Tryzelaar joining the Lutes/White practice and Saul Katz, and later, Robert Kramer, joining the Hiebert/Morton practice. Dr. Kramer began his medical career as a family practice physician in Steamboat Springs, Colorado after training in internal medicine and family practice. He then decided to pursue a surgical career and enrolled in the surgery residency at MMC. Intrigued by the blossoming of cardiac surgery here, he went on to complete cardiothoracic surgery training in Toronto and returned to join the MMC program. He became a major contributor to the Northern

New England Cardiovascular Disease Study Group and later succeeded Dr. Morton as Director of the Division of Cardiothoracic Surgery, then as Director of Cardiac Surgery Research and Quality Improvement. In spite of various rearrangements in practice groups, the cardiac surgery program as a whole advanced steadily, eventually becoming as large as any program in New England by volume, performing 1600 cases in 2001.

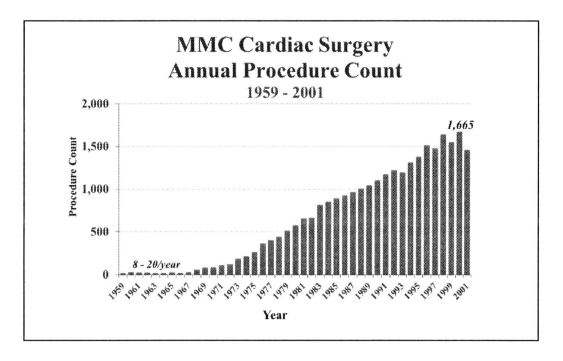

Coronary Angioplasty

In 1977, Dr. Andreas Gruentzig introduced the balloon angioplasty in which many of the obstructing coronary blockages could be expanded using a balloon on the end of a catheter and thus avoiding an operation. This and coronary stenting, which followed a few years later, along with demographic lifestyle changes and statins, significantly diminished the number of patients requiring coronary bypass surgery during the 1980's.

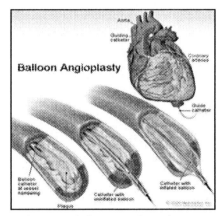

Illustration depicting a balloon angioplasty where a tiny catheter with an integrated balloon is guided into a coronary artery, the balloon positioned into the area of stenosis, inflated, thereby improving blood flow through that segment. This original procedure has subsequently been enhanced by the addition of drug-eluting stents that discourage restenosis of the vessel.
From: MedicineNet.com

Mitral Valve Repair

Concurrent with these developments, Dr. Alain Carpentier from Paris France introduced the technique of surgically repairing certain diseased mitral valves without having to replace them with mechanical valves. Several of our surgeons made the trip to Paris to learn the technique and returned to add it to their skill set here.

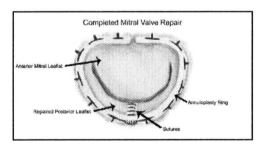

From heartlungdoc.com

Subsequently, Dr. Dominic Paolini, who trained in pediatric cardiac surgery at Boston Children's Hospital joined the staff to reinvigorate the congenital surgery program. A few years later was joined by Dr. Reed Quinn who trained at the Hershey program in Pennsylvania. He was recruited to join the program after completing a fellowship in congenital surgery at Boston Children's Hospital. Shortly after Dr. Quinn's arrival Dr. Paolini left and one of Dr. Quinn's former associates, Dr. Paul Weldner came on, initially to work with Dr. Quinn. During this same period, various implantable devices were being developed to support the failing heart of a patient awaiting a heart transplant or recovering from a severe heart attack or surgical procedure. Both Drs. Quinn and Weldner were trained in the use of these devices as well as transplantation.

Northern New England Cardiovascular Disease Study Group (NNE)

In 1987, when coronary surgery had stimulated the development of many cardiac surgery programs across the country in large community hospitals as well as teaching hospitals, the New York Times published a report using raw data to compare the outcomes of all the cardiac surgery programs in the State of New York. The article disclosed significantly different operative mortality figures among the various hospitals in the state, suggesting a widely variable level of expertise. The immediate response from the medical profession was that certain hospitals, academic centers in particular, were operating on much sicker patients than the other hospitals and that no effort had been made in the article to adjust for this. Dr. Steven Plume, a surgeon and Gerald O'Connor PhD, an epidemiologist from Dartmouth, recognized this as an opportunity to create a risk-adjusted formula which would accurately track the results of various programs and look for strengths and weaknesses. Recognizing the risk that competition among competing centers might interfere with accurate data collection, they decided to include only the four centers from Northern New England, each of which had distinctive referral areas: Dartmouth, Maine Medical Center, Catholic Medical Center in Manchester, and UVM in Burlington. Eastern Maine Medical Center opened their program and joined the group the following year.

The early meetings were largely organizational and included representatives from each institution: Steven Plume and Gerald O'Connor, from Dartmouth, Christopher Maloney and David Charlesworth from Manchester, Jeremy Morton from Portland, Larry Coffin from Burlington and Robert Clough from Bangor. Systems were developed in each hospital for accurate data collection and non-threatening reporting, modeled after W.E. Deming. Data was collected for nearly three years before enough cases were entered to create a prediction rule and test it for accuracy so that subsequent cases could be adjusted for risk and mortality comparisons made appropriately depending on how sick the patients were to begin with. The initial hypothesis was that there would be very little variation in outcomes between centers and among surgeons, once the patients we're adjusted for severity of illness. Surprisingly, it was discovered that although all of the outcomes were acceptable by national standards, there were significant differences between centers and among individual surgeons.

Suddenly, the purpose of NNE changed from demonstrating that all surgeons were above average to eliminating variability among surgeons and centers and thereby improving results overall. By this time, several surgeons from each institution were interested in the project and NNE generated reports showing where each institution and each surgeon stood relative to the others. To avoid embarrassment and reluctance to contribute more data, the data points on the reports were coded such that each surgeon knew only his own code and the code of his institution. Organized teams of surgeons, anesthesiologists and OR nurses from each institution visited each other's centers and observed surgery, looking for ideas and techniques which would improve results at home. These visits proved to be very productive, generated collaboration and companionship and brought the institutions closer together emotionally and cooperatively.

In the early 1990's, as coronary angioplasty evolved, the cardiologists joined the group and added their data and wisdom, greatly increasing the depth and significance of the organization. Over the ensuing 25 years, the NNE has accumulated outcomes and other data on well over 90,000 cases, greatly increasing the power of analyses and leading to numerous publications. The NNE group became a model for the Society of Thoracic Surgeons Database and for a number of other regional outcomes-monitoring and quality improvement initiatives in this country and Canada.

Physician Assistants

In the late 1970's, Dr. John Kirklin, a leading cardiac surgeon and innovator, spent two days at MMC as a visiting professor. He commented that MMC had a good program but that it was inefficient in that we still had two fully trained cardiac surgeons scrubbing on each case. He suggested that hiring a physician assistant trained in cardiac surgery to be a first assistant and to help in the care of the patients before and after surgery would improve efficiency as well as quality of care. The search for the perfect PA was begun by Dr. Morton. Physician assistants represented a relatively new entity in the health care field, growing out of the Vietnam war where a large number of well-trained hospital medics and corpsmen returned to civilian life without employment opportunities which would take advantage of their skills.

The first training program for PAs was started by Dr. Eugene Stead at Duke and by the early 1970s several more sites came on board and a credentialing process was put in place. Initially, the idea was to support the dwindling population of primary care physicians, but soon emergency rooms and specialty surgeons began to realize the value of these well-trained professionals in their practices. There were no PAs at MMC at the time and Dr. Morton was not certain how well the idea would be received. Rather than take the chance of an interminable period of deliberation and discussion amongst the staff and administration, he decided to seek forgiveness rather than permission and found a young, bright and energetic PA, Larry Adrian, at the Geisinger Clinic in Pennsylvania who had trained in Houston and at Maimonides Hospital in New York and was anxious to move to Maine. The deal was closed and he came on board.

Credentialing was challenging. The internists were afraid he would erode their pre-operative consultation volume; the chief nurse announced that she didn't want a PA telling her nurses what to do; the residents were afraid that he would usurp some of the procedures they were accustomed to doing. Nobody thought a PA was qualified to take an adequate history or do a proper physical examination, much less be a first assistant in a heart operation. This was a bit more resistance than Dr. Morton expected and tough start for Larry. Convinced that it would work, Dr. Morton encouraged Larry to stay on and put up with the inertia, which he very willingly did. Because of his skills and very captivating personality, he gradually convinced every one of the enormous added value a PA could bring to patient care. Shortly thereafter, Dr. Lutes hired Barb Heyl, PAC who became equally indispensable. Over the next several years, many more PAs came on staff in cardiac and other surgical specialties and the emergency room and many nurses went on to graduate training to return as nurse practitioners in both surgical and medical specialties. They now represent a vital segment of the health care delivery system.

Current Era

In 2009, MMC celebrated the 50th anniversary of the cardiac surgery program. The early cardiac surgeons created a foundation upon which was built the efforts of multiple generations of cardiac surgeons with more sophistication and technology and knowledge to reconstruct hearts, support patients with implantable devices and resuscitate patients with extracorporeal circuits.

The end of the 20th century brought significant changes in the practice structure and ultimately at the beginning of the 21st century, all of the MMC cardiac surgeons became hospital based and employed. Technology and training has brought delivery systems to replace valves through small incisions and advances in the science of perioperative management have made the experience safer for patients.

Nearly 45,000 cardiac surgery procedures have been performed since 1959 at MMC using evidence available to guide appropriate selection of patients, the technologic advances gained by the cardiopulmonary perfusionists, understanding of myocardial physiology, myocardial protection, vascular biology, secondary prevention, heart teams, and multidisciplinary teams of perioperative caregivers. The academic environment of MMC has fostered relationships with basic scientists as well as the hiring of clinician-scientists, adding translational research to the repertoire that five cardiac surgeons began in the 1960's and 1970's before some of the talented young cardiac surgeons now practicing in 2017 were born.

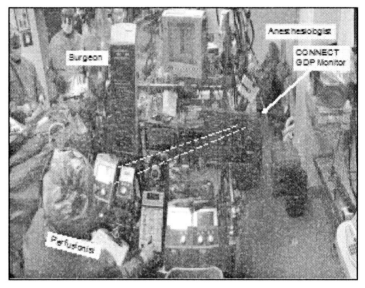

Heart-lung machine The cardiovascular perfusionist operating the pump is seated at the lower left. With permission from RC Groom, MS, CCP

CARDIOLOGY

By Mirle A Kellett, Jr. MD

Days of Change

The end of the 20th Century and the early 21st Century have been periods of explosive growth in the understanding of disease processes and have seen development of a range of tools to improve both diagnosis and treatment. Change occurred in different specialties at varying rates, with cardiovascular (CV) disease at the forefront of these changes. How a medical community, a hospital and the local practitioners, pick and choose what services to add to their community and who will drive the implementation differs in each community. This chapter will explore some of the key changes in CV medicine over these decades and how they were implemented in Portland, Maine, both at Maine Medical Center (MMC) and in its associated practices.

By the mid-1980's, cardiology in Portland was delivered by one large practice, Maine Cardiology Associates (MCA) - a small group practice, several independent practitioners, and a pediatric cardiology group. MMC had a Coronary Intensive Care Unit (CICU) and inpatient cardiology units supported by active cardiac catheterization, echocardiography and nuclear cardiology labs. Harold Osher MD was the hospital-employed Chief of Cardiology and Costas ("Gus") Lambrew MD was Director of the CICU and of the cardiology fellowship. There was a close relationship with the 9 CV surgeons. Most of the physicians in the community had completed their training before 1980.

At about the same time CV imaging evolved with the addition of 2D and then 3D echo, as well as stress echo (ESE) and transesophageal echo (TEE). Percutaneous coronary intervention (PCI), which revolutionized the management of coronary artery disease (CAD) and was first performed in 1977, was gaining broad acceptance by the mid 80's. Initially drugs and then PCI and other devices to limit heart attack (AMI) size were studied intensively in clinical trials and became the standard of care. The arrhythmia world saw the development of advanced pacing strategies, then the development of the implantable cardioverter defibrillator (ICD) and intracardiac techniques to ablate tissues that support arrhythmias using electrical and radiofrequency energy sources. How the community would implement these advances in CV medicine is the story of the development of the CV program at MMC into a nationally competitive program.

Cardiology

Before reviewing the implementation of specific programs, it is important to recognize several environmental factors that would facilitate or impede their adoption. By the late 80's and early 90's, there were two large and growing competitive groups, MCA and the newer and smaller Cardiovascular Consultants of Maine (CCM). Both groups were trying to develop large regional practices to compete with other centers and with each other. Outreach and new programs could either be developed by one group for competitive advantage or collaboratively for maximum program benefit. Gus Lambrew MD, the new Chief of Cardiology fostered a collaborative environment within the hospital. Leaders in both groups recognized that collaboration and ultimately merger were the best approaches to growth and program quality. While it took until 2014 for the practices to ultimately merge and be acquired by MMC, several merger efforts over the preceding two decades kept the groups talking and working together.

At the same time as the cardiology groups were trying to merge, the cardiac surgeons and the cardiologists approached the hospital to develop a "heart center." As these were bed and resource intensive specialties the relationship with the hospital was often strained. The consultant group APM was retained and the Maine Heart Center (MHC) was created in 1995. The board of the MHC made up of ten CV physicians and five of the senior management of MMC became the first of several iterations of physician-hospital collaboration. The MHC offered global fee products for multiple cardiac DRG's as part of MMC's participation in a national global fee cardiac initiative, the National Cardiovascular Network (NCN). The NCN tried to develop a network of high quality CV centers that could contract with national corporations for cardiac care. The emphasis on documented quality accelerated efforts to develop quality improvement programs and metrics to demonstrate the improvement in outcomes. Ten years later, MMC created a Department of Cardiac Services that brought CV surgery (CVS) and cardiology into a single department with administrative support. In 2012 this morphed to the current Cardiovascular Service Line which also includes vascular surgery.

A key factor in program growth and quality was the development of the Northern New England Cardiovascular Disease Study Group (NNECVDSG). This group was formed by CV surgeons from Maine, New Hampshire and Vermont in response to Medicare's plans to publish hospital outcomes for CVS. Facilitated by CV surgeon Steve Plume MD and epidemiologist Gerry O'Connor, both from Dartmouth, this group quickly expanded to include interventional cardiologists. An outcomes database for CVS and PCI was developed and regional quality improvement projects commenced. Portland's participation was spearheaded by CV surgeon Jeremy Morton MD and interventional cardiologist Bud Kellett MD. While the initial efforts were entirely physician driven, the MHC provided the ideal opportunity to explore a physician-hospital partnership. MMC enthusiastically supported the effort and funded development of a local data collection tool with a programmer and two nurse data coordinators. Using the data to fuel quality improvement, the MMC CV program developed a national reputation and received several national quality awards.

The other key environmental factor was the presence of a fledgling research program within the department under the leadership of Dr. Lambrew. Participation in the TIMI II Trial exploring the use of thrombolytic therapy to treat AMI was an early step in developing a robust list of NIH and industry sponsored trials investigating topics in almost all subspecialties of cardiology. Many members of the Department served as principal investigators for these trials. Participation in these studies allowed MMC and its providers to investigate novel and exciting therapies, making them available to the MMC patient community. In the interventional cardiology arena, Bud Kellett and the interventional physicians and research coordinators developed a reputation for research quality that provided MMC with access to novel therapies such as drug eluting stents, and to be positioned to get the next important study. Participation in research required compliance with protocols which had the added benefit of creating a culture of compliance with standards of care. Two NIH funded studies, BARI and SYNTAX, were instrumental in forming interdisciplinary teams of cardiovascular surgeons and interventional cardiologists. These studies, which compared the effectiveness of PCI versus coronary artery bypass graft surgery (CABG) in certain subsets of patients, required joint decision making between the two specialties. They fostered cooperation between the two specialties and presaged the era of percutaneous valve treatments for which Medicare mandated a team management approach. Participation in research had prepared the group to respond to these new requirements.

With this background in mind, we will now explore the implementation of some specific programs created during this era with particular emphasis on the physician inputs and environmental factors that influenced the ultimate success of the program.

Imaging

By the mid 80's, MMC and its affiliated practices had robust echocardiography capabilities including 2D, Doppler and color. Over the next decade the challenge would be how to add the evolving technologies of exercise stress echo (ESE), transesophageal echo (TEE), and 3D echo. Implementation of these technologies would require physician champions, the acquisition of new hardware, and a commitment to educate the technical staff. Two physicians, Peter Shaw MD and Karl Sze MD who arrived in Portland in the late 70's, were passionate about echocardiography and committed to having state-of-the art echo as part of their respective practices. They routinely attended the best echo courses and came home with a desire to add these advances to MMC's lab. They each pursued advanced training at other facilities which allowed them to become the physician champions while simultaneously stimulating interest in the other echocardiographers and the sonographers. When the physician champions had acquired adequate skills and generated support among their colleagues, they worked with the Cardiology Division Chief to make the case to the administration that this was an essential service for MMC and to purchase the needed equipment. The technical leadership of the lab provided by Norma Willis and Dennis Atherton were critical to the success of these new programs. They worked tirelessly to train their sonographers and supported the physicians who had problems adapting to the new technology. This partnership between a physician champion, the echo lab Technical Director, and the sonographers continues and has supported the standardization necessary for computer generated structured reporting. Having physicians like Karl and Peter with a commitment to a subspecialty, a desire to remain on the cutting edge of their area of interest, and the willingness to learn new skills while in practice has been a key factor in the evolution of MMC's cardiology program.

In the early 1980's radionuclide imaging was being developed to assess myocardial perfusion and ventricular function. No one in the Portland medical community had any experience in the new field of nuclear cardiology. Dr. Bob Morse from cardiology and Dr. Russ Briggs from radiology collaborated to start a program. Dr. Morse took a six month sabbatical at the Massachusetts General Hospital and returned to partner with Dr. Briggs, an experienced nuclear medicine physician. Cardiologists performed the stress tests, the scans were performed by the nuclear medicine technologists, and the physicians jointly interpreted the scans. The program was very successful. Most cardiologists hired after their pioneering efforts were trained in nuclear cardiology and the practices added this capability to their offices. Like any shared program, there were stresses and strains to accommodating program growth and reading schedules but the joint reading persists and has been the model to develop collaboration around cardiac CT and MRI procedures.

Interventional Cardiology

PCI was first performed in 1977 in Zurich, Switzerland by Dr. Andreas Gruentzig. The original procedure was performed with a relatively crude balloon catheter with a short fixed guide wire at the tip, and many cardiologists questioned the significance of the procedure. Initial adoption in the US was slow and largely confined to large academic medical centers. The first PCI's in Boston were performed in 1979 and 1980. Gruentzig and others cautiously educated new physicians in live demonstration courses, proctors helped new providers with their first several cases, and the procedure quickly became a standard of care for certain patients with CAD. To start a new program required buy-in from the CV surgeons who needed to provide "back-up" for complications in the lab and the purchase by the hospital of an expensive inventory of interventional angiography products. Starting a new program was a daunting endeavor. There were very limited options to recruit an experienced physician, so MMC physicians made the decision to learn on site. Drs. Richard Anderson and John Driscoll began the program at MMC, and over the next several years they were joined by Drs. Paul Sweeney and Warren Alpern. The program grew slowly and cautiously as the group attended live demonstration courses and worked together to maximize their experience.

The growth curve changed dramatically with the arrival in 1986-87 of two new physicians, Drs. Josh Cutler and Bud Kellett. On completion of their fellowship training, both Josh and Bud had stayed in junior faculty positions at large academic medical centers, Georgetown and Boston University respectively. In Boston there was a citywide PCI club where cases and experience were shared and which rapidly accelerated the pace of learning. By the mid 80's we were collaborating to produce large live demonstration courses. This type of experience not only advanced our skill set but gave one the confidence to continue to add new tools and techniques on your own. The six Interventionalists at MMC did cases together and met regularly to share experience. Over the two year period from 1987-1989, the case volume grew by over 300%. Bud Kellett brought research relationships with industry, and the opportunity to join the Beth Israel Hospital in Boston in the NIH funded Bypass-Angioplasty Revascularization Investigation Trial (BARI). This increased the credibility of the program because of its participation in an NIH trial and access to the newest devices which were appearing at a rapid rate. The equipment improved rapidly with lower profile and stronger balloons, a family of steerable guidewires and an ultra-low profile balloon-on-a-wire. In this era of two practice groups often behaving competitively, the PCI group committed to sharing these new technologies. Enhancements in technology increased the complexity of the cases which were appropriate for PCI. All of these factors contributed to the improving reputation of the program which led to increased referrals from Maine and New Hampshire hospitals and the ability to recruit a cadre of Fellowship trained Interventionalists including Drs. Tom Ryan, David Burkey, Paul Vaitkus, Mary Fahrenbach, Bill Dietz, Peter Higgins and David Butzel. By the end of the 1990's both the PCI and CABG programs had grown to become the largest in New England. The addition of the NNECVDSG data in the early 90's allowed both programs to know their outcomes and become early adopters of quality improvement. This led to recognition of MMC's program quality by such external agencies as Healthgrades, Solucient, and US News and World Report.

Maintaining the volume and quality of the program required constant attention to obtaining excellent results, managing referral relationships and having access to all latest techniques. The group met every week at PCI conference to review outcome data and individual cases. Every new technique needed a champion from each group to start the program with a commitment to proctor each other so that every member of the team had all the tools at their disposal. With the Cardiology Division offices on the floor of the cardiac cath lab, every physician was encouraged to ask for second opinions or to call a colleague to share a learning moment. This team approach allowed the physicians to share cases and deliver a consistent product to their colleagues when they were on call. This collaborative approach served the program well when expensive new therapies such as drug eluting stents or the glycoprotein IIb/IIIa receptor antagonists became available. Appropriateness criteria were developed and reviewed frequently which lead to a phased-in cost-effective adoption of the new therapies. PCI continues to evolve and the MMC physician providers continue to provide an excellent service.

Acute Myocardial Infarction (AMI)

At the same time that Andreas Gruentzig was performing his first PCI, cardiologists were beginning to understand the role of plaque rupture and subsequent thrombus formation as the proximate cause of ST elevation AMI (STEMI). If clot caused the STEMI, then it was hypothesized that clot removal could limit or prevent the damage. This paradigm shift in STEMI care led to a series of research protocols using thrombolytic drugs and mechanical strategies to clear the artery. MMC participated in numerous AMI trials, initially under the leadership of Dr. Gus Lambrew and then Dr. Bud Kellett and always in close collaboration with our Emergency Department (ED) colleagues under the leadership of Dr. Bud Higgins. By the late 1990's, evidence was building that emergency PCI performed within 90 minutes of ED arrival would be superior to thrombolytic drugs delivered within 30 minutes of ED arrival. Despite significant doubt that MMC could achieve those standards, the ED and PCI groups collaborated to create a new protocol which would allow MMC to participate in the GUSTO II trial and answer this question.

The old protocol for STEMI patients involved the ED assessing the patient and calling the clinical cardiologist on call to come to the ED and assess the patient. Only after the assessment was complete, could the treatment start. The new protocol empowered the ED physician to interpret the electrocardiogram (ECG), make the diagnosis and simultaneously call the interventional cardiologist and activate the cath lab. The interventional cardiologist would often meet the patient as they were arriving in the lab. While this sounds like a simple change, the obstacles were significant. To make this work, the ED team had to hone their ECG skills, be willing to screen patients for inclusion and exclusion criteria for the treatment, and get the patient's consent to treatment. The interventional cardiologists had to learn to trust the ED physician's judgments and engage that physician in a productive dialogue if there were differences of opinion about the diagnosis or appropriateness of therapy. Internally within the cardiology practices this meant the interventional cardiologists managed all the STEMI patients and needed to have a separate and more frequent on call schedule. With the protocol refined and in place, STEMI patients were being treated in under the 90 minute goal and STEMI mortality dropped by 3%.

By the early 2000's, MaineHealth asked the interventional cardiologists to develop a health system wide strategy for STEMI care. Dr. Bud Kellett chaired a working group that initially included cardiologists from several MaineHealth hospitals. Given the geographic distances separating some of the hospitals, a strategy that combined the use of thrombolytic drugs in remote hospitals with emergency transfer to MMC for later PCI with direct PCI for patients who were either ineligible for thrombolytic drugs or close enough to meet the 90 minute goal was agreed upon. The task force then expanded to include system wide ED physicians and nurses in order to operationalize the protocol. A set of performance metrics was developed and shared at semi-annual working group meetings. To further improve the speed and effectiveness of treatment, the team reached out to Emergency Medical Service (EMS) providers, who received advanced training in ECG interpretation and were empowered to activate the cath lab through their local EDs. In his role with Maine EMS, Dr. Matt Sholl led the EMS education efforts. Named the AMI-PERFUSE network, the program is now directed by Dr. Tom Ryan. This collaboration involving providers from EMS, Emergency Departments, and inpatient CV caregivers has had a huge impact on CV mortality in the MaineHealth service area. Since its inception in 2004, over 4,000 patients have been treated and over 120 fewer patients have died from STEMI then would have in the days prior to this protocol.

Electrophysiology

Electrophysiology (EP) was another subspecialty of cardiology that experienced remarkable growth beginning in the 1980s and continuing to the present. Dr. John

Love was the first fellowship trained electrophysiologist to come to Portland and he had to convince his new employers, Drs. Bernie Givertz and John Driscoll that EP could add to their practice. Dr. Love joined Dr. Fred Poulin who was implanting pacemakers. With assistance from then Chief of Cardiology, Dr. Harold Osher, Dr. Love was able to get a used *E for M* recorder and stimulator and began doing HIS bundle studies and VT stimulation studies. Patients requiring treatment were referred to Boston. He then partnered with Dr. Johann Tryzelaar to do intraoperative mapping during LV aneurysmectomy. In 1987, Drs. Love and Tryzelaar went to Minneapolis for training in epicardial ICD placement and shortly after their return implanted MMC's first ICD. Based on their pioneering efforts, MMC became a referral center for ICD's in Maine. This program continues to grow and currently implants over 300 ICDs per year.

During the late 1980's and early 90's, academic medical centers were pioneering new ways to treat supraventricular tachyarrhythmia's (SVT) using mapping techniques to identify the pathway, which was subsequently ablated with either radiofrequency or direct current. In 1991, Dr. Joel Cutler was completing his training at the University of Oregon in such a program and wanted to return to Maine to practice. Much like Dr. Love, he had to convince his future partners and the Medical Center that this was a valuable treatment option for patients and that MMC should start a program. Dr. Cutler started the program and worked in partnership across group lines with Dr. Love to create a very successful SVT ablation program. Over the next two decades they were joined by Drs. Charles Carpenter, Andrew Corsello, Hank Sesselberg, Michael Field, and Brooke Ritvo. Working closely with the device industry and participating in a number of EP clinical trials, the program grew and is supported by three EP labs and a dedicated staff.

Atrial fibrillation (AF) remained the most challenging SVT to treat with multiple centers developing a range of ablation strategies with varying levels of success and a complication rate that was much higher than other SVT ablations. The MMC EP program wanted to be a full service EP program but had strong referral relationships with Boston teaching hospitals with excellent outcomes, and struggled to justify starting a program. The solution was to actively seek out a physician well trained in AF ablation to start MMC's program. Dr. Michael Field was hired from the Brigham and Women's Hospital in Boston to start the program. He began slowly taking difficult patients back to Boston and doing cases there with his mentors. He also did all his cases at MMC with one of the other EP physicians in Portland so the entire group benefited from his experience. The AF ablation program grew quickly with outstanding success and a very low complication rate. By the time Dr. Field left Portland to pursue an academic career, MMC's EP group had developed an outstanding reputation and was confidently adding new programs such as laser lead extraction, ventricular tachycardia (VT) ablation and a new left atrial appendage occlusion device program with the Watchman device.

Congestive Heart Failure

In all of the subspecialty areas of cardiology, the addition of new treatments and technologies was driven by the interest of one or more physicians in the group pushing to develop the service. The one notable failure of this approach was in the area of advanced care of patients with congestive heart failure (CHF). Advanced CHF care evolved slowly as a specialty. There was no defining diagnostic tool or procedure available to the general clinical cardiologist. When Medicare started measuring CHF hospital outcomes, MMC approached the groups to recruit a CHF specialist. Several attempts were made to recruit a CHF specialist in the early 2000's, but several very talented and interested candidates were concerned about the two group model and how they would fit into the community. As the groups moved towards merger and acquisition by the hospital, Dr. Joe Wight obtained his CHF boards and spearheaded the effort to recruit additional physicians. Today, under the leadership of Division Chief Dr. Doug Sawyer and CHF physicians Drs. Esther Shao and Sam Coffin, MMC has developed a large advanced CHF program including mechanical support for the acutely failing heart and destination ventricular assist device (VAD) therapy.

Percutaneous Valve Treatments

Cardiovascular medicine has been at the leading edge of the incessant push to make treatments less invasive, lower risk and available to a broader range of patients. In the last decade, this has resulted in the availability of non-surgical options to treat both aortic and mitral valve disease. At this point in time percutaneous mitral valve repair and aortic valve replacement are reserved for patients felt to be at excessively high risk for open surgical procedures but still able to achieve significant benefit from the procedure. Starting a high risk valve program was a daunting task and required a great deal of preparation on the part of any center wishing to start a program. Many of the attributes of the MMC CV program described above that led to the start of successful programs were instrumental in MMC's development of this program. Key issues included an excellent relationship with device manufacturers developed by outstanding participation in their research studies, a history of physician champions who brought programs to completion, and in the case of the valve program, demonstrated collaboration between the Divisions of CV Surgery, Cardiology and Cardiac Anesthesia. MMC was able to demonstrate prior success in each of these areas, develop a "valve center" and successfully gain access to the Edwards balloon mounted aortic valve prosthesis and the E-Valve MitraClip device for percutaneous mitral valve repair. The original valve center team consisted of CV surgeons Drs. Reed Quinn and Paul Weldner, interventional cardiologists Drs. David Butzel and Bud Kellett, echocardiographers Drs. Mylan Cohen, Marco Diaz and Dr. John Lualdi and cardiac anesthesiologists Drs. Angus Christie and Paul Lennon. This outstanding team used this opportunity to build on previous levels of interdepartmental cooperation and take it to the next level. A patient being evaluated at the Valve Center received the shared input of the entire team, assuring the patient the best and most individualized treatment plan. Currently several hundred high risk patients are evaluated each year and the treatment outcomes have been exceptional.

Conclusion

The last three decades have seen incredible change in the diagnostic and therapeutic tools available to treat patients with cardiovascular diseases. The adoption of most of these advances has largely been driven by committed physicians who followed their passion, convinced their colleagues and MMC of the benefits to patients and provided leadership resulting in successful implementation of programs of excellence in CV care.

Dermatology

By J.Michael Taylor MD

Dermatology In Maine -- 1950 To 2015

The dramatic transformation of dermatology in Portland and in Maine must be presented against the background of the scientific and clinical advances in dermatology in the US and worldwide.

Broad View of Dermatology in the 20th Century

Although dermatology residencies are now the most sought-after slots for medical school graduates, the discipline had historically been considered the "weak sister" of the medical specialties with the surgical subspecialties residing nearer to the top of the hierarchy. In pre-WWII Europe, it became the specialty of the Jews since they were denied access to the more prestigious specialties. Dermatology in the US reaped the benefit of this prejudice in the 1930's and 40's with the migration of Jewish academics and professionals. Most of the medical school dermatology departments were populated and headed by German Jews who brought scientific rigor to what was then, in the US, a more often anecdotal discipline.

Scientific advancement in medicine, and dermatology in particular, began to accelerate after WWII. The National Institutes of Health (NIH) had existed for almost 100 years before WWII with a primary interest in the study of infectious diseases. The NIH then refocused its research priorities toward military concerns during WW II. The passage of the Public Health Service Act in 1944 guided the direction of US (and international) research from that time to the present. The NIH budget expanded from $4M in 1947 to more than $1B in 1966. The Division of Arthritis, Musculoskeletal, and Skin Diseases was only created in 1980, with dermatology clearly an afterthought. In 1995, Stephen Katz MD,PhD a dermatologist, was named to head this NIH Division

Dermatology in Greater Portland and Maine from 1950

Just as dermatology at the NIH lagged behind other specialties in the US, it also did so in Portland. Some physicians declared that they were "specialists" in dermatology even though they were not educated in the specialty. Allergists claimed special knowledge probably because of the shared interest in eczema and allergic skin reactions. Fully-educated and Board Certified dermatologists began to slowly arrive with the way being paved first in the mid-1950s by Harvey Ansel from Boston University (BU) and soon thereafter by Don Cole and Bob Sommers from Dartmouth. Dick Stevenson, a general surgeon, joined the pack performing skin surgery. Then came Joel Sabean from Dartmouth. Joel settled in South Portland. Mary Morse, also from BU joined Harvey Ansel, but after a few years started her own practice. Below is a rough chronology of dermatologists who contributed to the early years of growth:

- Ron Rovner, from Hershey and a former pediatric resident at MMC, opened his practice in the 1980s;

- Michael Taylor joined Mary Morse when he completed residency at UCSF and returned to Portland in 1982. They established Dermatology Associates (DA);

- DA was joined by Lucinda L Wegener from Oregon. Lucinda is married to cardiologist Joel Cutler;

- Brian O'Donnell joined the practice and then went out on his own to practice the new sub-specialty of Mohs Surgery;

- Julia Harre arrived in Portland and established a solo practice;

- K. Eric (Rick) Kostelnik from Dartmouth joined Dermatology Associates;

- David Baginski from Iowa joined DA;

- Jennifer Bragg, born and raised in Bangor, the daughter of Dr Frank Bragg, an internist, joined DA after her residency at NYU;

- DA was joined by Carrine Burns, a Mohs surgeon, who had completed her residency in Family Medicine at MMC and then completed a residency in dermatology at the University of Rochester. Carrine came with her husband Peter Bauman who set up his dermatology practice in Lewiston which at that time had no practicing dermatologist;

- Rob MacNeal joined the DA practice as a Mohs surgeon when Carrine Burns left the practice to join her husband in Lewiston; and

- Intermed began adding dermatologists to its roster.

As of 2017 Dermatology Associates has 13 dermatologists and 2 nurse practitioners. Although the practice is based on general dermatology, there are two Mohs surgeons and two dermatopathologists. It is the largest dermatology group practice in Northern New England, including Dartmouth and the University of Vermont.

If it sounds as though Dermatology Associates was the primary center for dermatology in Portland during the '80s, '90s, and the first decade of this century, that's because it was. We founded the Maine Dermatology Association, initiated the annual skin cancer and melanoma screening, launched twice yearly academic meetings, instigated the partnership between Harvard Medical School's dermatology residency and the Aroostook Medical Center, taught and managed the MMC Outpatient Dermatology Clinic, taught in the MMC Family Practice Residency Program, and volunteered in the annual Fishermen's Forum performing screening exams for the fishermen who gathered at the Samoset. Dermatology Associates now has satellite practices in Biddeford, Brunswick and Scarborough.

Dermatology in Greater Portland and Maine is seeing a mini-explosion with the addition of two, soon to be three, dermatologists at Intermed. Martin's Point is looking for a dermatologist. Maine Medical Center is actively recruiting a dermatologist. And close by there are new dermatologists in Biddeford, Brunswick, and York. There were two and now one dermatologist in Camden. The Family Practice Residency Program in Augusta has recruited its own dermatologist. The Togus VAH now, for the first time, has its own full-time dermatologist. Bangor has two dermatologists and Belfast one. I suspect I may be unaware of others since I have been retired for 5 years at this writing.

Why the Explosion?

Medical practice seems to create its own demand. How else can one explain the fact that there were 4 dermatologists in Portland in the early '80s and we are now closing in on 20. Or could it possibly be that dermatology has advanced from an anecdotal "weak sister" to a full-fledged science based specialty? Or both?

Scientific Advances

Mohs Surgery

During the 1950s and 1960s, Frederick Mohs, a dermatologist at the University of Wisconsin/Madison, first working with laboratory mice, developed microscopically controlled surgery to completely remove skin cancers while limiting the sacrifice of adjacent normal tissue. Although it appears at first to be "frozen sectioning" which has been used by plastic surgeons for decades, the novel staining, the 360-degree examination of the margins (instead of sampling), and the fact that the surgeon - in this case usually a dermatologist - also is his/her own pathologist so that there is no possible communication error between the surgeon and the pathologist - has increased the accuracy of the excision. While preserving as much normal tissue as possible, the Mohs technique has demonstrated a lower recurrence rate than standard surgery or frozen sections. Dermatology, a specialty that had limited itself to punch biopsies and small incisions, now removes more skin cancers than do plastic surgeons; a major transformation. Greater Portland has three Mohs' surgeons and will soon have four. And Carrine Burns is in Lewiston. The development of Mohs' technique has also been dermatology's gift to plastic surgeons and ear/nose and throat surgeons since these specialties have incorporated the technique into their practices. General pathologists have learned the technique and are encouraging its use more and more widely.

Lasers

Another gift from dermatology to other specialties is the clinical use of lasers. The early research and development of clinical lasers took place at the Massachusetts General Hospital (MGH) Wellman Center for Photomedicine. This research has been lead by dermatologist R . Rox Anderson and his colleagues. The annual Harvard Laser Clinical Conference was established and led by two dermatologists, Kenneth Arndt and Jeffrey Dover, with a large audience of clinicians from a variety of specialties and from all over the world. Up-to-date information has been shared generously and openly with other specialties for more than 20 years.

Although dermatology was on the forefront of research in clinical laser applications, practicing dermatologists - most of whom had limited experience with hands-on treatments - were slow to incorporate expensive lasers into their practices. In contrast, plastic surgeons were quick to see the benefits and incorporated them into their practices. This was true in Portland as well as nationwide. It should be noted that there were significant regional differences in laser incorporation into practice with West Coast and Florida being the most rapid adopters.

Starting in the late '80s, Dermatology Associates developed a contract with a mobile laser unit based in Boston and performed destructive procedures such as tattoo removal, wart ablation, and removal of vascular lesions such as birthmarks, telangiectasias, angiomas and rosacea. As more physicians purchased their own lasers, the mobile company went out of business. We purchased our own small portable destructive laser to treat warts and benign skin growths and referred our vascular patients locally or to Boston. A vascular laser was purchased in early 2000. The use of lasers became more "cosmetic" and less disease based and our practice made a deliberate decision not to follow the road into a cosmetic practice. We felt strongly that we were educated to prevent diseases and to cure sickness. Dermatology Associates is one of the few large groups nationwide to hold to this standard.

Cosmetic Dermatology

One of the Greater Portland Dermatologists, Joel Sabean, was at the forefront of incorporating cosmetic dermatology into his practice. Dr Sabean had lasers, performed collagen injections, performed dermabrasions, and more. He was an excellent general dermatologist as well as a leader in cosmetic procedures, but retired in 2016. None of the remaining dermatologists in Portland have taken up his cosmetic mantle. In fact the Laser Center, established by a D.O. Proctologist has become the local leader in cosmetic procedures, not merely limited to the use of lasers. A pediatrician in Falmouth offers a variety of cosmetic choices. Plastic surgeons also provide a range of cosmetic procedures.

That is not to say that dermatologists in Portland perform no procedures. Dermatology Associates has a vascular laser used primarily to treat birthmarks and rosacea. Dr. Jennifer Bragg learned to use Botox for the treatment of hyperhidrosis, but also uses it for some cosmetic procedures. Still, cosmetic procedures represent a minor deviation from the primary purpose of treating people with skin problems at DA.

Phototherapy

Phototherapy had been used by dermatologists for several decades, mostly at academic centers, for both inpatient and outpatient treatment of psoriasis, eczema, lichen planus, and photo-dermatitis. It was slowly brought from the academic centers to

Dermatology

private practices and was introduced to the Greater Portland area in the late 1980s. At first limited to the Portland area, there are now phototherapy units in Biddeford and Brunswick and elsewhere in Maine. Although its value may decline because of newer treatments for psoriasis and eczema, these units still have a place in the offices for years to come.

Biologics

The newer treatments for psoriasis, the biologics, have upended the old saying that dermatologists can treat but never cure. The development of these new immune therapies has resulted in 80% to 100% 'cure' for psoriasis and other chronic illnesses. These new biologics came to dermatology largely from rheumatology where they have revolutionized the treatment of rheumatoid arthritis and its cousins. Dermatologists now have powerful medicines at their disposal to replace topical steroids, topical Vitamin D, and systemic methotrexate which carries with it certain well-known risks.

Accutane

Although it is used less now than when it was introduced three decades ago, Accutane (isotretinione) was a breakthrough in the treatment of acne. Instead of years long treatment with oral antibiotics, topical benzoyl peroxides, Retin-A, and topical antibiotics with usually limited control, Accutane cleared the patient's acne in 4-6 months. For 80% of patients skin remained clear after cessation of treatment. It was seen as quite miraculous at the time, despite the costs and inconvenience (regular visits and blood tests). However as the risks of therapy - birth defects and a reported increase in suicides – became apparent, its use is now more limited. It is still used for severe cases of scarring acne under tight monitoring.

Dermatopathology

Academic dermatology departments began incorporating pathologists in the 1970s. Soon thereafter dermatologists were educated in skin pathology which is now a recognized sub-specialty of dermatology. Having a clinically educated dermatologist also reading the pathology has been a major step in advancing research and increasing clinical diagnostic accuracy. Dermatology Associates recruited a dermatopathologist,

Carmen Rinaldi, early in the 21st century. His presence moved the practice from a "community outpost" to a more scientifically focused discipline. His arrival was the single best recent addition to dermatology in Portland.

Change is the only certainty

When I returned to Portland in late 1982 to practice dermatology there were four dermatologists, all in solo practice. In 2017 there may be a single solo practitioner. I know of no one, anywhere, who has opened a solo practice in dermatology in the past decade. The trend toward group corporate practices has affected dermatology as well as all of medicine. Changes in reimbursement away from procedure oriented to global reimbursement are certain to have an effect. The challenge is to have a personal relationship with the patient while being tugged in the direction of a business model. We are still seeing this evolve.

Emergency Medicine

By George L. Higgins III MD

The Birth, Evolution, and Life of Emergency Medicine as a Recognized Specialty at Maine Medical Center

As I reflect upon the emergence and maturation of the specialty of emergency medicine, both nationally and here at the Maine Medical Center (MMC) during my personal medical career, I am truly proud. After all, I was swept up in this rather challenging yet rewarding House of Medicine journey from its inception, and I am happy to announce that I have been privileged to contribute to emergency medicine's development here at MMC. Let me start at the beginning of this journey.

I first stepped foot in MMC's Emergency Department in 1972 when I was a third-year medical student at Tufts University School of Medicine in Boston. Tufts was affiliated with MMC at that time and allowed sixteen of us to spend our entire third year in Portland. Although this experience was subtlety (and occasionally bluntly) described at that time as "limiting any chance at an academic career" by my Boston-based professors, I jumped at the chance. And I've come to value this as one of the bravest and best decisions I've ever made. Believe me, today there is no limit to academic advancement at MMC.

But before I continue my personal reflections, let me briefly describe the status of emergency medicine that existed in many other areas of the country at that time. Importantly, there was no officially recognized specialty of emergency medicine. There were no training programs in emergency medicine. There were no emergency medicine textbooks or peer-reviewed journals. In fact, the practice of emergency medicine was defined by its typical physical space within the hospital: ER (emergency room) doctors practiced in the ER. And what an eclectic and interesting group these ER docs typically were. Many had left their more traditional specialties (e.g. pediatrics, family medicine or internal medicine) because of their attraction to the broad, diverse, never predictable and fast-paced nature of emergency medicine. They were hired without any type of certification. Others had dropped out of their practices because of burn-out, attracted to the appeal of "just working shifts, clocking in and clocking out". Because of this culture, the quality of care provided in the ER was understandably variable, ER docs were routinely criticized by their specialist consultants (fairly and unfairly), and practicing in the ER was referred to as "living in a fishbowl". To be fair, even with its limitations, this mosaic model was an improvement over the model practiced in prior decades. Back then physicians of all specialties were expected to "do their time in the Emergency Ward" as a requirement for being granted hospital privileges.

Fortunately, because of thoughtful and courageous leadership, emergency medicine at MMC was already in its early transition toward its eventual and deserved destination when I presented to the Emergency Department on the very first day of my very first clinical rotation as a third-year medical student (who had been sequestered in classrooms for the prior two years). I had no idea what an absolutely thrilling and energizing adventure I was embarking upon.

MMC's Emergency Department was then capably led by Dr. Frank Lawrence, who had assumed the leadership reins from Dr. Daryl Thorp, one of the very first Chiefs of Emergency Medicine in Maine. As Chief, Dr. Lawrence's natural charisma, endless energy and healthy competitive spirit were infectious. Most importantly, he made it a priority to recruit an outstanding group of physicians. These young professionals were genuinely attracted to emergency medicine. Doctors Phelps Carter, Michael Lamb, Meredith Bennet, David Getson, and Richard Chandler, among others, measurably elevated the level of care delivered at the bedside. Dr. John Saucier, the first Emergency Medicine trained physician in Maine, soon joined them. Their collective efforts were invaluable to the early emergence of emergency medicine as a respected specialty at MMC.

Dr. Lawrence also ensured that he sat at tables with institutional leaders and other Chiefs where important institutional clinical decisions were made. He recognized that this cooperative strategy was an essential ingredient in the early development of emergency medicine at MMC. Facility upgrades of the Emergency Department and expansion of the attending physician staff resulted.

When I first encountered the physical space of MMC's Emergency Department in 1972, it was typical of hospital ED's around the state: located on the ground floor to allow easy access to incoming ambulances arriving at the back of the building; one fully equipped and one partially equipped critical care room; two "quiet rooms" (for patients requiring behavioral health intervention); one OB/GYN room; one ENT/Eye room; six patient care cubicles, each separated by curtains; and one multipurpose chair for treating ambulatory patients with various complaints. X-ray films were reviewed on "view boxes" mounted on walls in strategic locations throughout the Department.

All multidisciplinary documentation was captured long-handedly on a single, two-sided, triplicate paper form. Often a single sentence from the medical provider captured the entire history, e.g. "Chest pain one hour ago, radiating to jaw, now gone".

Emergency Medicine

Physical exam findings were recorded with similar brevity. Medical decision making was rarely captured. A single diagnosis was recorded with finality. Alternative diagnoses that were obviously considered by the clinician were not shared. Although this type of documentation would not be remotely acceptable today, somehow it got the job done with impressive efficiency and favorable patient outcomes.

The open and inclusive culture of education that existed throughout MMC in 1972 allowed us "third-years" to essentially function at the level of resident physicians. We were encouraged to attend conferences and were invariably invited to the homes of our mentors. This type of medical student status was uncommon back in provincial Boston, as I painfully learned during my final year of medical school. There the time-honored caste system of hierarchical advancement was alive and well. Medical students spent much of their time in the clinical wards drawing blood and collecting urine samples. Fortunately, this archaic model no longer exists in American medical schools.

Another important fundamental residency training tenet that was alive and well at MMC and hospitals across the nation undoubtedly contributed significantly to the eventual emergence of emergency medicine as a specialty: the rotating internship. During the first year of post-graduate training all residents (identified as "interns") rotated through the traditional specialties, including internal medicine, surgery, pediatrics, and psychiatry. Electives in cardiology, anesthesiology and others were available. These rotations kindled interest in a subgroup of young clinicians who preferred a broader patient experience. To this day, training programs in emergency medicine continue to emphasize this type of diverse exposure and learning.

Now that I've painted the picture of what emergency medicine was like at the beginning of my career, let me quickly share some of the more significant milestones that have brought us to where this specialty is today at MMC.

The first emergency medicine residency was established in Cincinnati in the mid 1970's. There are now over 200 programs in the United States, including our own program at MMC. Emergency medicine as a specialty was finally recognized by the House of Medicine in 1979. This past year, MMC received over one hundred competitive applications for each of its ten first-year emergency medicine positions, and the overall quality of these young professionals is most impressive. Our graduates are now practicing in communities all over the country, with a significant percentage of them electing to remain here in Maine, their adopted state. As a result, the level of emergency medicine provided in a number of Maine's emergency departments and communities has never been higher. It is worth mentioning that currently MMC has the only emergency medicine residency in the Tufts University School of Medicine, our academic partner.

Along the way, my passion for emergency medicine has rewarded me with many opportunities to contribute to the advancement of this specialty at MMC. Let me share a few of those I consider to be most memorable to me.

Due to my continued interest in emergency medicine, I left my internal medicine practice and joined MMC's Department of Emergency Medicine in 1981 as its physician educator. In addition to my clinical duties, I was responsible for providing didactic and written educational materials to all rotating interns. These young trainees came from all existing MMC residencies, such as internal medicine, pediatrics, surgery and psychiatry. This was the first small step in the transformation of the Department of Emergency Medicine from a purely clinical experience to a more robust educational one. This injection of structured learning was embraced and practiced by both physicians and nurses within the department. Patients and families benefited as a result.

When Dr. Lawrence retired, I became Chief of the Department in 1986 and accelerated this departmental transformation by recruiting and hiring outstanding graduates from highly regarded emergency medicine training programs. Collectively they worked tirelessly to advance the Department to collaborative and respected academic status. MMC's emergency physicians began to have a presence on institutional committees and work groups, further advancing collaborations and professional relationships.

The next major milestone was, without question, the essential one that has earned the Department of Emergency Medicine at MMC the deserved reputation as being academically outstanding. Dr. Mark Fourre joined our faculty right out of training and quickly established himself as a gifted teacher and clinician. One day he approached me proposing that he take on the Herculean task of developing an emergency medicine training program at MMC. I promised him all the support from within and from without the Department that I was capable of mustering. Needless to say his huge investment of time and effort was successful, and the residency was officially recognized by the Board of Emergency Medicine in 1992. This was a once in a lifetime achievement that Dr. Fourre will forever treasure. The first year of the program we had six first-year emergency medicine residents. Today there are thirty, ten in each of the three years of the program. I would also add that there are currently over thirty members of the emergency medicine faculty who, in addition to their other administrative duties, ensure that each of our graduates are exceptionally well trained and patient-centered.

In 1994 MMC and the Osteopathic Hospital of Maine (OHM), also located in Portland, merged. Understandably this rather major event initially generated pockets of controversy within both medical staffs. However, emergency medicine leaders in both hospitals embraced this as an opportunity for improvement. The outcome of focused strategic planning resulted in the transformation of OHM's Emergency Department into a twelve-hour free standing acute care facility, Brighton First Care. Dr. Jonathan Karol, Chief of Emergency Medicine of OHM, remained at BFC as its director. Several OHM emergency physicians joined the staff at MMC and became much more involved with post-graduate training. Patients quickly learned to self-select which facility best met their needs, resulting in a better patient experience. Today nearly 100,000 patients entrust these two facilities with their care.

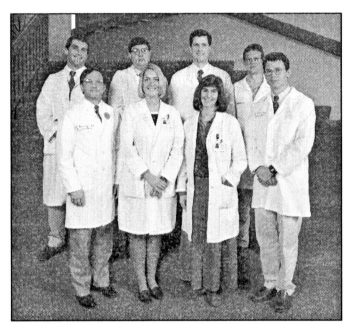

Emergency Medicine Residents – 1997

I would be remiss if I didn't take a moment to highlight just a few of the other advances I've witnessed during my career in emergency medicine at MMC that were inconceivable when I started practice, and each of which has significantly improved the care we collectively provide to our patients who entrust us with it.

- Continuously available and life-saving imaging techniques such as CT-imaging, MR-imaging, and bedside ultrasonography;

- Collaborative interdepartmental interventions such as Trauma Team activation, Stroke Team activation, Critical Care Team activation, Pre-hospital Cardiac Catheterization Lab activation, Difficult Airway

Response Team activation, Pediatric Intensive Care Team activation, interventional neurology, interventional cardiology, interventional radiology, and endovascular intervention;

- Amazing procedural and team training at MMC's state of the art simulation lab;

- Electronic health record systems that provide comprehensive documentation and point-of-care decision support tools;

- An onsite landing pad for medical helicopter crews to quickly deliver the sickest and most injured patients to our care;

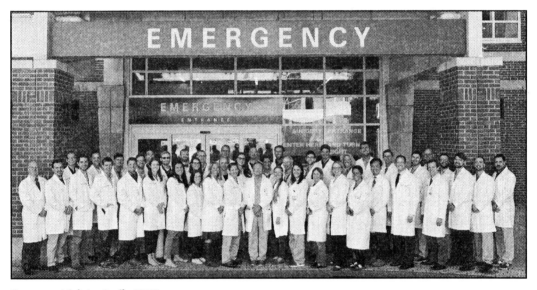

Emergency Medicine Staff – 2017

- A major renovation of the Emergency Department resulting in six critical care rooms; twenty three acute care rooms; seven ambulatory adult rooms; ten pediatric rooms, including a child-specific critical care unit; six behavioral health rooms; eight clinical decision support rooms; two CT scanners in addition to traditional radiology and dedicated ultrasound capability; an eight bed Clinical Decision Unit that provides expedited care for patients too sick to discharge, but not sick enough to require hospital admission; separate triage areas for both ambulatory

and ambulance transported patients; and on-site
decontamination capabilities;

- The vision and skilled leadership of Dr. Michael Gibbs and, currently,
  Dr. Michael Baumann who succeeded me as Chiefs
  of the Department. They have continued to capably integrate the
  specialty of emergency medicine at MMC into the vibrant healthcare
  system known as MaineHealth; and

- MMC's innovative collaboration with Tufts University School of
  Medicine that has produced the very successful Maine Track program.

Let me end my reflections by recognizing perhaps the most meaningful advancement
I've been privileged to witness during my career: the incorporation of authentic patient-
centeredness into every day practice.

When I was in training all those years ago, it was not uncommon to label and stigmatize
patients the second they crossed the threshold of the emergency department. This
was initiated by the triage nurse and carried through the entire encounter by the care
team. Derogatory terms such as "drug seeker", "frequent flyer" and "worried well" were
quickly attached to individuals and remained stuck to them during future Emergency
Department visits. Patients in the waiting room were often ignored and only brought
into a care area when it was convenient for staff. Patients who elected to leave before
an evaluation because of prolonged wait times were not viewed as a failure of the
system but as less work to be done. Too often the focus was on the providers and not
on patients and families. This toxic culture, I am happy to announce, no longer exists
at MMC.

Through dedicated team training and mentoring, our emergency medicine physicians,
nurses, advanced practice providers, residents and support staff now view the patient
to be the center of all we do together. Decision making is always shared equally with
the patient and family. Patients waiting for care are given priority, and the waiting
room is kept as empty as possible. We are flexible rather than dogmatic as we develop
management plans that best meet the patient's personal goals without compromising
safety. We raise the possibility of palliative and hospice care without being asked
when we believe the patient and family will benefit. By honoring this patient-
centered commitment each and every clinical shift, we ourselves are rewarded with
greater professional satisfaction and the keen awareness that what we do as physicians
really matters.

Thank you for allowing me share these personal reflections and memories with you. The positive changes I have witnessed and participated in during my career at MMC have been many and meaningful. I now pass the baton to my younger colleagues and will celebrate the inevitable improvements they will undoubtedly contribute to our dynamic healthcare community.

ENDOCRINOLOGY

By S. Thomas Bigos MD

Origins of the Endocrine Division

Today we take many standard endocrine laboratory tests for granted. Automated high speed laboratory procedures are readily available to most physicians. However this was not the case at the end of the 1960's and even into the early 1980's. The changes that led to today's complement of services largely began with the steroid chemistry work that emanated from centers such as the Worcester Foundation in Shrewsbury, Massachusetts which led to FDA approval of the oral contraceptive in 1960. This announced the dawn of modern endocrinology.

Endocrinology abruptly advanced in the late 1960's and early 1970's with the discovery and refinement of immunochemistry. This work formed the basis for nearly all subsequent advancements in the field. In 1977 the investigative work of Rosalyn Yalow PhD, a physicist; Roger Guillemin MD; and Andrew Schally MD represented the critical development of immunochemistry and resulted in their sharing the Nobel Prize for Medicine and Physics.

Dr. Yallow's work with Dr. Solomon Berson MD refined development of the in vitro immunoassay methodology which enabled identification of the antibody to the insulin polypeptide in human serum. This discovery demonstrated that it was possible to measure small amounts of substances in human serum by creating specific antibodies to a discrete polypeptide in an animal immune system and then using that antibody to search for the given substance in human serum. They succeeded in identifying methods to measure human parathyroid hormone, adrenocorticotropin, gastrin and growth hormone. These demonstrated that it was now possible to identify and measure virtually all hormones in vitro – thus creating the ability to investigate the behavior of substances that were previously unmeasurable.

It is important to emphasize that although these discoveries were revolutionary, immunochemistry techniques did not immediately become available as refined and useful clinical tools. Rather, they remained principally research tools confined to academic institutions. A great deal of work and refinement was needed on many fronts in order for them to become universally available to clinicians since most of the assays that physicians now use every day in endocrinology were either in their infancy for clinical application – or simply not available at all. The facilities for producing the new technologies and contributing to the growing fund of information in endocrinology were mostly available only through established academic medical research laboratories. Those were also the programs which were training the physicians schooled in the most advanced techniques of immunochemistry and competitive protein binding assays. Maine Medical Center (MMC) would need to recruit such physicians to its staff to be able to offer a modern and fully capable endocrine service.

Whereas MMC had particular practical advantages for a timely entry into the field of modern endocrinology in the 1970's it also had some deficiencies. As the largest hospital in the state it had the greatest number of patients and the most modern medical facilities in Maine. It was sufficiently removed from other large medical centers that it could develop at a controlled rate designed to meet the needs of the region without competitive outside pressure. Finally, it had an inquisitive, thoughtful and well-educated physician staff coupled to a burgeoning relationship with Tufts Medical School in Boston. Yet two elements required for success were still missing from MMC. First, a broader presence of specialty medical services was required. Fortunately this deficiency coincided with a period in which subspecialist physicians were beginning to move away from the traditional larger centers such as Boston and New York. Second, MMC was deficient in its informatics capabilities as it was not an academic center when the medical information explosion was born. Advanced informatics capabilities were central to endocrinology and the development of steroid chemistry and the new immunoassays. For MMC to have a successful endocrine program it would need to satisfy these conditions.

Following completion of his internal medicine residency at MMC in the 1960's, Dr. Hugh Johnston pursued a fellowship in clinical and research endocrinology at the Peter Bent Brigham Hospital in Boston. This was followed by an additional interval of steroid research at the Worcester Foundation in Shrewsbury, Massachusetts. He then returned to the MMC with a vision for a modern endocrinology department. His idea involved creating a new endocrine immunoassay laboratory that could serve the patient base and at the same time contribute to the medical literature while meeting the needs of a clinical service. In 1969, with the forward-looking support of then Chief of Medicine, Dr. Albert Aronson, he was encouraged to form the Division of Endocrinology (DE) within the Department of Medicine.

Recognizing the advantages offered by MMC, the new Division of Endocrinology could participate directly in the development of new assays and be involved in the groundbreaking advances of the time. Since it was undertaken locally, this effort could be driven by the clinical priorities of MMC physicians and patients. At the time, the emergence of such a division outside of a major medical research center was both innovative and a large commitment. The required components – in particular the antibodies required for immunoassay - were not readily available. Developing them required animal inoculation with a given agent, harvesting the serum, titering antibodies that were generated against the target antigen, determining the avidity of the resulting antibodies for their target, evaluating cross reactions with other substances that could possibly result in erroneous results and then evaluating the antibodies in sera of patients with varying illnesses to establish a test's clinical utility. The laboratory required skills in the preparation of radioactively labelled tracer agents required for immunoassay procedures. Finally the effort required that an investigator establish collaborative efforts between one's own laboratory and other research laboratories working on similar projects. In this way it could contribute to progress in the field without becoming an insular entity.

Beyond establishing the laboratory, the Division had the additional important responsibility of providing a teaching program for medical students and residents in the Department of Medicine as well as an educational program for staff physicians. At the same time it needed to provide a comprehensive clinical consultation program. Years later when a more well-developed endocrine physician staff was in place, the DE was also called upon to provide a post-residency fellowship program at the request of the Department of Medicine.

The Endocrine Laboratory initially provided urinary steroid assays, a competitive protein assay for serum cortisol and an immunoassay for the gonadotropins LH and FSH. After two years additional help was needed to develop other areas of the laboratory as well as to meet expanding teaching and consultative services.

To that end, in 1974 Dr. S. Thomas Bigos was recruited from the Massachusetts General Hospital (MGH) in Boston. He came with specific clinical interests in thyroid and parathyroid diseases and contributed the components necessary to advance laboratory capability in those fields. He was generously supported by the Dr. Farah Maloof's thyroid unit and laboratory at the MGH. Dr. Maloof provided the gift of the antibodies that permitted the MMC endocrine lab to build its own TSH assay as well as a new free-T4 assay which utilized equilibrium dialysis. Both were the standards in the field of thyroidology at the time. Dr. John Potts, Chief of the MGH Endocrine Unit, gifted the antibodies necessary to develop the first parathyroid hormone (PTH) assay at MMC.

Other services that grew with Dr. Bigos' arrival included the capacity for the Division to deliver radioactive iodine therapy to patients with thyroid cancer and hyperthyroidism. The Division became one of the nine North American academic medical institutions collaborating to provide data on the care of patients with thyroid cancer. Over the three decades that followed the Division participated with these other centers in the formation of the National Thyroid Cancer Treatment Collaborative. This group was responsible for publishing a number of scholarly articles on thyroid cancer which described the creation of a thyroid cancer staging system, a prognostic index, surgical recommendations and the definition of thyroid cancer patients who were or were not candidates for radioactive iodine treatment. It also participated in defining radioiodine as a diagnostic tool, differentiated from its use as a therapeutic tool.

In 1977 Dr. Richard Eastman's hiring completed the early development of the DE. His arrival from the Clinical Research Center at the National Institutes of Health was critical to the development of expertise in pituitary disease, adrenal function, and gynecologic endocrinology. He contributed significantly to the expansion of the educational services of the Department of Medicine as well as the expansion of endocrine service to outlying clinics.

Together, Drs. Johnston, Bigos and Eastman delivered comprehensive specialized laboratory, educational and clinical services to the MMC medical community. By the late 1970's their efforts resulted in the development of outreach clinics elsewhere in Maine. The first of these was a teaching and clinical program at Saint Mary's Hospital in Lewiston. This progressed from monthly to weekly and eventually to multi-day per week sessions. Later, clinics were installed at the Kennebec Valley Medical Center in Augusta and at the Thayer Hospital in Waterville, which eventually merged and became the Maine General Medical Center.

Over time the Endocrine Laboratory compiled a large banked catalogue of serum samples from normal persons and from populations of patients having various endocrine as well as non-endocrine diseases. These samples and their accompanying clinical data made it possible to rapidly evaluate the quality of later modifications of its own assays. They also allowed the Division's lab to trial and assess the clinical quality of commercial assays under development by other companies. Through such collaborative efforts the Endocrine Laboratory learned the limitations of upcoming commercial products, accessed advances in antibody production and made further improvements to its own assays. Examples of such collaborative services included work with entities such as Corning Biomedical Laboratories in Needham, Massachusetts, Abbott Laboratories in Lake Forest, Illinois and the Endocrine Metabolic Center at St. Joseph's Hospital in Oakland, California as well as with other academic center laboratories.

In 1985 Dr. Daniel Spratt joined as the Division's fourth member. He contributed to the further development of gynecologic endocrinology. He also pursued investigation of pituitary function in the setting of acute illness from non-endocrine disease.

Endocrinology

These studies provided information regarding the clinical interpretation of endocrine laboratory testing in patients with non-endocrine disease. These findings emphasized the importance that context played in the interpretation of endocrine testing given the pliability that the normal endocrine system displayed as it responded to non-endocrine illness.

An example of these efforts was the observation of abrupt thyroid, cortisone and sex steroid hormone loss to urine during cardiac surgery resulting from the displacement of these hormones from their carrier proteins when plasma volume was expanded with the Hespan infusion that accompanied going on bypass pump. The result was a massive loss of these molecularly small hormones. Further investigations described the period required post open-heart surgery for these losses to be corrected and establish more normal protein bound hormone levels. Another study described the pituitary function changes that accompanied the catabolic events occurring in special care unit patients as they adjusted to the metabolic stresses of their illness.

Other collaborative efforts that proved academically and clinically productive are described below:

Laboratory experience at MMC with the development of the heelstick method of measuring serum TSH levels in newborns led to collaboration with Dr. Marvin Mitchell at the Massachusetts State Laboratory, Dr. Reed Larson of the Peter Bent Brigham Hospital in Boston and others in the successful development of the New England Congenital Hypothyroid Screening Program.

In the era prior to the advent of computerized axial tomography (CT) and magnetic resonance imaging (MRI) scans, in conjunction with neurosurgeon Dr. Jules Hardy of the Notre Dame Hospital in Montreal, Canada, the MMC DE published the first reported cure of pituitary-determined hypercortisolism ("Cushing's Disease") in a patient with a normal sella turcica. Dr. Hardy was the pioneering neurosurgeon who developed the transsphenoidal approach to the sella turcica which was followed by a microscopically directed exploration of the pituitary gland. The patient in this case had a radiographically normal sella turcica but all the clinical hallmarks of hypercortisolism. At surgery the patient was found to have an offending ACTH secreting pituitary microadenoma, defined as less than 10 mm diameter, which in this case was five millimeters. Selective resection of the microtumor resulted in the patient's cure with no other subsequent pituitary deficits. This case report helped confirm the microadenoma origin of hypercortisolism for many patients with so-called "Cushing's Disease."

This experience then led to a later report that was one of the two early reported series of patients with pituitary-determined hypercortisolism who were treated surgically by transsphenoidal microsurgery. The patients for this surgical publication came from Dr. Hardy's combined experience derived from patients referred by the MMC DE and the Notre Dame endocrine department. The microscopic minimally invasive central nervous system intrusion that was pioneered by Dr. Hardy resulted in more complete visualization of the pituitary gland, more complete micro and macro tumor removal, no traditional craniotomy, no disruption of the frontal lobes or to the base of the brain, no postoperative cognitive disruption for the patient attributable to the procedure, fewer complications and shorter hospital convalescence. Today this is the preferred surgical route for management of most types of pituitary tumors.

A further literature report was generated by the combined experience of Dr. Eastman and his associates at the NIH. Together they reported the particularly elevated perioperative hemorrhagic risk that accompanied the use of transsphenoidal surgery for removal of a macroadenoma (tumor greater than 10 millimeters maximal diameter).

Dr. Bigos collaborated with Dr. Bruce Nisula of the National Institutes of Health detailing the utility of the use of cyclophosphamide in the management of advanced thyroid eye disease. and with Dr. Clark Sawain and others at the Boston Veterans Hospital reporting on the measurement of TSH and anti-thyroid antibodies in describing thyroid function changes that occurred in the elderly.

The Division of Endocrinology, by virtue of its laboratory capacity, identified a young female patient with delayed puberty resulting from her lack of the hypothalamic releasing hormone GnRH (gonadotropin releasing hormone) which was necessary for the release of pituitary luteinizing hormone (LH) and follicle stimulating hormone (FSH). Once defined, puberty and physical maturation were only possible through the daily administration of estrogen and eventually the addition of progesterone as well, both in pill form. This process was overseen by Dr. Bigos. She was managed medically through puberty into adulthood. When she became pregnant, she was referred to the MGH Reproductive Unit where an innovative program for administration of GnRH through a subcutaneous pump was available to stimulate the patient to secrete her own pituitary LH and FSH and thereby ovulate. This resulted in the first successful pregnancy by this method in the United States.

The Division helped to usher in the modern era of fine needle aspiration (FNA) as the preferred approach for thyroid biopsy. The MMC experience comparing the utility of FNA vs. cutting needle biopsy was reported in conjunction with Dr. Walter Goldfarb of the MMC Department of Surgery and Dr. Ronald Nishiyama of the Department of Pathology. This work expanded the support in the medical literature for the use of fine needle aspiration biopsies as these could be performed by non-thyroid surgeons under topical anesthesia in a standard outpatient examining room. Also, the FNA had the additional advantage of permitting biopsy of smaller nodules – ultimately leading to the wider use of FNA for the evaluation of thyroid nodules. Fine needle aspiration of the thyroid has now become a routine component of thyroid care.

With the development of accurate serum measurement of pituitary growth hormone levels, the use of timed stimulated sampling for the diagnosis of growth deficiency in both children and adults became feasible. This led to collaboration with Genentech Corporation (San Francisco) to develop the concept of a regional pituitary testing center that included updated investigation of growth hormone deficiency as part of its offerings. This allowed individual practitioners outside of a research center to refer their patients for complete endocrine testing without dealing with the delays then associated with traditional academic centers.

By combining MMC's bone biopsy results and laboratory PTH results from its renal, pathology and endocrine sections with similar data from Dr. Hartmut Malluche of the renal service at the University of Kentucky Medical Center and information from Drs. Reitz and Weinstein at the Endocrine Metabolic Center in Oakland, California the three centers were together able to construct the first nomogram in the United States used specifically for the measurement of PTH levels in chronic dialysis patients. The bone histology of these patients could then be plotted against their serum PTH levels. The resulting nomogram assisted in tracking the course of accelerated parathyroid activity in patients on dialysis and their susceptibility to a particular form of metabolic bone disease. It was then used as an important part of the decision in these patients regarding who was a candidate for parathyroid gland removal. As a result, over time, fewer patients with renal failure on chronic dialysis were found to be candidates for parathyroid surgery as part of the management of their bone status. This decision preserved more normal parathyroid function and improved medical management of bone health for the dialysis population. It also helped the later medical management of patients who underwent renal transplantation. The

PTH and histology data base thus generated was later submitted by the MMC Endocrine Lab to the NIH following a request from the NIH that it be made available to be included in their accumulating data base for patients on chronic dialysis.

In the late 1980's and early 1990's, the Division became a participant in the multicenter trial of calcitonin as a therapeutic agent for the treatment of osteoporosis. Part of the cost of a new dual energy bone densitometer required by the study was covered by the calcitonin study grant itself. Collaboration with the Division of Rheumatology led by Dr. Paulding Phelps at that time became a very important part of the Division's development in the area of metabolic bone disease. Dr. Larry Anderson from rheumatology generously and effectively led the collaborative effort with the rheumatology practice's research and clinical needs dovetailing well with the Division's needs. His help assured the ability to together fund the needed densitometer without needing a MMC contribution. The densitometer was generously provided floor space in the rheumatology offices. MMC research and clinical patients were offered ready access for studies. Dr. Anderson's gracious assistance was greatly appreciated.

With the completion of the calcitonin study and the availability at that point of bisphosphonate and parathyroid hormone in addition to calcitonin as FDA approved therapeutic agents, treatment of osteoporosis became eligible for financial compensation. The call for densitometry in both the rheumatology and endocrinology divisions then reached a demand that permitted each unit to acquire its own machinery. That said, the cooperation between divisions remains an effective example of working together in medicine and something for which the Division remains grateful.

Finally, Dr. Bigos authored a chapter of the Clinical Laboratory Annual edited by Dr. John Batsakis of the M. D. Anderson Hospital in Houston, Texas and formerly the Chief of Pathology at MMC. It dealt with laboratory testing anterior pituitary function in children and adults.

In 1991 Dr. Jerry Olshan joined the Division from the endocrine program at the Children's Hospital of Philadelphia to help meet the burgeoning clinical need for pediatric endocrine services. He was later joined by Dr. Alan Morris in 1997. These two physicians, members of the future Division of Pediatric Endocrinology within the Department of Pediatrics, also were critical components of the Pediatric Diabetes Section (see later developments).

Endocrinology

Early in the evolution of endocrinology at MMC it had been agreed that the Division would remain within its original design parameters and not enter into competition with private practices in delivering diabetic care. However in 1991 the MMC Board of Trustees decided that a true medical center should develop its own comprehensive diabetes center. This was deemed necessary to preclude MMC patients from having to go to Boston or elsewhere to receive the truly specialized care needed by some patients. This mandate was passed from Dr. Hillman, who was then Chief of Medicine, to the Division of Endocrinology. Discussions were held with the local private practices that delivered diabetes care. Although offered a directorship position, the practitioners elected to restrict their participation in the new center to serving in the clinic as part of its care delivery activities.

At that point, given that administrative, research, clinical care and teaching responsibilities required for directorship of a diabetes clinic, Dr. John Devlin was recruited from the University of Vermont's Fletcher Allen Medical Center (now the University of Vermont Medical Center). At that time he was a participant in Dr. Ethan Simms' diabetes-centered endocrine program. Dr. Devlin agreed to assume leadership of a new Diabetes Center at MMC in 1991.

By the end of the 1991 the Diabetes Center (DC) was established. However, the kaleidoscope of continuous change in the medical world was well under way and accelerating. The DC taxed the Division's space. Not only was space needed for clinical room but it was needed for the inclusion of Dr. Devlin's NIH funded research program. Further resources were required to extend care for the pediatric diabetes population - that factor becoming one of the most important drivers for the creation of dedicated space for the Diabetes Center. This was initially accomplished by acquiring additional facilities at the bottom of Congress Street adjacent to the MMC parking garage.

Relocation of a number of other MMC services was occurring at about the same time. New buildings were being purchased and old ones repurposed. The Osteopathic Hospital of Maine was subsumed under the auspices of MMC. As described in a separate chapter of this book, the old K-Mart site in Scarborough was purchased and converted into a new medical campus - redesigned for use by the Radiation Therapy Center, the Maine Center for Cancer Medicine and the MMC Regional Laboratory. Space was also included for the DE which by then also included the DC. Eventually, in the early 2000's, the endocrine and diabetes services were moved together to a single building of their own further south on Route 1 in Scarborough from the MMC campus. The DE and DC remain at this site to date.

Early in its evolution the Division of Endocrinology appreciated the importance of an electronic medical record (EMR). This occurred years before the issue became a public and political healthcare topic and before it was naively and falsely perceived as a near panacea for many, if not all, medical practice ills. At the time however, no such record was available. The earliest commercial EMR were plagued by a number of flaws. None was specifically designed for endocrinology. The first available EMR was difficult to manipulate and prohibitively expensive. It was obvious from the slow rate of development of a satisfactory commercial record that none was going to be available to the Division for many years.

As a result, within the limits of its desktop computer capabilities, the Division opted to try to create its own record. This placed it in the position of being one of the first specialty groups to become familiar with the practical limits and needs of an effective EMR designed for a specialty practice. Disease specific information was required to populate a record with the questions necessary to accumulate the appropriate clinical information for a given problem. Similarly, focus needed to be placed on the physical findings peculiar to a given disorder. Finally, an appropriate disposition list for a given differential diagnosis had to be generated. There were then medical confidentiality requirements as well as concerns about potential misuse of computerized records to be addressed.

The end result was the creation of a record system that although limited in design and features, incorporated most of the Division's short term requirements. It was adopted with the recognition that it was an imperfect solution and would remain as such until greater computer sophistication permitted a more complete version appropriate to the specialty to be obtained. By the mid 2000's there still was no commercially available system that could meet the Division's needs. With a series of internal modifications the Division continued to use its own record until MaineHealth adopted the Epic system after 2010.

Beginning around 2000 there were programmatic changes in the DE that were inevitable. The pediatric endocrine program became a service unto itself, physically moving to the MaineHeath facility in Portland as part of the Department of Pediatrics. Dr. Devlin remained with the DE until 2006 when he left to develop ancillary diabetes services for smaller hospitals in the region. Reproductive endocrine programs throughout the country came to be dominated by surgical training programs with integrated medical endocrine services. As a result most of reproductive endocrinology was eventually transferred to the Department of OB/GYN where a cadre of gynecologists was available to address endocrine issues. Dr. Daniel Spratt actually transferred from the DE to the Department of OB/GYN in 2000. These changes released critical space that the Division needed for other programs.

After running the fellowship program for a number of years the Division became overwhelmed by its clinical demands. In the prevailing economic climate it was unable to continue to devote the required amount of educational time to the fellowship program and therefore the program was closed.

Most of the outreach clinics were terminated after 2000 with the exception of the diabetes service provided through St Mary's Hospital and directed by Dr. Irwin Brodsky. The reason for closing the outreach services was mostly the development of various other programs. The Division was unable to support multiple locations with the equipment and personnel needed for thyroid biopsy, thyroid ultrasound, bone density and therapeutic infusion and testing services that had developed in the parent facility. Furthermore, as has been the case with medical specialty services throughout Maine, specialty endocrine practices of differing size emerged in other locales throughout the State. This was particularly the case in the Lewiston, Bath and Bangor areas.

In 1984 Dr. Eastman left the division to return to Georgetown as head of its endocrine section. He later returned fulltime to the NIH where he later became the Director of the Extramural Grant Program.

Drs. Robert Bing-You (1986), Daniel Oppenheim (1989) joined the Division to bolster clinical service. Dr. Bing-You has subsequently centered his later career in the Department of Medical Education.

To briefly summarize the progress of endocrinology in Portland, we again note that endocrine immunoassays were still in their infancy in the Division's early days. They required development and application to clinical use. As this happened a nationwide explosion of advances in assay methodologies occurred resulting in a plethora of new clinically important information. In addition, by the end of the 1990's methodologies that used radioactive components were dropped as assays became fully automated. By the mid 2000's the laboratory component had become well developed and automated. Academia by this time had turned its attention to the genetics and molecular biologic correlates of medicine. The clinical laboratory became less critical as a center for medical advancement. Rather, it represented a cost center for the health care system of

MaineHealth and was subsumed into NorDx. The role of the Division in laboratory efforts became one of an advisory position on the laboratory's board.

For this writer, it has been a distinct privilege to have been active in practice at a time that allowed me to be part of a generation of physicians who played important roles in many of the seminal advances in their chosen field of medicine in Portland and nationally. An intellectual challenge was always at hand, new issues were never lacking, growth and development in skills were there to be achieved provided the effort was given. Never was a patient denied care for lack of insurance or any other reason. For both professional and personal satisfaction I will always be indebted to Maine Medical Center. I hope that a similar experience is in store for physicians who follow in the future.

Family Medicine at MMC

By Ann K. Skelton MD

The history of family medicine at Maine Medical Center (MMC) parallels that of the specialty nationally. The evolution from general practice as the prevalent legacy medical delivery system, through the post-war period dominated by specialization, to the development of the discrete specialty of family practice (FP), and finally to distinction as family medicine (FM) was not without tension as the specialty differentiated itself. The Department of FM at MMC could not have been successful without the support of the institution and colleagues in many other specialties.

The 60-year history of the Department has seen it following national trends toward specialization within the discipline through fellowship training while retaining a firm base in primary care delivery. The outpatient setting has become an increasingly compelling focus for education. To that end, MMC has supported the development of high functioning model offices for patient care and learning. Department members developed new educational and clinical approaches, sharing their scholarly activity through national publication and presentation, and bringing MMC national recognition for excellence in family medicine.

The 1949 minutes of MMC's Medical Executive Committee (MEC) mentioned a magazine article about a hospital that expanded its structure to include a Division

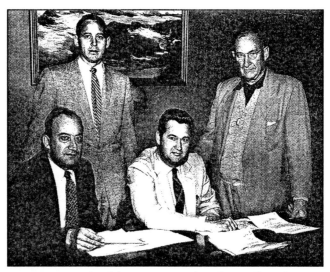

Dr. Branson, seated on left, Dr. Fogg on right and Dr. Hill standing in 1956. The identity of the other physician standing is unknown.

of General Practice (GP). The only division of GP known in the Northeast was in Salem Massachusetts. The MEC tabled the matter. In 1953 the issue of a possible Division of GP was again raised, and the MEC decided it should give further study to the matter. Finally in January 1956 the question was posed: "Should we establish a Division of General Practice at Maine General Hospital?" The general practitioners present identified several reasons to do so. The division would:

- Offer postgraduate medical education for themselves;

- Encourage interns and residents to practice in rural parts of the state; and

- Enable the medical profession to better serve the indigent in the hospital and through continuity in follow up after discharge from the hospital.

The consensus of those present was to establish a plan to develop a division. Comments were received from Drs. Marston, Geyerhan, McIntire, Branson, George and Charles Geer, Dyhrberg, Fogg, Finks, Hinckley, Stevens, Parker, Hawks and Thompson. In February, Dr. Philip Thompson chaired a GP committee to plan for such a division. By June, the MEC voted to establish a GP Service which would function as a service with an attending staff with all the rights, privileges, and responsibilities of active staff members. The members of the GP Division voted to recommend Dr. Sidney Branson as its first Chief. In 1957 Dr. Charles Geer was appointed Associate Chief. The members of the Division staffed the general medical clinic on Mondays and Fridays.

Dr. Branson published "On the Establishment of a Department of General Practice in a Large Hospital" in the Journal of the Maine Medical Association in 1957. In this article, he reflected on the process that included surveying chiefs of other departments to provide practical and didactic education to fit the needs of general practitioners, thus enlisting assistance of specialist colleagues from the Department's inception. In addition, Dr. Branson surveyed each general practitioner about his interest in participating in the service. Of 32 physicians questioned, 18 committed to spending at least eight hours weekly on Departmental work. One statement from Dr. Branson's article referred to the benefit that accrues from incorporating general practice within a hospital structure: "The presence of general practitioners makes for better balance in all phases of hospital mechanics." With that, planning was underway for a GP residency.

In 1958, Dr. Branson gained MMC approval for a two-year GP residency program. In the year prior 5 MMC residencies had been approved: medicine, surgery, radiology, pathology and anesthesiology. In 1958, the residency options expanded to include both general practice and cardiovascular diseases.

The clinical model for GP in the hospital clinic evolved. Access was changed to an hour per day every day, providing the availability to evaluate any patient who "came in off the street." By 1959, the residency was fully operational, with two residents per year in each year of the two-year program.

In 1962, Dr. Branson stepped down and Dr. Phillip Fogg came on as Chief. The screening clinic was renamed the General Medical Clinic with rotations of two months to provide continuity and follow up, rather than GP physicians screening patients then referring to other clinics for all follow up. In 1963, the Residency Review Committee for GP approved MMC's residency for two years of training. The attending staff numbered 21. Dr. Fogg resigned as Chief in 1964 to enter a psychiatry residency. Dr. Fogg and the department members recommended Dr. Robert Pawle to serve as Chief, and he was confirmed.

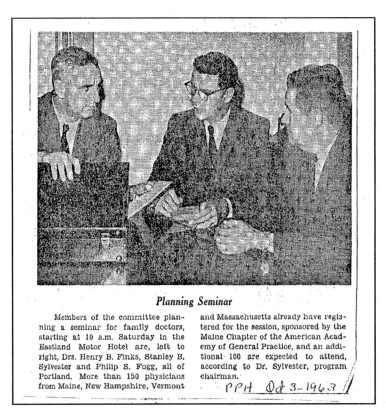

Planning Seminar

Members of the committee planning a seminar for family doctors, starting at 10 a.m. Saturday in the Eastland Motor Hotel are, left to right, Drs. Henry B. Finks, Stanley B. Sylvester and Philip S. Fogg, all of Portland. More than 150 physicians from Maine, New Hampshire, Vermont and Massachusetts already have registered for the session, sponsored by the Maine Chapter of the American Academy of General Practice, and an additional 100 are expected to attend, according to Dr. Sylvester, program chairman.

PPH Oct 3-1963

Planning Seminar in 1963. Drs. Henry Finks, Stanley Sylvester & Phillip Fogg

Issues during Dr. Pawle's tenure reflected the struggles faced by general practitioners operating in specialist dominated hospital environments nationally. At MMC, tensions were most marked with obstetrics and internal medicine. One example of such a conflict was a 1966 rule requiring consultations for inductions planned by non-obstetricians. The rule was developed by the department of obstetrics and challenged by Dr. Pawle. After review by the MEC the rule stood, but to improve communication a new policy was approved: "If a Chief of Service is considering a new policy pertaining to his service but affecting others he should first discuss it with members of his service and then forward it to MEC for approval. The MEC will notify those affected." The tensions with internal medicine were evident in the struggle to develop an inpatient family medicine service for adult patients.

The American Board of Medical Specialties initially recognized the specialty of family practice in 1969. In MMC's division, discussions were underway to prepare for change in the specialty name to family practice. Those already in practice could sit for Family Practice boards until 1978 without residency training. Anticipating the conversion of the GP Residency to FP, Dr. Pawle brought forward some of the national training requirements for FP, including the requirement for a "model Family Practice Unit" in which physicians assumed responsibility for the care of a family. He felt that establishing a community medical program would address many needs.

By 1972, MMC and the City of Portland were planning for a FP Clinic on Munjoy Hill. Planners anticipated that the clinic would be open to all income groups, coordinated with MMC specialty clinics and the emergency and inpatient services. Jointly, they identified 4 principles for the clinic.

1. They should provide comprehensive health care with top-level services and should stress preventive medicine;

2. The ability to pay principle should prevail with a sliding fee scale from usual fees to no charge whatsoever;

3. There should be one standard of medical care regardless of ability to pay; and

4. Care should be continuous rather than episodic and should be achieved by appropriate relations with the faculty at the MMC.

From the start, planners recognized the importance of addressing issues beyond the strictly medical and therefore included dentists, nutritionists and social workers.

Not everyone at MMC supported the advent of a FP residency. The Director of Medical Education and Internal Medicine Department Chief at the time thought family practice would come and go… "A fad like women's hats."

Fortunately, others had more foresight. In 1972, The Area Health Education Center (AHEC) provided a $4.9 million grant to Tufts School of Medicine to recruit physicians to practice in a rugged corner of the country in a state without a medical school – Maine. The press article about the program was titled "Being Sent to Siberia" and described 16 third year students going to Maine for a year of clinical training, with some fourth year students pursuing electives in Maine. The grant included support of faculty development for physicians, and to support the building of the "model Family Practice Unit" as a first step toward developing a FP residency. At the time, Maine had one physician per 1100 people; Boston had six per 1000. Discussion of development of a clinic on Munjoy Hill continued. The outcome of "being sent to Siberia" was positive. Surveys of the medical students who had rotated at MMC revealed very positive experiences and many revealed that they had plans to stay in Maine.

In 1973, MMC established two new departments: The Department of Community Medicine and the Department of Family Practice. Dr. Robert M. True was recruited to direct a new Family Practice residency. He was a Bowdoin graduate, who left a Massachusetts practice to return to Maine where he had family.

In April, Dr. Douglass Walker, Medical Director of MMC included a letter of intent and proposal to the State planning board regarding a Department of Community Medicine and a Model Family Practice Unit. The Family Practice Unit was designed to provide care to residents of Munjoy Hill and the Casco Bay Islands that would be:

- Family oriented and personalized;
- Comprehensive;
- High in quality; and
- Low in direct cost to patients.

Importantly, the site was to be designed to provide an "ideal learning experience for family physicians who will take the experience to their own practices in Maine."

Augmenting the AHEC grant, a Robert Wood Johnson Foundation grant provided $359,000 for three years of support to develop and test improved practice and educational patterns to expand access to ambulatory services and primary care in Maine rural communities.

In December 1973, an inaugural meeting was held of the newly established Department of Family Practice at MMC. Dr. Robert True served as Chief, with Dr. Robert Caven as Associate Chief. Meeting minutes reflect discussion of privileges, and encouragement of those present to change from courtesy to active in order to participate in teaching at the model unit.

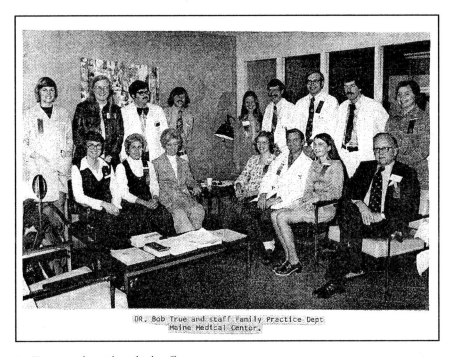

Dr. True, on right, with medical staff

The Model Family Practice Unit opened in 1974 at the corner of Congress and India Streets. A Community Advisory Board for the FP Unit was established in June 1974, 5 months before opening ceremonies. For patients needing hospitalization, Dr. True outlined policies regarding admissions in conjunction with medicine, surgery, pediatrics and obstetrics, and defined the roles of FP residents and attendings and those of other services. Dr. True and his colleagues were also busy identifying a curriculum for the FP residency. In November, the Department discussed affiliation with Mercy Hospital on teaching internal medicine to FP residents. This was driven in part by decreased bed availability at MMC and surgeons' migration to Mercy in response. The MMC MEC voted to approve the philosophy of FP residents rotating through Mercy with Mercy's MEC approving the concept as well.

According to the AHEC report, the FP residency had 11 residents in training in 1974, the Model FP Unit was functioning and Robert True had been working for one year as its director. The residency received Residency Review Committee approval in 1974. The 1974-75 resident roster listed Drs. Haskell, Hogan and Morgan as second year residents with Drs. Kitfield, Reed and Saffer as first year residents. Dr. Haskell reflects: "When it began in the early 1970's there were only 7 programs nationwide. Residency opened in 1974 as a 3 resident per year program. Through a glitch, six residents matched in the first year. Despite views to the contrary, all were allowed to continue in the program." In the early days of the residency, the program attracted pioneers, becoming more mainstream with time.

By 1975, affiliation was in place with University of Vermont, with MMC officials interviewing medical students from Maine in an annual Burlington visit. The following year, the residency had a full quota of 12 residents. The FP Unit was accommodating 1,000 patients monthly. Two senior residents were rotating at Mercy. Planning was underway for a Peaks Island Health Center staffed by a family nurse practitioner who worked there most of the time, and at the FP Unit one day weekly, backed up by FP physicians. Dr. True faced opposition as he endeavored to reestablish a FP inpatient service. The members of the FP Department signed a letter to Dr. Al Aronson in his role as Director of Medical Education, to resolve the issue of the FP Inpatient Service. They outlined a process for FP admissions to each service, supervised by FP attendings and cared for by FP residents. The Department of Medicine opposed an independent inpatient Family Practice Service.

In 1975, Dr. Haskell, one of the first class of graduates, opened his practice in Yarmouth. Subsequent graduates, including Dr. Jeffrey Saffer, joined local practices and became the vanguard of the new FP community. Most of the graduates remained strong contributors to the program as teachers in the hospital or FP Unit. There was great loyalty to the Department and collegiality among its members.

In 1977, still headed by Dr. True, the Department was active in the development of the Casco Bay Health Station on Peaks Island and provided support to Sacopee Valley Health Center, the Steep Falls clinic and the Chebeague Island health care program. Ian MacInnes was chosen as Assistant Chief after Dr. Caven joined the military service.

In early 1977, Dr. True forwarded an American Academy of Family Physicians publication relevant to the FP inpatient service to Dr. Walker. "… If a clinical Department of FP is to be established in a hospital, it must be treated as any other clinical department…" The final responsibility for recommendations on clinical privileges shall reside with the clinical department of FP."

Dr. True requested a consultation from the Family Practice Residency Assistance Program. The consultant wrote in his April report, "There seems to be a feeling on the part of the administration and the faculty leaders that the family practice center and its curriculum are something "out there" which is different from the objectives of the institution. He recommended the creation of an inpatient service on which family physicians' patients are followed by residents. Additional suggestions included additional faculty, consideration of increasing to six residents per year, adding didactic conferences and recruiting more diverse patients (i.e., those of higher socioeconomic status). Also suggested was administering and accounting for the model FP Unit as a practice, not as a hospital unit and, in fact, to stop using the term "unit."

On January 9, 1978, Dr. True died suddenly and unexpectedly. His widow Marilyn shared his great love of family practice with his colleagues. In his honor, she provided funding for the Robert M. True Symposium, an annual faculty development conference attended by residents, faculty and family physicians from all over Maine. For years, this was the premier continuing medical education conference for family physicians.

Dr. MacInnes, the newly arrived Assistant Chief, became the Acting Chief. In June, the search committee voted to recommend Dr. MacInnes as permanent Chief, a position he accepted. However, he resigned in October to reunite with his family that had stayed behind in Edmonton, Alberta.

Recruited from Minnesota, Dr. Harley Racer became Chief and Residency Program Director in 1979. That fall, discussion of relocation of the Family Practice Center focused on a broader patient mix, increase in number of families and individuals treated, and the potential to increase from four residents per year to six. Dr. Racer left in 1980 to return to Minnesota. MMC recruited Drs. Donald Abbott and Charles Belisle from their practice in Yarmouth to serve as acting Director and Associate Director for the residency.

In 1980 the MMC Board of Trustees voted to share the cost of the FP residency with Mercy – which had housed the FP Inpatient service since 1976 -- and to develop a new FP Center at the Central Fire Station, sponsored by MMC and the City of Portland. A detailed proposal included needs assessment and design documents. The City Council voted to accept the proposal. However, 1981 saw the "demise" of the Central Fire Station as a potential site for the new Center.

In the same year, Dr. John Randall was named Chief. Dr. Belisle stayed on as his associate chief. Recruiting Dr. John Randall as Chief and Program Director provided the Department and residency with its first long period of stability. He was trained as a pediatric infectious disease specialist and well respected for his clinical skill. When he arrived, there was still major tension about what Family Practice should be and how much jurisdiction family physicians should have in patient care, especially in the hospital. At one point, Dr. Randall challenged the Director of Medical Education, to "decide whether MMC really wants a residency program." The response was affirmative, and MMC provided support for four residents annually.

Dr. Randall found Mercy "very hospitable" with the missions of Mercy and the residency being complementary. In 1982, the teaching faculty included many loyal community physicians: Drs. Abbott, Bonjour, Burnham, Ciampi, D'Andrea, deSieyes, Haskell, Hill, Hinckley, Knapp, Paulding, Rowland and Saffer. New conversations about relocating the FP Center focused on the North School on India Street. The ribbon to the new center was cut by George L. True, father of the late Robert True. Photos of the new center include one of Charlie Belisle, Associate Chief, with Ann McDonough, RN, head nurse.

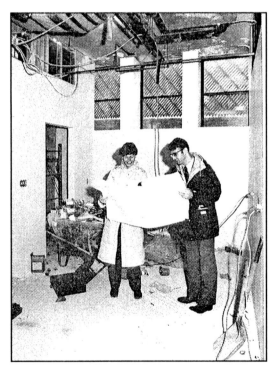

Ann McDonough, RN and Dr. Charles Belisle check plans
for India St. Clinic in 1984

Over the years, the Department was characterized by great loyalty and camaraderie. One of the events that fostered that camaraderie was an annual departmental retreat. A 1985 rental agreement secured a Girl Scout camp for a long weekend in October. Eventually, thanks to Dr. Richard Rockefeller's generosity with his island near Acadia National Park, it became the annual retreat site. Generations of family physicians, their families and their staff enjoyed walking, kayaking, mushrooming, collecting mussels, and singing on Bartlett Island.

Dr. Randall stated that greater acceptance of FP as a specialty within MMC coincided with Dr. Rockefeller's arrival in our medical community. Dr. Rockefeller not only "legitimized" the specialty in the eyes of many, he also brought innovation and research to the Department. A photo of Dr. Randall pictures him in front of a computer, using "Problem Knowledge Couplers," an early medical decision making tool developed by Larry Weed MD, and piloted with support of Dr. Rockefeller.

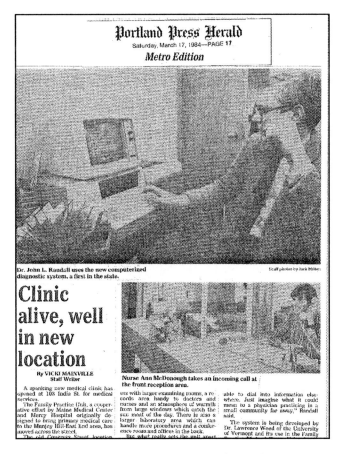

Dr John Randall checks out new computer at India St. Clinic

Another factor in the growing respect enjoyed by the Department within the medical community was Dr. Randall's recruitment of Dr. Joel Botler to serve as the FP Inpatient Service Director. Joel was a recent graduate of MMC's internal medicine residency. Along with his private practice, he covered the critical care patients at Mercy Hospital with the Mercy pulmonary and critical care group and enjoyed the respect of those colleagues. His presence and oversight assured the highest quality of care was delivered by the FP residents and attendings on the FP service. He built bridges between FP and Internal Medicine. For years, his white coat read as we saw him: "Joel Botler MD, Family Practice." The FP inpatient service modeled interprofessional practice with rounds attended by social workers, occupational and physical therapists. Specialists supported the residents' education; with a cardiologist and a critical care physician attending morning report each day, and the whole team reviewing each admission. The FP residents and teaching attendings had the full support of the Mercy pulmonary and critical care physicians, and the hospital's administration.

After serving for 10 years, Dr. Randall stepped down to become Chair of the Department of Family and Community Medicine at Jefferson Medical College in Philadelphia and Dr. Robert McArtor was recruited to serve as Chief and Program Director. Dr. McArtor' s tenure coincided with increasing interest in primary care as health maintenance organizations were developed in the 1990's. It was literally and figuratively a time for growth and building in FP. Dr. McArtor leveraged the appetite for primary care to develop new facilities and programs and to expand the thriving residency. Wanting to integrate more fully into the MMC, he moved the FP administrative offices from a brown house across Bramhall Street into MMC itself. A symbolic move, it came to represent his tenure and its legacy - solidifying FP's position of contribution within MMC.

Dr. McArtor requested a dedicated residency program director after years of the Chief serving in that role as well. Dr. Ann Skelton became the Program Director in 1995. In the same year, the University of Vermont developed a required clerkship in FP and Dr. Peggy Cyr was named to direct the experience in Maine.

The 1995 True Symposium featured "Cyriax Musculoskeletal Diagnosis and Treatment" as its annual conference. Interest in this course spawned others and led indirectly to the development of a fellowship in sports medicine.

In 1995, with the merger of the medical staffs of Brighton Hospital and Maine Medical Center, the potential for conflict with Mercy arose. The Department moved the FP teaching service from Mercy back to MMC. Questioned at first, this proved an important step in providing greater visibility for the Department through its best ambassadors – its bright, collegial residents and attendings who provide excellent care in the hospital.

Dr. McArtor obtained a grant to provide education in three domains: Quality improvement, Community oriented primary care, and rural health. The residency expanded to six residents per year, eventually expanding to seven per year under his leadership. By the end of his tenure, the faculty had expanded from four to ten.

In 1996, Dr. Branson wrote a letter to leaders of the American Academy of Family Physicians that made its way back to Dr. McArtor. The article was titled "First and Foremost." In it, he states, "we established the first family practice department and residency at MMC in 1956. There were no other programs in New England, perhaps the country. "I went before the Board at MMC with a plan for such a department. I was approached by the Governing Board and the Medical Staff and we got going in the summer of 1956."

In 1997, the True Symposium on Alternative and Complementary Medicine presaged future endeavors in integrative medicine. Looking for a broader patient base and more space for the growing faculty and residency – now recruiting seven residents annually - MMC opened a second FP Center in Falmouth. It was staffed in a new model, in partnership with Family Care Associates. Drs. Harper and deSieyes moved their new practice and their associate, Dr. Vicki Hayes, to the new facility. They saw patients side by side with residents, and eventually several additional faculty members joined the Falmouth crew.

A national trend in specialization within primary care disciplines was evident in MMC's Department of FP. Some of its physicians obtained certificates of added qualification in geriatrics. A second area of specialization was sports medicine. Dr. McArtor recruited Dr. William Dexter to return to Maine and establish a primary care sports medicine fellowship, which was accredited in 1997. The first resident entered the program in 1998. Dr. Dexter's leadership, including his tenure as President of the American College of Sports Medicine, and his positioning of faculty and residents in prominent national roles allowed for expanded national recognition for MMC in the sports medicine community.

Dr. McArtor's impact on growth and integration is reflected not only in the move of the administrative offices to within MMC and the new practice site in Falmouth, but also in the building of a new family practice center. The new building rose on the same site as the original 1974 building, twenty five years later. The opening was a community event, celebrated with a block party and a ribbon cutting ceremony performed by a husband and wife who had received care from and taught generations of residents.

The merger of Brighton Medical Center with MMC brought many osteopathic family physicians to the FP department. By 1997, a Division of Osteopathic Manipulative Medicine (OMM) was approved by the MEC. It was chaired by Dr. Donald Hankinson, its members providing neuromusculoskeletal medicine consultations to an average of over 25 patients a day. The name of the Division changed to Neuromusculoskeletal Manipulative Medicine (NMM), and the by-laws were changed to permit NMM to be the only specialty not formally recognized by the American Board of Medical Specialties to be eligible to practice at MMC.

During Dr. McArtor's tenure, there was increased focus on scholarly activity. National grants were secured to improve curriculum in rural medicine, quality and community-oriented care. Dr. Neil Korsen was named the Co-Director of the Dartmouth Cooperative Primary Care Research Network. Dr. Alain Montegut involved faculty, residents, and curriculum consultants in the development of family practice as a specialty in the country of Vietnam, an effort supported by grant funding. Further funding supported the introduction of "informatics" as the internet developed and point of care decision-making tools became available.

The FP Center changed under Dr. McArtor's leadership. As suggested in the Residency Assistance Program consultation years prior, the Center changed from administration as a hospital "unit" to a model office practice. He recruited Dr. Jacquelyn Cawley, who effected that change, along with a new practice manager, Deborah Lovley and Ann McDonough, FP's head nurse.

The practices of family physicians in greater Portland changed during the 1990's as more physicians moved from "onesies and twosie" practices to form larger group practices. The largest of these were Bowdoin Medical Group, InterMed, Martin's Point Health Care, Scarborough Family Physicians, and Casco Bay Physicians (the MMC faculty group). Despite those changes, a significant number of physicians remained "independent" and practice that way today.

In 2000, Dr. McArtor assumed responsibility as Chief Medical Officer for the newly developed MaineHealth system, and Dr. Ann Skelton was appointed Chief of the Department.

A National Institutes of Health grant supported the integration of Complementary and Alternative Medicine (CAM) into the FP curriculum. As with other originally educational endeavors, this area of focus soon affected clinical services delivered as Department members partnered with community practitioners including osteopathic physicians, acupuncturists, homeopaths and mind-body specialists.

Within the hospital, a Maternal Child Health Service became a part of the inpatient service, with residents and a small group of dedicated attending physicians providing care for pregnant women, newborns and hospitalized children from the FP Center and other local practices.

Dr. Alain Montegut, whose Vietnam education project was completed with full support of the FP Department, came on as Residency Program Director. In that capacity, he continued to provide international linkages for residents and faculty.

Dr. Craig Schneider, recruited after completion of an integrative medicine fellowship in Tucson, AZ to serve as faculty leader for the CAM project, remained on after the grant's conclusion. In 2005 MMC supported the development of a fellowship in integrative medicine. Through the fellowship learners participated in on-site education in Tucson, distance learning, and in a fourth year of residency.

By 2005, Dr. Montegut's international work took him to Boston University, and Dr. Alison Samitt became Residency Program Director. On the national scene, in 2005 the specialty name changed from family practice to family medicine. MMC maintained a regional and national reputation for the FM residency program as a highly desirable educational experience.

In 2007 the MEC and MMC Board of Trustees approved a new Division of Community and Preventive Medicine headed by Dr. Jo Linder. The Division is a partnership among the Departments of FP, Pediatrics, Internal Medicine, Psychiatry and Nursing. It is housed within the Department of FM. Members include physicians, allied health professionals, administrators and others in those fields and others.

In 2007, MMC changed its educational partner from UVM to Tufts University School of Medicine (TUSM). Department members assisted in the development of the TUSM– Maine Track. The Maine Track required the development of a Longitudinal Integrated Clerkship as well as the traditional block rotation in FM for third year students. Dr. Peggy Cyr developed systems to support both third year options. She also wrote grants to AHEC, still supporting primary care initiatives, to introduce health professions to high school students in rural Maine, and to support medical students considering a career in FM.

Dr. Jeff Aalberg, who had served as Medical Director for the FM practices, continuing the innovative practice work begun through Dr. Cawley, moved on to a position at MaineHealth. Dr. Mark Bouchard became Medical Director. In 2011 the clinical practices of MMC were integrated with the growing ambulatory enterprise of Maine Medical Partners (MMP). Operations of the FM Centers were increasingly integrated with those of other MMP practices. By 2012 a Primary Care Medical Director position was created at MMP to oversee FM, internal medicine and pediatrics practices.

The FM Centers serve as a model for other educational programs, with a high degree of integration of the academic and clinical missions. They also serve as learning labs, producing innovations such as group medical visits for lifestyle medicine, open access appointment scheduling, transitional group visits and integrative medication assisted therapy for opioid use disorder.

In 2014 Department members developed an interprofessional education program based the interprofessional services offered at its "Hospital to Home" visits that serve practice patients transitioning out of hospital and rehabilitation facilities. The program includes home visits and provides opportunities for medical, pharmacy and social work students to learn from, with and about each other.

After twenty years of service as Sports Medicine Program Director, its founder, Dr. William Dexter, stepped down. Dr. Heather Gillespie assumed responsibility as Program Director in 2016, having returned from University of California, Los Angeles the year prior.

As population health became a more important component of the health delivery system, the Department sought and was awarded a $950,000 grant to plan and implement a residency in preventive medicine (PM). The PM residency was accredited in 2015, with Dr. Christina Holt as its Program Director. Through the program, residents who completed a primary residency in any specialty obtained a Masters of Public Health and learned from colleagues in public health, MaineHealth, and community partners. The focus of the residency was to serve vulnerable populations in Maine, namely elderly, rural, new Mainers and those with homelessness and mental health and substance use disorders.

Scholarly activity for the Department provided national recognition. Residents and faculty members worked with the research directors, Dr. Christina Holt and Amy Haskins, PhD to develop and disseminate new knowledge. The prolific work of Drs. Cyr, Dexter, Hayes and Holt, and Ms. Julie Schirmer ensured several national publications and presentations annually. In addition, many of FM's talented physicians contributed as leaders in larger institutional and MaineHealth systems. Leadership positions included Drs. McArtor and Botler serving as CMO for MaineHealth and MMC respectively, Dr. Cawley' s service as Chief Information Officer for MaineHealth, and Dr. Aalberg' s service as Senior Medical Director for MaineHealth Clinical Integration.

Dr. Charles Belisle was a Department leader deserving special recognition. He served in a variety of roles from the 1970's forward and became the Department's "master preceptor" - using his vast knowledge and experience to teach the next generation. His longevity provided extensive institutional knowledge and stability during times of change. Charlie's character, altruism and sincere interest in the people with whom he worked made him an invaluable asset. Charlie was singular in his service to the Department, its patients and learners. He earned well-deserved state-wide recognition as the Maine Family Physician of the Year in 2010.

The FM Department's greatest outcomes have been the quality of care provided to patients, and the impact of its graduates on health care locally, statewide and nationally. The majority of graduates remained in Maine, from York to Fort Kent. Others went as far as Alaska, and through development of FM as a specialty in other countries, touched medical care in international settings. To a greater and greater degree, MMC and other academic institutions became aware of the needs of the populations seen within their walls and undertook responsibility for their community health needs. The Department of FM has long worked in this domain. It evolved as a more and more valuable partner for MMC, its specialty colleagues, and the community as a whole. Its educational programs have proven to be outstanding and focused on meeting the mission of "education for societal needs."

Gastroenterology

By Douglas A. Howell MD

"The Tunnel at the End of the Light" - Peter B. Cotton

The story of our recognized excellence in gastroenterology (GI) at Maine Medical Center (MMC) begins with Laban W. Leiter MD, Maine's first gastroenterologist. First let me explain that our GI specialty is very large with a vast list of ailments, symptoms, and diagnoses, perhaps the longest in medicine. Our division overlaps every specialty and subspecialty with diseases from the esophageal inlet to the very bottom itself. We diagnose and care for cancer, infections, autoimmune, congenital, and degenerative disorders in both sexes from childhood to 100+ year olds. In the 1970's, Bockus' Textbook of Digestive Disease was seven volumes and today there are more than 150 chapters posted in UpToDate GI - more than any other specialty. This quick review of our division helps explain why gastroenterology CPT codes remain the second most common associated with admission to MMC. This does not include many CPT's that are our responsibility for initial diagnosis, admission or referral yet are eventually coded for other specialties, such as colon and pancreatic cancer or surgical codes like perforated ulcer or cholangitis.

A great medical center must have a great GI division to accurately diagnose, attract referrals for surgical care and train future physicians. We have accepted the responsibility to care for challenging cases, teaching and carrying on clinical research to document quality care - measured by accurate, prompt diagnoses, advanced procedural expertise and superior patient outcomes. These are the "three hats" of medicine – excellent clinical patient care, teaching and research. Our division has been recognized and honored locally, nationally and internationally in the past and up to the present for each of these "hats."

The question is only partially how did we accomplish these but more importantly who made this happen.

Laban W. Leiter MD received his MD from Harvard at the close of World War II. He met and married Eva Fearon, RN, from Brownville Junction, Maine. After military service he did a stint at the Manchester, NH VA and then came to the Maine General Hospital in 1954. Our Chief of Surgery at that time was Isaac Webber MD also from Brownville Junction and a graduate of Bowdoin Medical School for which Maine General was its medical campus.

Laban and Iva produced 5 wonderful and successful children, several of whom went into medicine as doctors, nurses and health administrators in our state and elsewhere. Laban practiced out of the front half of his home at 175 Vaughn Street for nearly 50 years, seeing office patients after his morning rounds and procedures at both Maine Medical Center and Mercy. His amazing routine was to stop seeing patients at 6:00 PM, exit through the back office door into his kitchen and have family dinner. After dinner, his "constitutional" was to walk over to the hospital to check on his inpatients before returning to his desk for paperwork and phone calls to the patients who had left a call back request. He always worked with one nurse and one receptionist. His work life never included an on call schedule or a vacation beyond a family event. He even kept this routine during summers from the family's beach front cottage on Pine Point Beach.

His clinical skills were incredible - especially considering that half of his practice was general internal medicine. He purchased the first semi flexible gastroscope with his own funds and established colonoscopy as a gastroenterology procedure here at Maine Medical Center. His early expertise was accomplished with great skill, beginning a pattern of statewide referral for GI cases that we enjoy today. His practice included all forms of GI disorders from cancer to inflammatory bowel disease to liver disorders and for all ages from pediatric to geriatric.

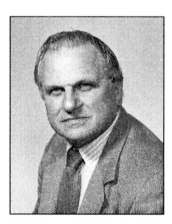

Dr. Laban Leiter MD

Beyond his clinical practice, Dr. Leiter was also very active in administration, serving on the MMC Board of Trustees, as Chief of Medicine and as Chief of the Division. By the mid 1970's his practice was heavy with physicians and family members – all as patients whom he refused to bill. His tiny waiting room often looked like the Doctor's Lounge.

In the late 1960's, Laban recruited Newell Augur MD from Columbia Physicians & Surgeons Hospital in New York as Maine's first GI fellowship-trained gastroenterologist. Newell had been summering at Prout's Neck at his family's summer house but was convinced that partnership with an individual of Laban's character would ensure his similar life goals. Newell brought his training and his teaching skills to raise the Department's range of procedures and teaching conferences to a new height while also serving on the MMC Board of Trustees and as acting Chief of Medicine. His wonderful family also excelled with his children becoming a physician, lawyer and legislator.

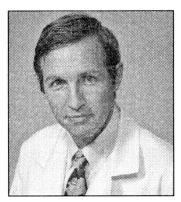

Dr. Newell Auger MD

In 1978, these two remarkable competent and inspiring physicians recruited me to join them as the third Maine Medical Center gastroenterologist. My training at Dartmouth encouraged me to interview at academic institutions. The great Thomas P. Almy, M.D, "father of gastroenterology," was then the Chief of Medicine at Dartmouth He introduced me to several of his former GI fellows who had risen to academic chiefs throughout the northeast. My interview here in Portland was encouraged by my wife, Sharyn, as her aunt and uncle were living in Cape Elizabeth. They had lived all over the world but retired to Portland and were very impressed with some recent medical care there. My first trip, principally hosted by Laban, found me walking and talking with him for hours – all about quality medicine and the responsibility beyond our practice to offer the most up to date modern GI care to the whole state.

I had the overwhelming feeling that a center filled with physicians of his caliber and with the potential to really impact the entire state's needs, more than compensated for leaving behind the prestige of big city medical school academia.

At Dartmouth, I discussed my interviews and my favorable impressions with Tom Almy, seeking his advice. He explained that individual commitment is more important than prestige. He encouraged me to take the position with its financial freedom and schedule flexibility. He agreed that private practice could permit my own decisions to balance my future. In the end, he agreed that I would have a better chance to craft a practice and wear all three hats here at Maine Medical Center.

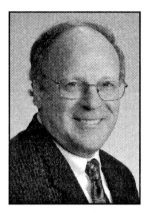

Dr. Douglas Howell MD

At Dartmouth I then began to pursue cutting edge training in procedures not yet available in Maine, focusing on endoscopic treatments of biliary and pancreatic disorders. After an introduction through Newell, I sought training by Dick Norton MD at Tufts, who had just returned from Niigata, Japan. He was the only physician in Boston, and one of the first in America, to remove a common bile stone endoscopically. I attended conferences in Toronto and New York and insisted that a Dartmouth attending, Jack McCleery MD, train with Dick as well.

On my final interview in mid-1977 with Newell and Laban the position was offered. I agreed, shook hands and said Sharyn and I would need to meet a realtor. Since there had been no discussions about finances, salary or contract, I asked Laban "what price range should we look at?" His response of "nothing too expensive" ended the conversation and I replied that I would start as of September 1, 1978. A handshake was our contract.

In brief, my career at Maine Medical Center has been remarkable, enjoyable, productive and wildly successful, largely due to the excellence of our physicians welcoming me, especially the radiology, pathology and surgical faculty. My ability to bring new technologies, new procedures, acquire and even develop new equipment, all contributed to improved patient outcomes. The range of unusual pathology presented to me from throughout the state, permitted some early clinical research projects which I encouraged medical and surgical residents to join in the absence of a formal GI fellowship.

After a number of original journal articles and presentations at regional and then national meetings, a medical resident, John "Jay" Bosco MD suggested I start an advanced interventional GI fellowship at Maine Medical Center. He would return for an extra year beyond the standard two years of fellowship at Lahey Clinic in Boston. I objected – there was no support, it would not be ABIM approved, it had not been established by our specialty societies, there was no available housing.....etc. - but I could try.

After a trial of a private practice supported part-time fellow, Al Muggia MD we were able to secure a full-time fellow's salary from industry. This was based on our clinical research presentation at our annual Digestive Disease Week. The institution agreed to the position and it was accepted with two years of funding.

From 1992 to the present, we have had the great privilege of hosting 25 consecutive years of advanced fellows who chose to train with us for one additional optional year. This year of training heavily emphases newer "cutting edge" procedures formerly performed by surgeons using open surgical techniques.

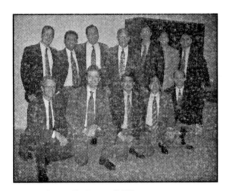
Group photo of advanced fellows

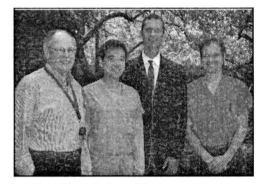
Drs. Howell, Low, Stefan and Bosco

Surgical common duct exploration quickly became endoscopic sphincterotomy with stone extraction. Post-op bile leaks were increasingly and now exclusively treated with endoscopic sphincterotomy and biliary stent placement.

Obstructive jaundice from cancer could be treated initially with plastic and later metal indwelling stents placed at ERCP. Eventually we have been able to incorporate ampullary adenoma resection, pseudocyst drainage and even transgastric retroperitoneal debridement for necrotizing pancreatitis. It was a strange and exhilarating ride in the bowels of the radiology department at Maine Medical Center.

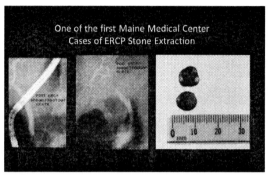

Early stone extraction

Through this time the Department has been able to recruit and retain specialty trained gastroenterologists to fill all the needs of Maine GI patients. Dr. Alan Kilby, with his special interest in liver disease, Dr. John Erkkinen in esophageal disorders, Dr. Benjamin Potter in inflammatory bowel disease, Dr. James Morse in nutrition and GI cancer genetics, Dr. Gordon Millspaugh in endoscopic ultrasound (EUS) related disorders, and Drs. Thalia Mayes and Kate Kennedy in irritable bowel disease and colon cancer screening - especially in women, Dr. Daniil Rolshud in advanced endoscopy with a focus on therapeutic EUS. Dr. Michael Roy and Dr. Andreas Stefan have excelled in their specialty interests and have added dedication to administration and teaching. Dr. Michael Roy, our partner for many years, took over as the Chairman of the Department of Medicine four years ago and Dr. Andreas Stefan has been Chief of the GI Division as well as President of our large and expanding GI group practice.

Overall, and with great confidence, I can say we are one of the great GI divisions practicing in the USA today! This fact has been recognized by our national society, The American Society for Gastrointestinal Endoscopy (ASGE), beginning with their fellowship support grants in 1994 and 1995. Our contributions to the field of endoscopy were recognized in 2002 when we received the prestigious Mater of Endoscopy Award given to one member of the society of over 10,000. Recognition of our outstanding, and in some ways, unique fellowship training followed in 2015 with the ASGE Annual Distinguished Educator Award. Finally, we just received the ASGE 2017 Distinquished Endoscopy Research Mentoring Award.

These awards spanning the three hats of medicine proclaim and confirm that GI services at Maine Medical Center are measured with the best in the world. We all owe our deep thanks to our forebears – Laban Leiter, Newell Augur, John Gibbons, George Sager, Walter Goldfarb, Clem Hebert, Emerson Drake, Chris Lutes and many many others who came to Maine and made Portland a great medical center.

General Surgery
and the Department of Surgery at MMC

By Carl E. Bredenberg MD and David E. Clark MD

The movement to subspecialization and the development of the academic medical center

Introduction

General surgery is a specialty with particular focus on abdominal and GI diseases, diseases of the breast and soft tissues, surgical diseases of the thyroid and parathyroid and the management of multiple trauma. The basic clinical general surgery residency is 5 years in duration, although some academic programs may require an additional 1 to 3 years in laboratory research.

The 5-year general surgery residency is also a prerequisite for subspecialty fellowships of 1 to 3 years duration in cardiothoracic surgery, pediatric surgery, colorectal surgery, vascular surgery, trauma and critical care surgery, and plastic surgery.

As with the other major specialties, general surgery since the 1960's has undergone progressive subspecialization. At Maine Medical Center (MMC) this process was initially characterized by general surgeons on the attending staff who developed their own special interests and skills. Starting in the 1970's, some individuals with formal subspecialty training and certification came to MMC on their own initiative, often although not exclusively graduates of the MMC general surgery residency (who will be denoted by "MMCGS" and the year of their graduation). Only since about 1990 has the stability and authority of the Department of Surgery leadership allowed for formal institutional planning and recruitment.

Increasing subspecialization has been a nationwide trend manifest by the increasing variety of fellowships open to graduates of general surgery residencies and by an increasing number of subspecialty boards and "certificates of added qualifications". The drivers of this nationwide trend among residency graduates are vigorously debated but include both the desire to have a more limited field to thoroughly master as well as the practical advantage of obtaining a "ticket" of special skill to make the newly minted surgeon more valuable and employable in a competitive marketplace.

General surgery at MMC historically developed through individual private practices. A full-time salaried chief for the entire Department of Surgery was not hired until 1972 and the salaried position of Residency Program Director was not established until the late 1980's, at which time trauma surgery was also established as the first hospital-supported surgical subspecialty.

The Department of Surgery has benefited in having stable leadership since 1990. The two decades prior to this had seen a total of six Department Chiefs, while since 1990 there have been only two, Dr. Carl Bredenberg and the present incumbent, Dr. Brad Cushing. During this same time interval, there have been only three General Surgery Residency Program Directors: Drs. Albert Dibbins, Michael Curci, and James Whiting (the current Director). During much of this interval, Dr. Walter Goldfarb headed the Division of General Surgery. All of these Departmental leaders shared a vision for a quality training program based in a department of diverse and well-trained, academically-oriented practicing surgeons.

Along with the development of surgical subspecialization, the last decade has seen many more private practices join the hospital as "full-time" salaried hospital-based practices, including neurosurgery, cardiac surgery, urology, and several general surgery practices. This has further facilitated the recruitment of subspecialists in all the surgery specialties and has helped to provide the additional financial support often required to establish new subspecialists.

General Surgery Residency

The General Surgery Residency at MMC was approved in 1947. This was one of the historical markers of MMC's becoming an "academic teaching hospital." More recently, the primary urology practice has joined the hospital and initiated its own residency program. In 2015, vascular surgery also inaugurated its own fellowship. Neurosurgery and Plastic surgery have also had residents rotating from residencies based in other academic and university hospitals. These resident training programs encourage academic subspecialization and also provide an inducement which helps attract high-quality surgeons to Portland.

In 1998 Dr. Jon Dreifus started a small simulation project for general surgery residents in what was at best a large closet across the hall from the departmental offices. Although initiated primarily to provide pre-clinical training in laparoscopic techniques, it quickly expanded to include basic open operative skills. This experience and the value of expanding it was one of the drivers that led to the multi-specialty Simulation Center now located at the Brighton Campus. Simulation centers have nationally become essential elements in procedural training in multiple specialties.

General Thoracic Surgery

General thoracic surgery (surgery of the chest other than cardiac) has a long history at MMC. In addition to his role as an early cardiac surgeon in Maine, Dr. Clement Hiebert was internationally recognized particularly for his contributions to surgery for benign and malignant diseases of the esophagus. Dr. Bredenberg trained at Johns Hopkins and came to MMC in 1990 after 18 years on the faculty of SUNY Upstate Medical University in Syracuse. He was Board Certified in Thoracic Surgery as well as general surgery and also had Certificates of Added Qualifications in both Vascular Surgery and Surgical Critical Care. In addition to Dr. Bredenberg, the cardiac surgeons in the past, particularly Dr. Seth Blank, have also done general thoracic procedures with varying degrees of frequency.

It was not until the last few years, however, that the Division of General Thoracic Surgery was formally established within the Department of Surgery with appropriate support personnel. Dr. Gary Hochheiser (MMCGS 2001) returned to MMC in 2016 to head this Division, after training for 3 years in thoracic surgery and practicing several years at the Baystate Medical Center in Springfield, Massachusetts. A second general thoracic surgeon will be joining Dr. Hochheiser later in 2017.

Vascular Surgery

Until the late 1980's, peripheral vascular surgery at MMC was practiced as part of general surgery or cardio-thoracic surgery. Nationally, the 1970's and 1980's saw an increased focus on vascular surgery as its own discrete specialty. This was highlighted by the creation of a Certificate of Added Qualifications in General Vascular Surgery during the 1980's.

The current vascular surgery program at MMC was the outgrowth of one private general surgical practice that dedicated a substantial part of its activity to peripheral vascular surgery, and progressively added selected graduates of the general surgical residency. Drs. Philip Lape (MMCGS 1950) and Ferris Ray (MMCGS 1959) initiated this focus and were subsequently joined by Drs. Robert McAfee (MMCGS 1965), Dick Dillihunt (MMCGS 1967), Bill Herbert (MMCGS 1981) and Bob Hawkins (MMCGS 1987). Dr. Dillihunt led vascular surgery from 1995 to 1999.

Dr. Jens Eldrup-Jorgensen joined the vascular group in 1988 coming from the faculty of the University of Illinois, Chicago. His general surgery residency was at New England Deaconess and his vascular fellowship was at Tufts New England Medical Center. He was the first surgeon in Maine both to have completed a vascular fellowship and to be Board Certified in vascular surgery by the American Board of Surgery. By 1999 when Dr. Jorgensen assumed the leadership of a formal Division of Vascular Surgery, general surgeons (other than the few named above) and the cardiac surgeons had limited activity in vascular surgery.

With a high volume of vascular surgery and fellowship trained subspecialists, the setting was right for establishing an MMC vascular surgery fellowship which was accomplished in 2015 and headed by Dr. Chris Healey who completed his vascular fellowship at Tufts New England Medical Center in 2008. Dr. Paul Bloch who trained at the University of Minnesota and Elizabeth Blazick who came from the general surgery residency and a vascular fellowship at the Massachusetts General Hospital added to the size and diversity of the Division.

The establishment of vascular fellowships and a full-fledged American Board of Vascular Surgery in 1998, along with the introduction and development of endovascular procedures in the 1990's, finally distinguished vascular surgery as a separate specialty both nationally and at MMC.

In 2017, Dr. Jorgensen stepped back from his role as Division Director and Dr. Brian Nolan was recruited from Dartmouth to lead the Division of Vascular Surgery, now consisting of 6 attending surgeons plus vascular fellows.

Transplant Surgery

The first kidney transplant at MMC was performed by Drs. Ray and Dillihunt in October of 1971. During the early years, kidney transplants were performed by the vascular surgeons with the assistance of the urologists for the ureteral re-implantation. Much of the para-operative immunosuppression was managed by the transplant nephrologists. The preparation and training of the team was thorough and from the beginning, the results were excellent.

In 2000, Dr. Jim Whiting was recruited from the faculty of the University of Cincinnati as the first full time transplant surgeon and added pancreas to the transplanted organs. Dr. Whiting's general surgery residency training had been at the Brigham and Women's Hospital in Boston and his transplantation fellowship at Rush Presbyterian St. Lukes in Chicago. The resource demands of liver, heart, or lung transplantation were and still are too great to justify inclusion in the transplant program at MMC, given the low expected demand based on the population of Maine.

In 2013, Dr. Juan Palma Vargas (MMCGS 2004) returned after a fellowship and several years of practice in San Antonio, Texas, to strengthen the MMC Division of Transplantation.

Pediatric Surgery

Dr. Albert Dibbins came to MMC as a solo practitioner in 1973, devoting himself exclusively to pediatric surgery. Dr. Dibbins had trained in general surgery at Yale, completed a pediatric surgery fellowship at the University of Pittsburgh, and remained on the faculty at Pittsburgh for several years. After a few years, he was joined by Dr. Michael Curci, who had also trained at Yale and Pittsburgh. The dedication and teamwork of this pair would have a major influence on all MMC general surgery residents from that time forward, as well as establish high-quality pediatric surgery for the state of Maine. In addition to being busy clinical surgeons both Dr. Dibbins and Dr. Curci served as General Surgery Residency Program Directors. Please see the chapter on Pediatric Surgery.

Divisions of Trauma Surgery and Surgical Critical Care

Dr. David Clark (MMCGS 1980) returned to MMC after a fellowship at the Shock Trauma Center at the University of Maryland Hospital in Baltimore, inspired in no small part by the example of the MMC pediatric surgeons. Up to this time management of multiple trauma was the responsibility of the general surgery staff with much of the actual care delivered by the resident staff. The years after the Vietnam War saw a nationwide effort underway to improve the quality and organization of trauma care. Dr. Clark was a leader in the development of a statewide Emergency Medical Services system in Maine in which MMC has played a crucial role.

Dr. Clark was joined in 1987 by Dr. Bill Horner (MMCGS 1972), who also had completed a trauma fellowship. Their expanded effort required salary support from MMC, since trauma care was becoming more non-operative for which reimbursements rates were low. Dr. Horner left for a position at EMMC in Bangor in 1989 where he became valuable in collaborating on further development of a statewide trauma system. Dr. Horner was replaced by the recruitment of Dr. Melinda Molin from the University of California, San Diego and Dr. Roy Cobean from the University of Vermont and

Harborview Hospital in Seattle. Dr. Molin was instrumental in expanding the coverage of the trauma service to include surgical critical care.

When Drs. Molin and Cobean later turned their clinical activities to non-trauma specialties, Dr. Brad Cushing was recruited from the University of Maryland to lead the trauma service and Dr. Gene Grindlinger from Boston Medical Center to lead the surgical critical care part of the service. Under Dr. Cushing's leadership as Division Director and subsequently from 2004 as Surgeon-in-Chief, the trauma and surgical critical care services expanded to their current prominence. The Division is now led by Dr. Joseph Rappold who has had extensive trauma experience serving as a naval surgeon with Marine combat units in Iraq and Afghanistan. The Division also includes Dr. Lee Hallagan (MMCGS 2013) who returned after a Trauma Fellowship at Beth Israel Deaconess and eight other surgeons. In 2016, Dr. Damien Carter was recruited from the University of Washington to be the director of a newly created burn and soft tissue service and to reinvigorate MMC's Burn Unit.

The American College of Surgeons has certified MMC as the only Level I Trauma Center in Maine and the (MMC) Barbara Bush Children's Hospital as the only Pediatric Trauma Center in the state.

Surgical Oncology

Surgery for cancer has long formed a substantial part of general surgery. At MMC, Dr. George Sager (MMCGS 1954) was a leader among the general surgeons in participating in institution and statewide oncology programs and activities. His contributions and the success of establishing gynecologic oncology encouraged the hospital to recruit and support a specialty trained surgical oncologist in general surgery. Following a two-year surgical oncology fellowship at MD Anderson Cancer Center in Texas, Dr. Marc Demers (MMCGS 1990) returned as the first surgeon at MMC to focus exclusively on surgical oncology. However, after two years, Dr. Demers left to practice in Florida.

Encouraged by this experience, the private Maine Surgical Care Group, with the support of the hospital and departmental leadership, in 1996 recruited Dr. Dougald Macgillivray from the full-time staff at the University of Connecticut to serve as head of a Division of Surgical Oncology at MMC. Dr. MacGillivray was joined a few years later by Drs. Lisa Rutstein (MMCGS 2001) and Justin Baker (MMCGS 2010). After Dr. Baker left to practice in Minnesota, Dr. Timothy Fitzgerald was recruited from the faculty of Eastern Carolina Medical School to head the Division.

Colorectal Surgery

Certification by the American Board of Colon and Rectal Surgery (ABCRS) requires a two-year fellowship following a 5-year general surgery residency. Nationwide, many general surgeons still consider colon and rectal surgery to be an essential part of "general surgery."

In 1990 Dr. Cathel McLeod came to MMC as the first surgeon both certified by the ABCRS and who limited his practice exclusively to this area of surgery. The son of a distinguished MMC cardiologist, Dr. McLeod received his subspecialty training at the University of Minnesota. He established an active practice despite the continuing involvement of other general surgeons in this area. He was subsequently joined by Drs. M. Parker Roberts and Sara Mayo (MMCGS 2000), both fellowship trained colorectal surgeons.

Surgery of the Breast

Dr. Melinda Molin had been recruited to join the trauma service from UC San Diego in 1990. As she was then the only woman general surgeon in Portland, Dr. Bredenberg suggested that she add care of women with diseases of the breast to her practice. Shortly thereafter there was a surge of interest in the community for a dedicated breast service. The hospital responded with the necessary support and infrastructure for both outpatient care as well as an inpatient service.

Dr. Molin subsequently left the trauma field and was hired by Mercy Hospital to start a breast service there. Over subsequent years several women surgeons in private practice have focused in breast surgery at MMC. In 2016 Dr. Paige Teller (MMCGS 2008) was recruited by Maine Surgical Care (by now a part of MMC) to lead the breast service and serve as Co-Director of the MMC Breast Care Center. Following a fellowship in surgery of the breast Dr. Teller held academic positions in Boston and at the Medical University of South Carolina in Charleston prior to returning to MMC. The Breast Care Center provides multidisciplinary consultation and treatment as well as important links to support groups for patients and families.

Bariatric Surgery

Bariatric surgery in its current iteration began through the initiative of Dr. Roy Cobean with infrastructure support from MMC. Surgery to reverse morbid obesity by restructuring the patient's GI track has been around since the 1960's. It fell into disrepute as the long-term morbidity of the early operative procedures became clear.

The high mortality and morbidity of morbid obesity has been well documented. Despite all attempts, achieving and maintaining significant weight loss in these patients by non-surgical means is rarely successful. This almost total failure of non-operative management, combined with the development of better operative procedures that have few long-term complications, has led to a nationwide development of bariatric surgery programs and to its growth at MMC.

Acute Care Surgery

The progressive subspecialization within general surgery created a paradox both at MMC and nationally. Once a few years separates them from their initial general surgery training, those surgeons whose clinical practice had become limited to a narrow subspecialty may no longer feel that they have the breadth of skill and current experience to manage basic general surgery emergencies that present to the hospital Emergency Room or as in-house catastrophes. As a consequence, subspecialization had led to the development of a new subspecialty: "acute care surgery." Ironically acute care surgery is a reincarnation of the original concept of the "general surgeon."

The nucleus of the acute care surgery group at MMC, as in most institutions, consists of the trauma and critical care surgeons. The daily practice of these subspecialty surgeons includes a broad array of medical and surgical management issues. Both trauma and critical care surgery provide a relatively small volume of operative experience making these surgeons eager for additional opportunities to work in the Operating Room. At MMC, they are joined by a small core of other general surgeons, including Drs. Fred Radke (MMCGS 1981) and Jon Dreifus (MMCGS 1995) who continue to take pride in their broad experience in managing acute intra-abdominal and soft tissue emergencies and are perhaps the only true "general surgeons" remaining at MMC.

Other Changes

The past 50 years have seen progressive development in the MMC Department of Surgery and increasing subspecialization within general surgery. Coinciding with this trend has been an increase in academic activity marked by an increase in the size of the general surgery residency and the addition of formal training programs in urology and vascular surgery.

Academic publication has long been part of the activities of the Department of Surgery. These publications have been clinical investigations for the most part, but there has also been basic laboratory work and outcomes research with collaboration with the scientists at Maine Medical Center Research Institute (MMCRI) and the outcomes research group at MMC.

Outreach activities within general surgery and the Department of Surgery more broadly, like those of the other departments at MMC, have yielded more than just increased patient referrals from around the state. Members of the Department including those under the broad rubric of general surgery have played leadership roles in state, regional, and national professional organizations. Drs. Drake, Hiebert, Dibbins, Goldfarb, and Radke have each served as President of the New England Surgical Society, and Drs. Morton and Curci have each been Vice-President. Drs. Dibbins and Curci have furthermore each received the New England Surgical Society's Nathan Smith Award for their distinguished contributions to surgery in New England.

Drs. Bredenberg and Jorgensen have each served as President of the New England Society for Vascular Surgery. Dr. Jorgensen now leads the nationwide quality improvement effort of the Society of Vascular Surgery.

Drs. Hiebert, Dibbins, and Whiting have been Directors of the American Board of Surgery. Dr. McAfee has been President of the American Medical Association.

Dr. Radke and Bredenberg have each served 6-year terms on the Board of Governors of the American College of Surgeons. Dr. Clark has been a member of its Committee on Trauma. Drs. Curci, Radke, Roberts, and Bredenberg have each been elected President of the Maine Chapter of the American College of Surgeons.

The participation of physicians in national and regional professional leadership roles is an important characteristic of academic medical centers and of major regional medical centers.

Summary

The course of general surgery and the Department of Surgery at MMC over the last several decades has in many ways mirrored that of other disciplines. This has included increasing subspecialization of clinical activity, often leading to formally structured divisions within the Department of Surgery. Other critical features have been the focus on academic activity, including increases in residency and fellowship training programs and leadership roles of MMC surgeons in regional and national professional societies.

Another structural development, particularly in the last decade, has been the transformation of most of the private practices in the fields of general surgery (as well as those in neurosurgery, urology and cardiac surgery) into hospital owned entities. This shift has facilitated the financial support and recruitment of surgeons with specific expertise and academic interest.

Thus, the development of MMC over the last several decades as a regional referral center for surgery and its subspecialties has paralleled MMC's broader progress in becoming a regional referral hospital and a true academic medical center across multiple departments and specialties.

THE HISTORY OF INTERNAL MEDICINE IN PORTLAND

By Robert A. Sturges MD

The medical landscape of the greater Portland community was very different in the 1970's – indeed it was primitive by the current standards now forty years later. The majority of primary care was delivered by solo general practitioners most of whom had only one internship year after medical school graduation (one year was minimal requirement for a license to practice at that time). These general practitioners usually did not have night or weekend coverage arrangements nor answering services. Virtually all care delivered after hours was in the emergency rooms. There were several small fledgling internal medicine practices, including those of Ed Hardy and Bill Taylor in Falmouth; Winton Briggs, Steve Larned, and Jim Halle in Cape Elizabeth; Philip Whitney, Norman Saunders, and Dan Bryant in Portland; Jack Davy, Mike Batt, and Jane Pringle in Portland; and David Scotton, Charles Thurber, and George Higgins in Scarborough. This is not an all-inclusive list.

In 1978 Jim Calderbank and I established Westbrook Medical Associates as a two-person practice. It was the first internal medicine practice west of Maine Medical Center (MMC) and east of Bridgeton. During our residencies at MMC many specialists, especially in cardiology, lamented the fact that they had no full-service primary care internal medicine practices for continuing care of their patients west of Portland. Our first answering service - shared with plumbers and electricians - was in the basement of a residential house. This change in the nature of primary care to practices that featured residency-trained internists with board certification and 24/7 coverage was very well-received and we were quickly successful as this became the standard for all medical practices. The same upgrade was occurring in pediatrics and family practice, but we all remained individual small practices until the 1990's (as discussed elsewhere in this book).

I first arrived in Portland as one of sixteen third-year medical students from Tufts University School of Medicine on Labor Day 1971 in a new program under which we spent the whole academic year at MMC. This was the program's second year and was MMC's first attempt at extending medical education to include medical students. We came in spite of many classmates who expressed doubts about the quality of education that we would receive outside of Boston hospitals. To the contrary we all felt we were treated well by attending staff and hospital staff. If we wrote an order for blood work someone from the lab would actually come and draw it (instead of ourselves). We were also much more active in medical care, not relegated to the back row watching procedures. We then returned to Boston for our fourth-year rotations.

I returned to Maine Medical Center for my internship July 1973 (as did George Higgins who eventually became Chief of MMC's Emergency Department). This was the last year of the "rotating internship" under which a trainee was not guaranteed a spot for second or third year residency. Unfortunately of the fourteen interns that year, ten wanted internal medicine (IM). But the program only had four openings. I was ranked #5 and was anxiously considering other programs when another intern decided to return to UVM, and I was given the slot to finish training at MMC. Currently there are thirteen positions in each year for R1 through R3 levels in internal medicine for a total of 39 residents in the IM program.

In reviewing memories of residency training in the 70's, a few anecdotes come to mind:

1) My first rotation as an intern was spending nights in the Emergency Department (7 pm-8 am). In those days the intern was alone from midnight to 8 am with a resident available to call for backup.

2) The first computerization at MMC arrived with the Technicon MIS system in 1974. It was mostly used for scheduling diagnostic studies, retrieving lab and x-ray results and creating orders with physicians encouraged to enter their own orders (a controversy at the time but the predecessor to current nearly universal CPOE systems). MMC was the fifth hospital in the country to install the system and the first to use it with pediatrics. The MIS system had no algorithms for pediatric medication dosing – a feature that our pediatric residents at the time had to develop.

3) The first "beepers" appeared in 1975. Prior to that the public address system was the only method of communication. Indeed, if a resident tried to go to sleep in an on-call room, a call had to be placed to notify the operator of the correct extension for receiving calls. The first beepers could not be called pagers as they did not even show a number.

Maine Medical Center changed its medical school affiliation from Tufts to the University of Vermont (UVM) in 1980. A new Chief of Medicine arrived in 1981 – Robert Hillman MD, a hematologist from University of Washington in Seattle. Under his leadership for the next 17 years the IM residency program grew exponentially as many new fellowships were added. These included critical care, nephrology, infectious disease and others. New specialty clinics were spawned in the Department including an HIV clinic under Robert Smith MD, a nutrition clinic under Philip Whitney

MD, and Lipid clinic under Len Keilson MD. The quality of teaching in medicine greatly improved with attending physicians throughout the Department still teaching voluntarily. Any patient care revenue generated by teaching attendings went to the Department for its projects. The "Silver Shovel", emblematic of superior teaching as voted annually by the UVM medical students on both the Burlington and Portland campuses, resided in MMC's Department of Medicine for 9 of the 15 years from the early 80's to late 1990's. Members of the Department also became heavily involved with research including oncology protocol projects with institutions in Boston, which helped support the founding of the MMC Research Institute (MMCRI) in 1988. MMCRI is now regularly awarded major NIH grants and has attracted prominent medical researchers from around the country to its Scarborough campus.

John Tooker MD served as the Internal Medicine Residency Program Director in the 1980's and early 1990's before taking a national position with the American College of Physicians. He is credited with starting an outreach program that recruited volunteer primary care physicians (PCP) from around Maine to join the Rural Practice Network. All second year IM residents now spend a rural month in the offices of these physicians which has proven to be a rewarding experience for most participants and has encouraged graduating MMC residents to set up practice in less urban areas around the state.

In anticipation of a looming shortage of primary internists and other primary care physicians, Peter Bates MD took the lead in reestablishing a closer affiliation with the Tufts Medical School in 2009 with a "fast track" program designed to help deserving Maine students overcome obstacles including tuition affordability. Currently 40 medical students per year are largely recruited from Maine and spend about half of their 4 years of medical school in Maine. The program features earlier integration of students with practicing physicians in the state with a goal of producing more PCPs for Maine. The first class graduated in 2013. The program is highly sought after by Maine students.

General IM practices remained mostly as small independent groups of 2-4 physicians until the 1990's. At that time the Clinton administration began promoting the concept of managed care and Health Maintenance Organizations (HMO). One of the first big changes was the closing of the Osteopathic Hospital of Maine because of the decline in demand for hospital beds. This occurred in 1992 and stimulated integration of osteopathic practitioners into allopathic practices, both in primary and specialty care. At the same time, the University of New England (UNE) opened an osteopathic medical school and began supplying more graduates who were increasingly accepted into allopathic training programs, including those at MMC, further blurring any degree distinctions between MD and DO.

Merger mania also took over medical practices throughout the medical community. Four independent IM practices from Westbrook, Falmouth, Cape Elizabeth, and Scarborough merged to form Greater Portland Medical Group (GPMG) in 1995.

Under the leadership of David Howes MD the Martin's Point practices were consolidated and InterMed was established by Tom Claffey MD and his colleagues. All of this activity was spurred by fears that insurers would increasingly negotiate physician contracts and that larger practices could have more favorable terms in agreements and bigger impact on the practice of medicine. GPMG formed for this reason as well as to maintain distribution and geographic access around greater Portland. All GPMG physicians also wanted an affiliation with MMC as a faculty practice to maintain continuity of their commitment to IM education in medical clinics and in-patient services. Teaching at the time was not reimbursed, therefore requiring a higher level of that commitment and discouraging some physicians from participating. Those who stuck with it felt that teaching and exposure to house staff and students served to keep us up-to-date and help in recruiting like-minded physicians. Most of us provided both office and hospital care although hospitalist medicine was emerging. Over time many physicians gave up hospital practice as they felt it to be inefficient and overly demanding.

Managed care in the 1990's presented many challenges to practices, especially in primary care. This was most evident with the advent of the primary care "gatekeeper" role. This greatly increased the office burden of extra phone calls and paperwork, mostly for referrals to specialists. Physicians found overhead to be rising and practice revenues falling. All of us had been small business owners trying to run our own practices. Many did not have the business acumen or interest to continue to be independent as the environment changed. This was particularly true for physicians more involved in the teaching programs at MMC. The development of Medical Services Corporation (MSC) as an extension of MMC was necessary to allow us to continue our commitment to teaching and treating all patients. This organization has now grown and expanded throughout the MaineHealth system as Maine Medical Partners (MMP).

Another movement to organize physicians throughout the area began in the early 1990's with meetings of a growing group of primary care physicians and specialists that took place at 6:30 AM. To deal with managed care, insurers, and many other issues, these concerned physicians engaged with the MMC administration in an effort that led to the establishment of the MMC Physician Hospital Organization (PHO).

The core principles of the organization included:

1) Offering single-signature contracts representing the hospital and a full panel of physicians to insurance plans;

2) Enhanced standardization and quality of care; and

3) A collective ability to monitor parameters of medical care to manage risk contracts and lower the cost of medical care.

Initially, the MMC PHO was inclusive of all physicians. As negotiations continued regarding structure of contracts that were binding, fee schedules, structure of governing boards and the relationship with MMC, several physician groups elected not to participate. Early on, Peter Wood signed on as CEO. He was instrumental in our initial and continued success. The MMC PHO lasted far longer than other PHO's around the country and grew over time as MaineHealth developed and expanded to include many local and regional physician groups, hospitals and other medical facilities.

One of the first issues for physicians was establishing a fee schedule using the Resource Based Relative Value System (RBRVS) and establishing a conversion factor which at the time varied with specialty. Keith Karunchek, a consultant from Charlotte, NC met with our new boards weekly eight times. An agreement was reached on having a single conversion factor for primary care and specialists. To the surprise of the consultant "no blood was shed" indicating that the involved physicians were cooperative, moderate, and had the common good of the community at heart as opposed to other more fractious physician groups he had dealt with on similar issues. The Community Physicians of Maine was the physician-run arm with a board composed of more than 50% PCP's whereas the PHO board was half physicians and half MMC representatives.

Through the years the PHO evolved with the times as quality of care became our leading purpose. Chronic illness registries were established, initially developing parameters for management of diabetes, then expanding to pathways for other chronic diseases. To help physicians achieve treatment goals, a Diabetes Care Manager Program was established for direct contact with patients to augment patient education and compliance. Although this service was not reimbursed by insurers it was the "right thing to do" as an extension of primary care offices. This PHO has further evolved to a MaineHealth Accountable Care Organization (ACO) in recent years.

One other innovative effort in primary care needs to be mentioned in any history of IM in our community - the development of the patient-centered medical home. This is a construct under which primary care offices utilize more teamwork among office staff members to enhance patient education and coordination of care beyond what the physician can do alone. For many practices this has meant expanding the role of nurse care managers, initially employed by the PHO exclusively for diabetes management. This project had been largely spearheaded by the late Richard Engel MD, an experienced internist, in his position as former Maine Governor of American

College of Physicians, and involved member of state level committees on medical innovations. Several pilot sites were started around the state, including Westbrook Internal Medicine and Westbrook Pediatrics.

Overall, the prospects are good for general IM to stay strong for the benefit of the general Portland community.

MEDICAL ONCOLOGY

By Tracey F. Weisberg MD

New England Cancer Specialists:
Our Origins and What We Have Evolved to Today

The Beginnings of Medical Hematology
and Oncology in Portland Maine

The specialty of medical oncology and the broader field of cancer care were essentially non-existent prior to the 1960's locally as well as nationally. There were few tools to manage this group of diseases so patients were largely cared for by family physicians and surgeons. Cancer staging was a crude system describing disease as localized, regional, or systemic as established by the American Cancer Society (ACS). This system was essentially devoid of any prognostic significance. Radiation therapy treatments for cancer were evolving from the use of 240Kv machines - which produced severe skin burns and maceration - to cobalt therapy which was only a bit better with respect to treatment-induced toxicities. There were few chemotherapy agents available in the 1960's. Among them were 5-fluorouracil, methotrexate, actinomycin D, vinca alkaloids, and a variety of alkylating agents such as nitrogen mustard, Cytoxan, Leukeran, and Alkeran. The librarian at Maine Medical Center (MMC), Eleanor Cairnes, was the physician's best friend. There were no oncology textbooks and few cancer journals other than Cancer, and Cancer Chemotherapy Reports. There were no computer based searches. Surgical subspecialty journals were the major source of information.

The medical oncology practice known today as New England Cancer Specialists, formerly Maine Center for Cancer Medicine, was founded in Portland Maine by Dr. Ronald Carroll in July of 1967 as a practice limited to Tuesday and Wednesday afternoons in the office of Dr. Donald Marshall on Bramhall Street in Portland Maine. Dr. Marshall was the Chief of Urology at MMC at the time and graciously offered the use of his space to Dr. Ronald Carroll. This collaboration lasted only three months after which the practice moved to 255 Western Promenade, Dr. Ronald Carroll's residence, where it occupied the first floor while his family lived on the second floor. It was understood by the rest of the medical community that this was an internal medicine practice limited to the practice of cancer medicine. There were no oncology boards.

The practice was staffed by a single assistant who also did all the patient scheduling, typing and billing.

A cancer clinic was also established on Friday afternoons at MMC for patients who had no means of payment. Dr. Stanley Herrick from the Nuclear Medicine Department at Maine Medical Center organized which volunteer physicians would attend. This model over time proved cumbersome for patients with cancer due to lack of patient care continuity. In the early 1970's with the arrival of Dr. Carroll's first partner, Dr. Brian Dorsk, all patients with a cancer diagnosis regardless of their ability to pay were managed in the private practice located at 255 Western Avenue. This provided all patients with a single attending physician who knew their case, reduced confusion for patients seeking urgent care and after hours care, and included an assistant who knew each patient and could update their specific details. This integration of "clinic" patients into the private practice has been sustained through the present at New England Cancer Specialists and continues to differentiate us from many physician owned practices across the United States. An arrangement was in place whereby MMC would replace the costly chemotherapy drugs used in the care of patients that had no ability to pay for cancer therapies. This was mutually beneficial since MMC no longer had to staff a clinic while the private practice could efficiently integrate this population into its scheduling and emergency coverage services. Surgical care for this population was provided by the surgeons in their clinics which also served as the focus of multidisciplinary consultations.

Nine hospital based cancer conferences in outlying areas of Maine as far north as Rockland were attended by Drs. Carroll and Dorsk on a monthly basis. Cases were presented and the Portland based oncologists provided education and guidance to the local managing physicians. Drs. Carroll and Dorsk were emissaries of the newest information with regard to cancer and cancer treatment. The understanding of cancer biology and medical oncology was thus spread.

After Dr. Dorsk's arrival the practice moved briefly to a building on Chadwick Street while a new building was being built at 180 Park Avenue specifically for cancer care. The practice on Park Avenue was known as The Maine Center for Cancer Medicine and quickly grew in patient volume and physician providers. Drs. Daniel Hayes and Delvin Case joined the practice at 180 Park Avenue followed by Dr. Thomas Ervin, Dr. Tracey Weisberg and Dr. Fred Aronson. Ethel Murphy was the first nurse to join the practice when it moved to Park Avenue and developed a highly professional nursing service that has grown and matured to be the lifeblood of cancer care and care coordination to this day.

Cancer care in Portland in the 1960's was largely dominated by surgery. The natural history of the different cancers was underappreciated; a dominant perception remained that local therapies alone were the mainstay of treatment. Medical oncology was largely limited to the manipulation of recurrent breast cancer with hormone and was done by an internist (Dr. Stanley Herrick) who ran a nuclear medicine department within the radiology department. After Dr. Carroll's arrival, medical oncology was provided for some children as well as for adults with close collaboration of Dr. Norman Jaffe at the Children's Cancer Research Institute (established by Dr. Farber, the precursor institute of the Dana Farber Cancer Center) and their local pediatrician. Dr. Stephen Blattner, a fellowship trained pediatric oncologist arrived in 1981 and assumed the care of children with cancer in a separate private practice that was the predecessor to the Maine Children's Cancer Program (see Pediatric Oncology chapter in this book).

Demonstrating the value of systemic therapy to the surgeons and radiation oncologists, particularly the use of adjuvant chemotherapy for early stage disease, was difficult. Attendance was sparse at discussions on pivotal clinical trials or on topics such as the seminal tumor growth models developed by Skipper, Schabel and Wilcox despite the fact that these studies done during the 1950's and published in the early 1960's demonstrated the conditions for the curative basis for adjuvant chemotherapy. The results of early clinical trials run by Dr. Bernard Fischer and surgical groups like National Surgical Adjuvant Bowel and Breast Project (NSABP) were required to convince the surgeons of the value of early systemic adjuvant treatment - but this came in the 1980s. The initial adjuvant study by Fischer used Alkeran and was memorably terminated prematurely when President Gerald Ford's wife developed breast cancer. The study's early results demonstrated a benefit and she was given the drug. There remained some continued opposition to the use of chemotherapy for palliation of cancer because of toxicities.

Cancer Research in Portland Maine

In 1982 a Request for Applications (RFA) was issued by the National Cancer Institute (NCI) to establish Community Clinical Oncology Programs (CCOP) that would officially extend cancer clinical trials into communities, thus making research opportunities available to those not living in proximity to a large cancer center. The Maine Center for Cancer Medicine under the leadership of Dr. Ronald Carroll successfully competed for CCOP grants for two four year periods. Through the 1990's clinical trials through the cooperative group Cancer and Leukemia Group B (CALGB) and many pharmaceutical drug company trials were supported by Maine Center for

Cancer Medicine practice. Dr. Delvin Case was particularly interested in hematology clinical trials. Barbara Wood R.N. supervised the research effort as a primary nurse to Dr. Case and then also functioned as the office's research coordinator.

In the 1987 three researchers came to Portland: Drs. EJ Lovett, Bruce Bagwell and Kenneth Ault. The MMC Chief of Medicine, Dr. Robert Hillman, was an advocate for them to pursue research development at MMC. These scientists provided flow cytometry technology which at the time appeared to be a promising technology for providing additional prognostic information in newly diagnosed cancers. The oncology practice by that time had acquired the entire building on Park Avenue. Laboratory research in cancer in the Portland community began in space in the Park Avenue building adjacent to the oncology clinical practice which had been occupied by Dr. William Holt, an ophthalmologist. Maine Center for Cancer Medicine provided a subsidy for Dr. Ault to do his research. Dr. Ault, in addition initiated the MMC bone marrow transplant/stem cell transplant program. In addition, Dr. Carroll raised funds in the community to support that work. This lab served as the basis for the development of the Maine Medical Center Research Institute (MMCRI) program that expanded to a John Roberts road location and then eventually a magnificent laboratory research building that is present on the Maine Medical Center Scarborough Campus and is a site of innovation and a source of pride for the Maine Medical Center community.

Research continues to be a prominent feature of this hematology and oncology practice, as physicians enroll patients on to cooperative group studies through the Dana Farber Cancer Institute (DFCI) Lead Academic Participating Site (LAPS) grant and perform many pharmaceutical trials of high clinical value to our patients. We have established a dedicated research staff including a Director (Patrick McLeary RN), physician lead (Christian Thomas MD), regulator (Charlotte Rice) and a full-time research coordinator to lead clinical research in cancer in our offices. To date, the oncology practice has participated in 468 clinical trials. 132 of these trials are cooperative group studies with the first being performed in 1988 with Dr. Case as the principal investigator. To date, the practice has enrolled over 1000 patients onto clinical trials in this community. Trials that enjoyed particularly high accrual included the pivotal phase III study that brought trastuzumab (Herceptin) to the market and revolutionized the outcome of treatment for patients with Her2 amplification in their breast cancer. Another trial with robust accrual was the STAR Study of Breast Cancer Chemoprevention.

The practice had a growing appetite to learn the molecular genetics of cancer and understood that this technology would have everlasting impact on cancer prognostics and therapeutics. Dr. Karen Rasmussen joined the oncology practice as a genetic counselor and worked to educate the physicians and staff about the molecular biology of cancer. She was later joined by Susan Miesfield MD who further expanded the cancer genetics program. Currently Jessica Cary, a genetics counselor, works in all of the practice sites performing genetic consultations and working in concert with physicians in molecular medicine. Christian Thomas is the lead physician at New England Cancer Specialists in the state-wide collaboration with Jackson Laboratory molecular genetics program which has been graciously been supported by the Harold Alfond Foundation.

The Managed Care Era

With the advent of managed care early in the 1990's the Maine Center for Cancer Medicine moved to Scarborough. Maine Medical Center had established the need to consolidate outpatient cancer services on to a single campus and asked Dr. Carroll if the group would like to have space on the property (which was a beautifully renovated former K-Mart building). In this site, Maine Center for Cancer Medicine had in close proximity colleagues from the Maine Children's Cancer Program (MCCP), Radiation Oncology, and Gynecologic Oncology. There were imaging services on site as well as blood transfusion services, thus making all the aspects of cancer care highly convenient for patients undergoing therapies. This was value-added to the insurers as well.

The practice went through further professional expansion as Dr. Jacqueline Hedlund joined upon completing a fellowship in hematology and bone marrow transplant at the Fred Hutchinson Cancer Center in Seattle. Dr. Kurt Ebrahim merged his osteopathic oncology practice (previously located on Brighton Avenue in the Osteopathic Hospital) with Maine Center for Cancer Medicine. Dr. Preston Dalglish and his solo practice in Biddeford Maine were acquired giving the practice an office in Biddeford Maine. Expansion of cancer services into Brunswick on the Mid Coast Medical Center campus was initiated with the hiring of Dr. Thomas Keating, later to be joined by Dr. Richard Polkinghorn. The first advanced practice clinician (APC), Lisa Wolfe PA was also added to the practice at the new Scarborough site. The practice worked to serve regional hospitals by running clinics and providing care at Memorial Hospital in North Conway NH, Stephens Hospital in Norway ME, St. Andrews Hospital in Boothbay Maine and Waldo County Hospital in Belfast ME. Patients were seen a few times a month by the MCCM physicians while much of the additional nursing and office support was provided by the office staff in Brunswick and Scarborough. Oncology physicians continued to participate in these rural hospital tumor boards to help local physicians coordinate cancer care. These programs allowed patients in more rural locations access to care without traveling long distances and saved the hospitals from incurring the expense of full-time oncology physicians.

Managed care required a change in billing practices, and a system for line item charges and reimbursement which required a significant effort by the business office. Northern Data Systems of Falmouth (Charles Stevens) introduced the first computer systems into Maine Center for Cancer Medicine's business office. Office manager Anita Kilborn provided management and oversight to the business office.

With the recognition that the future of cancer care hinged upon patient outcomes, cost-intensive data collection was sure to be mandatory. The partners agreed to purchase an electronic medical record. With the move to the Scarborough campus, IKNOWMED became a fixture - for better or worse - for the MCCM physicians. Over time the group migrated to a Varian product and then finally settled on the Flatiron OncoEMR for collection of data and documentation purposes. This resulted also in the development of an information technology department at Maine Center for Cancer Medicine (MCCM).

Also during this time the development of a radiation therapy unit to serve cancer patients in the southern portion of our state was under discussion. Heated discussions between MaineHealth and York Hospital resulted in the eventual placement of this new unit in Sanford. Maine Center for Cancer Medicine as part of this project, opened a small satellite office adjacent to the new radiation unit.

In the late 1990's an effort was made to extend the National Comprehensive Cancer Center Network and its guidelines into cancer care at Maine Center for Cancer Medicine as one of the first community affiliates of that enterprise. The hospitals (MMC, Mercy, Mid Coast and Southern Maine Medical Center) after an initial agreement to work collaboratively, ultimately declined and finally opposed the project. Their position was that cancer data was the work product of physicians. Physicians could collect it concurrent with care and provide the data to the tumor registry (and the National Comprehensive Care data base) but the hospitals would retain ownership of it. This period marked the beginning of divergent thinking between what is now MaineHealth and the Portland physician community.

An Era Passes and a New Beginnings

Dr. Carroll retired in 2001, succeeded by Dr. Hayes as President of what had become the Maine Center for Cancer and Hematologic Disorders. Additional physicians joining the practice included Drs. David Benton, Trudi Chase (Brunswick), Betsy Connelly, Eleni Nackos (Brunswick), Brian Haney (Brunswick), Helen Ryan, Mathew Dugan, Devon Evans, Christian Thomas, Chiarra Batelli, John Winters (Scarborough), John Ilyas and Patty Deisler (Biddeford and Sanford). The advanced practice clinician workforce also expanded for all sites of the practice to now number 14 APC.

By the mid 1990's a growing understanding evolved that the organization would benefit from a CEO. Thomas Polko was the first CEO of the practice and Steve D'Amato PharmD was the second and is the current CEO of the organization. Steve D'Amato's leadership has been instrumental to the practice's sustainability. His expertise in cancer pharmacy management changed the practices in drug procurement from individual contracts with pharmaceutical companies to working closely with a group purchasing organization (GPO), Oncology Supply. The GPO provides significant support to community based oncology practices through assistance with attaining pharmacy certifications (USP 797 and USP 800) as well as technology for storage and inventory management.

Over time this physician owned practice has grown to 160 employees and is run by a leadership team including CEO, CFO, Operations Manager, IT manager, Research Director, Laboratory Director, and Human Resources Director. By 2016 the organization had grown to see 1/3 of all adult cancer cases in the state, totaling 3200 new cancer patients and 48,000 patient visits in the three office sites of Scarborough, Brunswick and Kennebunk.

A New Name and Brand Identity

The relationship with Maine Medical Center in the early 2000's became "cordially strained" due to clinic drug replacement policies and the development of an oncology service line at Maine Medical Center and MaineHealth. Maine Medical Center was granted federal 340B drug status in the late 2000's. Two specific criteria are common to most of the 340B-eligible hospitals: the requirement for a "disproportionate share hospital (DSH) adjustment percentage" above a certain level and the requirement that the hospital provide care to a defined percentage of low-income individuals who are not eligible for Medicare or Medicaid. This program is intended to give hospitals funds to pay for services that the poorest people in America cannot afford. There has however been much controversy about the program, accounting practices for it, and the impacts it has had across our country on hospital acquisition of private medical practices thus "inadvertently" inflating the overall cost of care delivered in the hospital-based setting. With the advent of MMC's 340B status, the "clinic agreement" that had been arranged by Dr. Carroll years earlier and sustained through more than three decades of good relations became strongly contested. MMC had less and less interest in replacing drugs used to treat indigent patients in the private practice and more interest in creation of its own chemotherapy infusion suite.

As a result, MMC transitioned from our once trusted partner from 1970 through the 1990's (during which the practice had provided leadership for tumor boards, leadership in the development and daily management of combined modality clinics like the Maine Medical Center Breast Care Center, oversight of the inpatient unit on the Gibson pavilion, education to the MMC Medicine A residents and with whom we had freely shared research accruals in support of the hospitals' accreditation) to a large health care organization seeking to assimilate our practice. It became clear that we needed to establish an identity distinct from the hospitals and the MaineHealth system. In July 2014 Maine Center for Cancer Medicine was renamed and rebranded as New England Cancer Specialists. This coincided with the merging of the one-man Biddeford and Sanford offices into a beautiful Kennebunk office site that opened to see patients June of 2015. We established a robust internet presence, developed poignant ads, and established a presence on social media with Facebook and Twitter. Our messaging is Quality, Innovation, Patient First, and Best Outcomes. Our relationship with hospital administrators remains tenuous. Our commitment to referring physicians and patients remains steadfast.

Payment Reform and Medical Oncology

The group had long recognized that the cost of cancer care would eventually become unsustainable. To expect fee-for-service to be the payment model in the years to come likely would mean deterioration to a financially unstable model as third party reimbursements continued to decline. When Dr. Barbara McAneny, Albuquerque New Mexico, invited the practice to join her CMS innovations project COME HOME, the partners quickly rose to the challenges of such a transformation. Treatment pathways were developed by the group and integrated into the electronic medical record, urgent care pathways and triage systems were standardized, and extended hours on weekend were offered to cancer patients needing supportive care. Through the COME HOME model, the practice reduced emergency room visits from 34% to 17%. We also learned that the cost of care delivered in our office was sometimes up to 20% or more lower than the same service delivered in a hospital based cancer clinic. Palliative care services were established both inpatient and outpatient with the addition of Drs. Mark Wrona and Thomas Keating. Throughout this process, the practice was well positioned to become one of the lead organizations in the CMS Oncology Care Model that was launched in July of 2016 and will be the platform upon which cancer payments will be developed going forward until 2022.

As part of the growing commitment to providing patients with high quality, safe and effective cancer care, the practice became QOPI certified through the American Society of Clinical Oncology in 2013 as well as one of the first 12 community oncology practices in the United States designated as an Oncology Medical Home by the Commission on Cancer.

Community Outreach and Patient Advocacy

Dr. Carroll and the original partners of Maine Center for Cancer Medicine recognized that research dollars raised in Maine by national based organizations sometimes did not fully come back to serve the Maine population. Dr. Carroll and Maine Center for Cancer Medicine was instrumental in the development of Maine Cancer Foundation, an organization dedicated to cancer research and education in Maine. Many of our physicians have provided Board leadership to this organization and innumerable employees in the clinical practice have been volunteers at fund raising events for this organization. The New England Cancer Specialists cannot request grant funding from this organization due to its "for profit" status. However, many hospital-based programs across the state that our patients access as well as the Maine Medical Center Research Institute have benefited from grants from this organization.

Dr. Carroll together with other oncology leaders throughout northern New England created the American Society of Clinical Oncology State Affiliate chapter Northern New England Clinical Oncology Society (NNECOS). The membership of this society is cancer care providers from Maine, Vermont and New Hampshire. The society provides educational opportunities twice a year through their meetings but more importantly is a vehicle for communication with state legislatures on key bills that impact patients with cancer and organizations that care for patients with cancer. Members of NNECOS have participated on ASCO committees such as the Clinical Practice Committee and State Affiliates Council. Dr. Thomas is an author on the ASCO PCOP model of cancer payment reform. Steve D'Amato participates heavily in ASCO and NNECOS but also has held leadership positions with American Association of Community Cancer Centers (ACCC).

Conclusion

Dr. Carroll's solo oncology practice – founded in July 1967 in his Western Promenade home - has grown over the past fifty years to become New England Cancer Specialists. His vision has touched thousands of patients and families in our state affected with this disease. His vision and the practice's ongoing execution continue to affect most aspects of cancer care from direct patient care inpatient and in the outpatient setting, education throughout the state, research development, and advocacy. The practice has been successful in continued recruitment of highly trained and highly qualified physicians from some of the most notable and comprehensive cancer centers in America including Dana Farber Cancer Institute, Yale University, Fred Hutchinson Cancer Institute to name a few. These physicians have inspired Maine Medical Center resident physicians to pursue careers in cancer and then return back to Maine to practice and care for patients. The contribution of this early physician leader in Portland has significantly impacted the current landscape of cancer care locally as well as created some of the most respected community leaders in cancer care nationally.

Neonatology

By Doug Dransfield MD

History of the Newborn Intensive Care Unit at Maine Medical Center from 1975 to 1995

Until the late 1960's pediatric care had not advanced to provide intensive care for newborn infants. President John Kennedy's son, Patrick, was born five and a half weeks early in August 1963. He died 39 hours later at the Boston Children's Hospital because of respiratory failure. There were an estimated 25,000 infants that year who died for the same reason. A decade later, the cause of respiratory failure for premature infants was understood and effective therapies were being developed. Three decades later subspecialties in both maternal care and neonatal care would be organized in a system of regionalized care that resulted in dramatically improved outcomes not only for premature infants, but also term infants who were ill in the first month after birth. Maine Medical Center's Newborn Intensive Care Unit (NICU) developed in parallel over that same time to become the regional center for neonatal care for Maine and Southwest New Hampshire. In 1970, the infant mortality rate in Maine was exceeded only by two other states in the nation. By 1995 Maine's rate was not only a third of what it had been but was one of the lowest in the nation. This chapter describes some of the events that occurred to make that change.

Care for mothers and their newborns at Maine Medical Center (MMC) in the 1970's was provided on the fourth floor of what is now Pavilion A. Management was consistent with what was available in the majority of hospitals in the United States. That is, there was none of the present day specialized care and no intensive care for ill newborns. The MMC Departments of Obstetrics and Pediatrics each had a residency program so there were resident physicians in hospital around the clock. The attending physicians were in private practice and would come to the hospital as needed to care for their patients or to supervise the residents' care of the clinic patients. The Department of Nursing had a staff of both obstetric and newborn nursery nurses. Sick newborns were cared for, as possible, in the newborn nursery. Premature infants who did not develop breathing difficulty could be provided warmth with an incubator and given artificial feedings by nurses who cared for them, but any complications were often fatal.

To place the care at MMC in context it is necessary to describe what was happening nationally. Newborn infants died because of premature birth, congenital malformations, and complications either of pregnancy or of labor and delivery. Obstetricians did not have ways to investigate when an infant was due to be born except the mother's report of her last menstrual period and her physical examination. Therefore, infants were classified by birth weight. The understanding that some small infants were small but not premature (small for gestational age) was just emerging. It was the prematurely born infants who developed the breathing problem called Hyaline Membrane Disease (now Respiratory Distress Syndrome or RDS). Although it was known that birth at earlier gestation age carried a greater risk of respiratory failure after birth, it took most of the 60's for the pathophysiology of RDS to be recognized as related to developmental lack of surfactant in the lung. With this knowledge, in the mid 1960's attempts were made to try to support premature infants with a respirator for days at a time. Successful survival began to be reported in the late 1960's as many major academic pediatric departments started to offer this care in specific intensive care nurseries. In 1975 the American Board of Pediatrics conducted the first examination of the subspecialty Board of Neonatal and Perinatal Medicine. Fellowship trained neonatologists graduated and were certified.

At Maine Medical Center Dr. George Hallett was the Chief of Pediatrics. He began to address the changes in newborn care. Dr. J. Daniel Miller provides details of that time in his "A View from the Sun Parlor: A History of Pediatrics in Portland, Maine". Dr. Hallett had MMC hire Dr. John Serrage, a pediatrician in Portland who had taken one year of additional neonatology training before starting his general pediatric practice. At the same time Dr. Albert Dibbins, having completed his training in pediatric surgery and several years on staff at University of Pittsburgh in 1974, opened his practice in Portland. He was joined in 1976 by Dr. Michael Curci, also a pediatric surgeon trained at the University of Pittsburgh. These two dedicated and skilled surgeons had training and experience providing intensive care for infants after surgery for congenital malformations. They also provided the surgical support needed for complications that occurred during assisted ventilation of premature infants. The Department of Nursing identified nurses in the newborn nursery with interest in caring for infants who needed ventilation and special care. Pediatric cardiologists Drs. Edward Matthews and Richard McFaul were available to advise on congenital heart disease. The Department of Respiratory Therapy hired Charles Kettel from Boston Children's Hospital who trained respiratory therapists to provide the specialty respiratory care for neonates that was being described in the medical journals.

It became clear that attempting to provide assisted ventilation and special care for infants would be better done in a separate nursery with nursing staff dedicated to that unit. Maine Medical Center opened the Newborn Intensive Care Center (NICC) in 1976. Around that time national organizations for pediatricians and obstetricians were meeting to develop guidelines that would set standards for organizing and coordinating care of pregnant women, fetuses, and newborns. The result was a plan for regionalization of obstetric and pediatric services. Regionalization was a system that categorized hospitals in three levels based on the services provided. Level III was to be the hospital for a region that would provide the highest level of care. The criteria for what constituted such a center were described by 1977. The staffing by physicians and nurses and the support of respiratory therapy, laboratory, radiology, engineering, and social services were suggested. There also were expectations set for the center to provide education in the region.

The Maine Medical Center invested in making the newly opened NICC meet these guidelines. It was not just the physical space and equipment that were needed. To be a regional center there needed to be coordination of care from other hospitals (Level I and II nurseries) allowing the transfer of mothers with pregnancy complications and failing that, the transport of critically ill newborns. Obstetric care for referred high-risk pregnant women and complicated deliveries was taken on by Harry Bennert MD, Donald McCrann MD, and David Ernst MD. In the Department of Pediatrics, Drs. Hallett and Serrage hired pediatricians to work exclusively in the NICC. Neonatologists including Drs. Courtney, Ebaugh, and Wender were recruited but their stays were short and there were never more than two at one time. The pediatric residents added large responsibilities to their duties by providing continuous coverage for care in the NICC as well as at delivery of high-risk infants. There were several residents from that time who were important in the improvement of care for ill newborns in Maine. Drs. Patricia Bromberger and Dr. Jan Wneck staffed the NICC after their residencies. Dr. Bromberger later became a neonatologist and practiced in San Diego. The extensive training obtained in the NICC resulted in MMC pediatric residency graduates who were highly competent in the care of sick newborns. When they established practices elsewhere in Maine they brought with them the ability to stabilize and transport infants to MMC. Drs. Dana Goldsmith (practicing in Rockland), Michael Hoffman (in Skowhegan), David Poleski (in Presque Isle), and Drs. Larry Losey and Jan Wneck (in Bath-Brunswick) were most helpful and should share any credit for reductions in neonatal mortality for Maine. To support the organization of a regional referral system the State of Maine and the March of Dimes provided grants that funded staff at MMC to go to the referring hospitals to teach nurses and physicians how to care for both at-risk mothers and ill newborns prior to transfer. Local hospitals also received grant money for equipment and transport incubators. Shortly after the grant started, Alison Tito RN was the NICC nurse hired to implement and coordinate education efforts. The grant also provided for regular transport conferences at the referring hospitals where Ms. Tito and an obstetrician and neonatologist would meet with the referring hospital staff to review all the mothers and infants referred from that hospital and to give outcome reports.

As the NICC assumed the role of a regional nursery the number of infants admitted increased. More infants required many more nurses, respiratory therapists, and doctors. The Nursing Department expanded the number of nurses that could provide intensive care. Three neonatal nurses, Ann Carroll RN, Carole Messenger-Rioux RN, and Mary Weinstein RN who began their careers at MMC in the 1970's shared their memories of this expansion for this chapter. All three recounted how as young graduates they came to the NICC and were trained by the nurses already working there. The nursing staff expanded by this method, and nurses went to other Neonatal Intensive Care Units to train and brought skills back to teach to the other staff. Nurses Carroll, Messenger-Rioux, and Weinstein were at the very core of the expansion of knowledge and quality of care by nursing in the NICU.

It soon became obvious that the number of infants in the NICC and the frequency of high-risk deliveries requiring a neonatal team required an approach other than just pediatric residents and two neonatologists. This staffing problem was occurring nationwide. The answer was for selected nurses to assume new roles to deliver care previously provided only by physicians. The three previously mentioned nurses and a half-dozen others took the training and made the transition to being nurse clinicians. The nurse clinicians made it possible for the day to day census of the NICC to remain near its 12-bed capacity. They also participated in the care of infants in the delivery room. By 1985 national certification of neonatal nurse practitioners (NNPs) was established. The nurse clinicians at MMC became NNPs. There is no doubt that the expansion of services and level of care of the NICU was possible only because of them. Indeed the entire nursing staff has been a dedicated group and many have worked at MMC 30 years or more. The continuity this has provided and the wealth of skills and experience present is remarkable.

In 1982 Dr. Alistair G. S. Philip was employed by MMC as the Director of Neonatology. He joined Dr. Doug Dransfield who had been employed in 1981 and was the only other neonatologist when Alistair began. Dr. Philip had been a neonatologist at the University of Vermont with Dr. Jerold Lucey, the editor of the journal Pediatrics. He was a first-rate academic neonatologist who had published on many aspects of neonatal care and had many contacts across the country with neonatologists starting neonatal units. Dr.

Philip worked with the Medical Center administration to expand the neonatology staff and to develop a new space for the NICC with the intention of making a true Level III regional center. When he was recently asked why he had been willing to come to MMC, Dr. Philip mentioned the MMC affiliation with the University of Vermont as a teaching hospital and the work of two people that he felt showed the potential available. First, was the work Alison Tito had done in organizing the care in the hospitals in Maine. Perhaps most important was Dr. Walter Allan. Dr. Allan was a pediatric neurologist who had an interest in neonatal neurologic conditions, particularly intraventricular hemorrhage in premature infants. Dr. Allan had come to MMC in 1978 bringing the ability to study this problem using bedside cranial ultrasound. When Dr. Dransfield came from Children's Hospital of Philadelphia (CHOP) in 1981 he too had been very impressed to see Dr. Allan doing these studies particularly since just months before, at CHOP, the only infant to have been examined by cranial ultrasound had to be taken to an ultrasound machine located at the University of Pennsylvania Hospital. Dr. Philip recognized the opportunity to collaborate with Dr. Allan as an advantage that would improve the status of the MMC neonatal nursery and provide research opportunities.

Maine Medical Center underwent a major expansion with the construction of the Bean Building in 1985. A new intensive care nursery opened at that time and was named the Newborn Intensive Care Unit (NICU). There was a gradual increase in staffing by nursing, respiratory therapy and physicians so that the bed capacity increased over several years to 24. At the same time the hospital increased and modernized equipment to match the "state of the art" found nationally.

In 1984, Dale "Skip" Kessler MD PhD agreed to leave a regional NICU in Wisconsin and added his academic background, excellent clinical skills, and careful, thoughtful manner to the MMC staff. Doreen Morrow MD, following her fellowship at University of Pennsylvania and CHOP, became the fourth neonatologist later in 1984. Dr. Morrow added a confident and caring approach to the team. Her "hallmark" was her clinical skill and devotion to any infant under her care. In 1988, two neonatologists, Drs. Lucinda "Cindy" Dykes and Daniel Sobel, arrived. Dr. Dykes brought a sensitivity that added greatly to the care delivered in the unit. Dr. Sobel fostered an approach to analyze and examine the work being done to find ways to make it better. The Division of Neonatology physicians shared the commitment that in their rapidly developing subspecialty they needed to bring all the advances that were occurring nationally to MMC. Their other fundamental belief was that caring for a sick newborn really required supporting a family. This belief was shared by everyone working in the NICU. Susan Soule MSW, a MMC employee, and Renee Newman, a volunteer were noteworthy for their help and support for families. Susan Soule was the social worker who was available to help with needs both financial and emotional. She also helped establish a parents' support group. Renee Newman, and her husband Tom, had been parents of infants born prematurely, a daughter in the years of the NICC and then a son was in the NICU. After their daughter was born they donated generously to the Bean Building funding campaign for the new NICU. Both children are now successful adults. Ms. Soule later asked Ms. Newman to help with the parent group, and she became an invaluable addition.

To be a true Level III perinatal center more than an NICU was required. Another critical component was the presence of Board Certified obstetric specialists in maternal and fetal medicine. Dr. Alan Donnenfeld provided this for a short time. Michael Pinette MD followed and brought the credentials and skills in prenatal diagnosis and identification and management of high-risk pregnancies.

Excellent radiology and ophthalmology services specific for premature infants were also needed. In radiology, Drs. Andy Packard and Robert Isler initiated those changes after which Dr. Charles Grimes helped develop the full range of neonatal imaging services that were required. Ophthalmology treatment for the condition retinopathy of prematurity (blood vessel changes of the eye after a very premature infant survives ventilation) was being developed nationally. Drs. Peter Hedstrom and then Jeffery Berman arrived with those much-needed skills. Other areas of the hospital that had to adapt and change to meet the needs of the NICU included the laboratories (e.g. ability to perform chemical analysis on micro samples) and medical engineering (e.g. maintaining the increasing array of electronic equipment).

The Department of Pediatrics attracted new subspecialists in increasing numbers. To pediatric cardiology and pediatric surgery were added pediatric subspecialists in hematology/oncology, neurology, allergy and immunology, infectious disease, genetics, nephrology, pulmonary medicine, endocrinology, and gastroenterology. By 1995 the evolution of the Department of Pediatrics resulted in the establishment of the Barbara Bush Children's Hospital at Maine Medical Center. The NICU was now a part of that hospital.

In the late 1980's there was evidence that the MMC NICU was being recognized regionally and nationally for the quality of care it provided. The first indication of this was that the NICU at MMC was an original member of the Vermont Oxford Network (VON/Network). VON was formed in 1988 to bring together neonatal centers "to improve the quality and safety of medical care for newborn infants and their families through a coordinated program of research, education, and quality improvement projects" (https://public.vtoxford.org/about-us/). MMC's NICU could now measure itself against other units in the U.S. and the world. Membership in VON allowed MMC NICU to participate in the multicenter trial of Survanta, surfactant replacement, for the treatment of RDS. This trial resulted in FDA approval of this treatment in August 1990 and was a major turning point in treating premature infants resulting in increased survival and reduced complications. The Network invited the MMC NICU to participate in other studies of quality improvement in neonatal practices that changed care. Today Vermont Oxford Network has over a thousand participating centers and the MMC nursery continues as a member.

The largest, best funded study was a collaborative one with the NICUs at Yale University and Brown University. Drs. Philip and Allan, working with Dr. Laura Ment at Yale and Dr. William Oh at Brown, were awarded funding by the U.S. National Institutes of Health to conduct a randomized controlled trial of indomethacin to prevent intraventricular hemorrhage in premature infants. The randomized treatment phase was completed between 1989 and 1992, but Dr. Allan continued follow-up studies on the infants until age 21.

In 1989, the neonatologists formed a private practice group, Maine Neonatology Associates (MNA). This allowed the neonatologists to make staffing and care decisions they thought were needed. Additional neonatologists were hired. Perhaps the most important change for care in the NICU was to have a neonatologist constantly present in the NICU. Also, always available was an additional on-call neonatologist to be activated when multiple events required more staff. At the same time, changes in the national standard for pediatric residency certification reduced the amount of time residents were training in neonatal care. To meet the service need created by the absence of residents, MMC employed additional NNPs. Patient care improved by this combination of the NNPs and in hospital neonatologist. It also improved resident education because a neonatologist was available to offer clinical instruction at the time of care - day or night. Proof of this benefit was the hiring of Peter Marro MD in 1993. Peter had been a MMC pediatric resident who went on to the University of Pennsylvania neonatology program and returned to join MNA, eventually became Chief of Neonatology.

As the number of infants continued to increase, so did the need to find additional space for hospitalized infants who no longer needed the highest level of intensive care before being discharged home. Maine Neonatology hired Dr. Brenda Medlin as a dedicated in-hospital pediatrician to care for infants in other infant care areas. The 24 spaces in the NICU could then all be used for intensive care. Dr. Medlin helped MNA improve the system for discharge and referral back to local physicians which also added greatly to parent satisfaction.

The final step necessary to establish the NICU as the regional Level III nursery for Maine was the creation, in 1995, of a full-time dedicated neonatal transport system. The transport service was initially facilitated by a private ambulance company however collaboration with the City of Portland eventually became the best way to offer this service. As a result of creating the transport system, community hospital staff could concentrate on stabilization of the infant while the NICU Transport Team joined to facilitate and complete the transfer. The transport team included two Portland Fire Department EMTs, a NICU staff nurse, a respiratory therapist, a NNP, and if needed a neonatologist. Despite a very cooperative regional obstetric referral system for "at-risk" deliveries, the unpredictable nature of some deliveries required the regular use of this service. Soon a third or more of the NICU admissions involved the transport team.

The story of the twenty-year transition from newborn nursery to Level III regional newborn center at Maine Medical Center is only partially presented here. The size of investment by Maine Medical Center and the hundreds of dedicated people who gave of themselves to make the NICU successful cannot be given adequate credit in such a short summary. The author wants to express extreme thanks and praise for what was done in the twenty years he worked in the NICU and apologize for the failure to name and acknowledge more individuals than was done.

Nephrology

By Paul A. Parker MD

Nephrology at the Maine Medical Center

Background

Two milestones in nephrology occurred in 1945 on opposite sides of the Atlantic. Willem Kolff MD, working in the Netherlands under Nazi occupation, succeeded in constructing a crude hemodialysis machine and attempted to treat patients with acute kidney injury. His first fifteen patients all succumbed, but his sixteenth patient - a 67-year-old woman with acute kidney injury - awoke from her uremic coma and survived. That same year in Boston, Massachusetts at the Peter Bent Brigham Hospital, Charles Hufnagel MD staff surgeon assisted by David Hume MD an assistant surgical resident and Ernest Landsteiner MD, chief resident in urology (son of Karl Landsteiner MD winner of the Nobel Prize for developing the modern classification of blood groups) procured a kidney from a deceased donor in their hospital's morgue and successfully grafted the donor kidney into the antecubital vasculature of a uremic 29-year-old female. The kidney itself was left outside the body swaddled in saline soaked gauze. After just four days the transplant was rejected by the young woman's immune system but it had functioned long enough for her to survive acute kidney injury. Despite these two enormous achievements the creation of the first functional artificial organ and the first successful human organ transplant it would be decades before these breakthroughs could be brought into widespread clinical use.

By the early 1950's medical centers across the country, perhaps most notably the University of Seattle in Washington state, raced to produce a practical dialysis machine and the means to repeatedly access a patient's blood stream. It would not be until 1960 that Belden Scribner MD working with Wayne Quinton, an engineer, developed the Teflon shunt that would allow for relatively easy and repetitive arterial and venous access to a patient's blood stream. This breakthrough in bloodstream access made it possible to provide chronic dialysis therapy to patients with end stage kidney failure. By 1966 when the American Society of Nephrology was established there were only 1,000 patients receiving chronic dialysis therapy in the United States. Funding for their care came from a hodgepodge of Public Health Service grants, research funds and charitable donations.

Efforts at renal transplantation were hindered by the lack of immunosuppressive therapy capable of preventing rejection. Renal transplants lasted only days or at best a few months before failing due to transplant rejection. John P. Merrill MD at the Peter Bent Brigham Hospital in Boston sought and found a pair of identical twins, one with end-stage renal disease and the other healthy and willing to participate in the first living donor transplant. To test whether the donor kidney would be rejected a skin graft between the twins was done first and it showed no rejection. Despite these results there was intense criticism from his peers over the potential risks. However Dr. Merrill and his team proceeded and on December 23, 1954 Richard J. Herrick received a kidney from his brother Ronald L. Herrick, who lived in Maine. It functioned well without the need for immunosuppressive therapy and Richard would live for nine years eventually succumbing to complications of hypertension and heart disease. His daughter Marjorie would earn her RN and pursue a career as a home dialysis nurse in Portland, Maine's first outpatient dialysis center. Over the ensuing years Dr. Merrill successfully transplanted a series of identical twin renal transplants, but it wouldn't be until the early 1960s that a successful drug protocol for treating rejection was identified and deceased donor transplants would be possible. As with dialysis though this potentially lifesaving treatment remained experimental, underfunded and largely unavailable.

Maine Medical Center

William C. Austin MD had grown up in Cape Elizabeth, Maine, and graduated from Bowdoin College and the school of medicine at Cornell University. He completed his medical residency which included a cardiology fellowship at Maine Medical Center and subsequently pursued advanced training at Memorial Sloan Kettering Cancer Center in New York City. There he studied acid base and electrolyte physiology and was introduced to, and trained in, the operation of dialysis machines. He returned to MMC in 1960 as a renal physiologist and was there to accept delivery of the first dialysis machine in Maine given to the hospital by the Department of Health and Welfare. Working with Ferris Ray MD, a gifted general and vascular surgeon who had learned how to implant the new Teflon dialysis shunt, Dr. Austin was able to obtain vascular access in patients and in 1960 he successfully dialyzed two patients, one with methanol and the other with barbiturate intoxication and both survived. Over the next decade, handicapped by a chronic lack of funding, Dr. Austin was able to provide a very limited number of dialysis treatments on inpatients with dialyzable overdoses and acute kidney injury. He performed these treatments himself in room 180 on PIC. It wasn't until 1968 that he recruited Lucille Hunter RN, a former surgical nurse and friend of his wife, and Rita Menard RN, a recent graduate, to work with him as the first dialysis nurses. Plans were put in place for a formal dialysis unit if funding could be obtained; the goal was to provide both inpatient dialysis and training for outpatient home dialysis. Two home dialysis machines had already been donated to the Maine Medical Center - one by the Altrusa Club with money raised at a Fred Waring musical concert, and one from the Augusta Junior Women's Club which collected 600,000 General Mills Coupons which they redeemed (believe it or not) for a home hemodialysis machine.

Meanwhile Dr. Ray, with the assistance of Stanley Dienst MD (who would be recruited by the Henry Ford Hospital in Detroit, Michigan in 1968 to head their renal transplant program) and Richard C. Dillihunt MD, then a surgical resident at MMC, were available to provide not only dialysis access but were also working to support the fledgling transplant programs in Boston by surgically retrieving kidneys from deceased donors throughout Maine. When a potential kidney donor would be identified somewhere in the state of Maine they would travel emergently either by car or small plane and sometimes with Maine state troopers providing high speed siren screaming ground transportation. Once the surgery was completed they would place the kidney on ice and race it to one of the Boston transplant centers or the Jamaica Plain Veterans Hospital and sometimes as far as the Presbyterian Hospital in New York City. Circumstances permitting, they would accompany the donor kidney all the way to the operating room where they would study the surgical techniques required to perform renal transplantation.

Maine Medical Center, with the urging of Donald F. Marshall MD then Head of Urology, Dr. Ferris Ray, newly appointed Head of vascular surgery, and Edward McGeachey, associate Vice President of Maine Medical Center, hired a consultant to evaluate the situation with respect to the need for potential nephrology services in Maine. The report estimated that approximately fifty people per year in Maine would require chronic dialysis therapy, and judged the Maine Medical Center to have adequate facilities to develop and maintain a dialysis program. Armed with this information, these three leaders presented their case to then Governor Kenneth M. Curtis and the Maine State Legislature. Ultimately, they were granted a total of $500,000 to establish a program that would offer state wide availability for both dialysis and renal transplant services.

In 1969 the Richard's Wing had been completed and had effectively doubled the size of Maine Medical Center. Five rooms were allocated on the fifth floor for the creation of a Division of Nephrology and Transplantation and seven Travenol dialysis machines were purchased. Tragically Dr. Austin, who suffered from multiple sclerosis, found it necessary to withdraw from the program at that time and MMC employed Andrew Welden MD, a nephrologist from Johns Hopkins University in Baltimore, Maryland to serve as a visiting specialist while the Maine Medical Center worked to recruit its own full-time nephrologist.

Jan S. Drewry MD a recent graduate from the renal fellowship program at the University of Texas (Southwestern) Medical School was hired and appointed Director of Nephrology and Renal Transplantation in July 1971. With the firm backing of MMC and the financial support provided by the state legislature she was charged with developing a program to provide in center acute hemodialysis, home training for the purpose of outpatient therapy and renal transplantation. Drawing on the experience of Rita Menard RN and Lucille Hunter RN she quickly organized the dialysis unit on R5 and began providing both acute and chronic hemodialysis. Lucille Hunter was named the first Head Nurse of the new dialysis unit on the 5th floor of the Richards Wing. Rita Menard was sent to multiple leading dialysis centers around the country including Seattle, Chicago, Philadelphia and Boston to study their programs and bring back information. Simone Blanchette RN, a Maine native recently returned from California where she had received dialysis training, was placed in charge of a new five-station home dialysis training center located on the first floor of the old Ear Nose and Throat Hospital known as Holt Hall on the corner of Congress and Bramhall Street. A specialized group to maintain the dialysis machines provide laboratory services to the dialysis unit and to assist with organ retrieval throughout the state was created and staffed by Richard Benoit, Stephen Land, Ellie King, Bruce White and others.

Dr. Ray traveled to Boston and studied alongside one of the pioneering transplant surgeons Anthony Monaco MD and subsequently assembled the surgical transplant team at the Maine Medical Center consisting of three additional vascular surgeons, Richard C. Dillihunt MD, Robert McAfee MD and Wesley English MD and four urologists Donald Marshall MD, Fred Clark MD Hugh Robinson MD and Robert Timothy MD.

Theresa Sprague, a young woman who had begun hemodialysis in the spring of 1971 just two months before Dr. Drewry arrived in Portland, was offered the opportunity to be the first kidney transplant recipient in Maine. Her friends urged her to consider going to Boston to have her transplant but she chose to stay at Maine Medical Center stating that "the doctors and nurses at Maine Medical Center are my friends." Her sister J. Campbell had courageously offered to donate her kidney. On October 24, 1971 Drs. Ferris Ray, Donald Marshall, and Anthony Monaco, (who had had traveled to Portland to observe) performed the first kidney transplant at Maine Medical Center.

It was successful and Theresa Sprague enjoyed an additional 29 years of life with normal kidney function.

1972 brought significant changes to both the field of nephrology and MMC. Nephrology was recognized as a medical specialty and the first nephrology boards were offered in 1972. It was also in 1972 that the federal government passed the Social Security amendment of 1972 which made patients with end-stage renal disease eligible for Medicare coverage for their dialysis and transplant healthcare costs. Dialysis and renal transplantation were no longer considered experimental and therefore eligible for private insurance and Medicaid coverage. This timely legislation provided financial support for chronic dialysis therapy and renal transplantation when these programs at Maine Medical Center were still in their infancy.

Donald A. Leeber MD, also a graduate of the renal fellowship program at the University of Texas (Southwestern) Medical School, was hired in July of 1972 and brought, in addition to his training in nephrology and transplantation, specialized training in tissue typing. With his expertise and a generous donation of $26,000 provided by Albert D Conley it was possible to establish the Conley Tissue Typing Laboratory in 1972. Ellie King was chosen to head the tissue typing laboratory which was located adjacent to the home dialysis training center in Holt Hall. Pursuant to the mandate of the state's financial grant, Dr. Leeber worked with physician groups throughout the state to assist in the creation of hemodialysis programs particularly at Eastern Maine Medical Center in Bangor and Mid-Maine Medical Center in Waterville. He also provided education to emergency room and hospital physicians throughout the region to assist them in identifying potential deceased kidney donors. Dr. Leeber was particularly active in the New England Organ Bank and served for years on its Board of Trustees. He was subsequently elected Chairman of the Board and under his leadership streamlined the board and modernized its administrative procedures. He would remain an active member of the board until his retirement in 1996.

Drs. Drewry and Leeber held that it was the mission of the nephrology service to provide patient care, to teach and to do research. Together they established the renal teaching service on P1C staffed by a renal attending and two second-year medical residents who rotated on a monthly basis and provided inpatient care to all nephrology, dialysis and renal transplant patients. For many years the renal consultation service was an independent service staffed only by the attendings. More recently with the introduction of the hospitalist physicians and a separate renal transplant service, the renal service was retired and the renal consultative service was expanded to include renal fellows, advanced practice clinicians, residents, and medical students.

It was also in 1972 that Dr. Leeber made his famous and still relevant observation that it required at least three nephrologists to provide care for one chronic dialysis patient. With this in mind he approached T. James Hallee MD, an internist practicing in Cape Elizabeth, with the opportunity to be the first nephrology fellow at MMC. Dr. Hallee accepted the position and upon completion of one year of fellowship provided all nephrology consultation service at Mercy Hospital and cross covered with Drs. Drewry and Leeber on call while still maintaining his busy internal medicine practice in Cape Elizabeth.

The nephrology and transplant service grew rapidly over the next few years outstripping the MMC's ability to provide for the ever-growing population of chronic dialysis patients and the need for outpatient consultation and follow up care for patients with chronic kidney disease and renal transplants. In 1977 Drs. Drewry and Leeber opened a private practice office (Drewry and Leeber Associates - later changed to Maine Nephrology Associates in 1980) and simultaneously opened the first outpatient dialysis center the Southern Maine Dialysis Facility. Both entities were located across the street from the Maine Medical Center at what was then 13 Charles Street. Lucille Hunter RN was appointed Head Nurse of this new outpatient dialysis unit and by the end of the decade was providing care for 55 end stage renal disease patients. Simone Blanchette RN continued to direct the home training center which was moved up to R5 and took over as Head Nurse of the inpatient dialysis unit and would hold that position until her retirement. The Department of Pediatrics attracted Susan Williams MD (later Susan St. Mary MD) who opened a private practice in June of 1977 to fill a critical need in pediatric nephrology care. In July of 1979 Paul A. Parker MD, from the University of Iowa joined the Drewry and Leeber nephrology practice and introduced the technique of fluoroscopic guided renal biopsy to replace the unguided bedside biopsy technique previously employed. In subsequent years fluoroscopic guidance would be replaced by ultrasound guidance which greatly simplified the procedure and avoided the need to expose patients with reduced kidney function to x-ray contrast.

Jan Drewry chose to return to Texas in 1980 and T. James Hallee MD accepted the invitation to leave his internal medicine practice and complete his second year of renal fellowship at MMC and join Maine Nephrology Associates in 1981. Well-known and respected throughout the community as a "physician's physician" he brought a gift for teaching and a bedside manner that defined his career.

Jonathan Himmelfarb MD, an early graduate of the renal fellowship program which included a year of research at the Brigham and Women's Hospital joined Maine Nephrology associates 1988. In addition to his clinical responsibilities he pursued an aggressive research program publishing over 200 peer reviewed papers during his twenty-year career at MMC, and he assumed the role of Division Director of Nephrology at MMC upon Donald Leeber's retirement in 1996. In 2008 Jonathan accepted the opportunity to establish and direct the Kidney Research Institute at the University of Washington and was named to the Joseph E. Eschbach Endowed Chair in Kidney Research and is the co-director of the Center of Dialysis Innovation. In 2015 he was elected President of the American Society of Nephrology.

Dialysis

The outpatient dialysis population grew relatively slowly due, in part, to other dialysis facilities which opened around the state. The Southern Maine Dialysis Facility which treated 55 patients by the end of 1980 surpassed 100 patients by 1990. James Wasserman MD joined the practice in 1992 following a fellowship at Brigham and Women's Hospital in Boston where he worked in the molecular physiology laboratory isolating and cloning molecular tubular transporters. He would continue his bench research at the Maine Medical Center and in 1996 assumed the medical directorship of the Southern Maine Dialysis facility.

The 1990s were a period of rapid growth and would necessitate the building of three additional outpatient dialysis facilities not simply to accommodate the increased number of dialysis patients but also to provide them with better geographic access to dialysis care. The Coastal Dialysis Unit was built in Bath in 1995, jointly staffed by the Lewiston nephrology group and the Portland nephrology group with Stuart Abramson MD also from the Brigham and Women's hospital as its Medical Director. Soon afterwards the York County Dialysis Center opened in Biddeford in 1996 with Paul A. Parker MD as Medical Director. In 1999 the Casco Bay Dialysis Center was opened in Westbrook, Maine with Patricia Cantlin DO as its Medical Director. It would not be until 2002 that the fifth dialysis unit, the Damariscotta Dialysis Center was opened in Damariscotta with Stuart Abramson MD as its Medical Director. A sixth Dialysis Center is currently in development and scheduled to open in 2018. It will be opened and directed by Dr. Paul Parker. Gary DiPerna, DO will assume the directorship of the York County Dialysis Center. The new unit will be unique in that it will focus primarily on providing primarily home dialysis training while also providing transitional orientation to new dialysis patients just starting chronic in center hemodialysis and out patients recovering from acute kidney injury. It will be one of the first units of its kind in the nation. Maine Nephrology Associates currently provides dialysis care for approximately 400 chronic dialysis patients including 60 home patients. The state of Maine currently has a total of 15 dialysis units providing therapy for over 900 patients.

Transplant

The transplant program which began with only one patient in 1971 grew steadily to seven transplants in 1972, 16 in 1977 and 26 in 1980. Dr. Ray continued to perform vascular and renal transplant surgery until his retirement in 1986 at which time the program continued under the leadership of Richard C. Dillihunt MD with the support of vascular surgeons William Herbert MD, Robert Hawkins MD and Jens Jorgensen MD and urologists Andrew Iverson MD, Brian Jumper MD and Sam Broadus MD. By 1990 there had been 439 renal transplants and by 2000 that number grew to 846 renal transplants at the MMC renal transplant program.

In 1999 John P. Vella MD, an attending transplant nephrologist from Peter Bent Brigham Hospital in Boston, joined Maine Nephrology Associates. As Assistant Division Director he worked with the vascular surgery group and in 2000 coordinated the hiring of James Whiting MD, a transplant surgeon, who was trained to perform both the vascular and urologic components of the transplant surgery. In 2005 a separate renal transplant service was created on R5 to care for all inpatient renal transplants and to provide consultative support for all solid organ transplants. A new outpatient office specifically for renal transplants was opened at 19 West Street in Portland. A defined medical transplant team included John Vella MD, Mark Parker MD (who assumed the Division of Nephrology and Transplantation Directorship in 2008 following Dr. Himmelfarb's move to Seattle, Washington), Payson Oberg MD, Mike Akom MD and Ana Rossi MD and Deb Hawks PA-C. A second transplant surgeon Juan Palma Vargas MD joined the surgical transplant team in 2013 and has been able to increase the availability of living transplant donors by facilitating participation in the Paired Kidney Exchange program. By 2017 a total of 1750 renal transplants had been performed with a success rate of greater than 95% both with deceased donor and living related transplants after the first year.

Interventional Nephrology

Creating and maintaining a suitable access to the bloodstream to provide chronic hemodialysis continues to be a significant challenge. Fistulas are prone to develop stenosis and not infrequently thrombose which in the past always required surgical intervention and frequently the placement of temporary tunneled internal jugular catheter access. In the late 1990s pioneering nephrologists learned the skill of interventional radiology and began performing interventional radiologic procedures focused primarily on maintaining dialysis bloodstream access. In 1999 Brad Schimelman MD an unusually gifted interventional nephrologist from Loyola University Medical Center joined Maine

Nephrology

Nephrology Associates and established a renal interventional access service. Initially operated at MMC and subsequently moved to the Scarborough Surgical Center, it has significantly improved the performance and maintenance of arteriovenous fistulas and grafts and greatly reduce the need for surgery and hospitalization. As the need for this service increased Robert Zimmerman MD was trained. When Dr. Schimelman left the service to work as a nephrologist at the Veterans Hospital in Togus, Maine, Dr. Zimmerman assumed the Directorship and trained Mahai Cosmo MD to share the work with him.

Teaching

The renal fellowship program, established in 1972, has graduated 42 fellows - of whom seven have joined Maine Nephrology Associates. There are currently six fellows in training. From 1972 until 2005 the renal service provided training for medical residents in nephrology and renal transplantation. In 2005 the renal consultation service was expanded to provide teaching for medical residents, medical students and renal fellows and the renal transplant service was made into a separate service also to provide training for renal fellows, medical residents, surgical residents and medical students.

Over the years every member of the Department has participated in providing specialized lectures on a variety of nephrology topics and renal attendings have been regular participants in the department of medicine's morning report.

The practice is especially proud of Mike Tranfaglia PA-C who joined Maine Nephrology Associates in 2009 after working in the varied fields of general medicine, dermatology, cardiology and vascular surgery. MMC chose to honor him in 2017 by creating an annual award in his name to be presented to the APP recognized for superior clinical acumen, compassion, dedication and professionalism. In 2012 Eric Holmes PA-C created an opportunity for physician assistant students to rotate through the renal service gaining experience in clinical nephrology, dialysis, transplantation and interventional radiology according to their preferences and in 2003 Mark Parker MD was awarded the Attending Physician Award for Teaching Excellence by the department of medicine.

Research

The goal of pursuing meaningful research began as early as 1961 with Dr. Austin who focused primarily on fluid and electrolyte disorders and the dialysis of toxins and contributed 41 publications over the course of his career. The work of Jonathan

Himmelfarb MD has been detailed above and he continues his research as Director of the Kidney Research Institute in Seattle Washington. Eric Taylor MD joined MNA in 2009 and has divided his time between clinical nephrology and NIH grant supported research into nephrolithiasis. Dr. Wasserman has had a particular interest in the medical benefits of exercise and has developed research programs designed to incorporate exercise and general physical development into the dialysis regimen. As Medical Director of the Southern Maine Dialysis Facility he has provided exercise, physical therapy and tai chi to patient's while on dialysis demonstrating their benefits and publishing his results.

Conclusion

Maine Nephrology Associates celebrated its 40th year of operation in 2017. It has grown to include 12 nephrologists and four APPs: Mike Tranfaglia PAC, Eric Holmes PAC, Emily Snow NP and Sara Rosa NP. From the very beginning it has been most fortunate to have an outstanding staff to assist in its growth and development and to provide the hands-on patient care and support that ultimately define any medical practice. Polly Bragdon our first office manager took a small private practice group from one IBM typewriter and a copy machine with a billing system consisting of index cards to an efficient modern computerized 21st century practice. Cheryl Merrill RN our first office nurse, fresh out of nursing school, learned nephrology and renal transplantation on the job and throughout her career set a standard of competency and compassion that continues to inspire us. We mourn her untimely death from pancreatic cancer in 2015. And a word of special recognition for Karen Kennie, the Division of Nephrology and Transplant secretary who for three decades has with grace and skill coordinated the myriad of tasks and personalities that have come her way.

Neither time nor space can permit an adequate review of all the individuals who have made a meaningful contribution in the service of nephrology at Maine Medical Center over the past six decades, but let me take this opportunity to thank each and every one of them.

Neurology

By Walter C. Allan MD, John Kelly Sullivan MD
and Richard L. Sullivan MD

Charles Kunkle was the first neurologist to choose Portland, ME for his practice. He came from a successful academic career at the Duke Medical School and had written the chapter on headache in Harrison's Textbook of Medicine. His specialty was headache, and he was known to spend several hours with a new patient obtaining and documenting the history and conducting a very complete neurologic exam. Charles retired from his practice in 1974 and supervised neurology education at Maine Medical Center until his full retirement in 1986.

Cornelius "Neil" Toner came to MMC for his medical internship and residency in 1958. After his neurology residency he returned to Portland in 1963. He left unexpectedly in 1967 and settled in Springfield MA where he spent the rest of his career. To replace Neil Toner, William ("Bill") Leschey was recruited by MMC in the early 1970s. As an inducement the hospital offered Bill and his family a house at the site of the Dana Education Center where they lived until they moved to Cape Elizabeth.

Around this same time began a dramatic expansion and improvement in diagnostic and treatment opportunities in neurology. Neurologists had experience and skill in diagnosing common as well as obscure brain diseases but treatment options were limited. Diagnostic procedures involved sticking angiogram needles into the carotid arteries, injecting air into the spinal canal and turning the patient in a somersault, and injecting oil-based contrast into the spinal canal for myelogram study. Any contrast that could not be removed at the time of the procedure would remain to float around the brain for life. Diagnoses were often made at brain cutting. The few available medicines included phenytoin, amitriptyline and prednisone - all cheap generic drugs.

The first CT scanner arrived at Maine Medical Center in 1976. The images were small and fuzzy and the patient had to lie still for 60 minutes. Nevertheless this allowed one to see large tumors and other mass lesions as well as congenital malformations and many other abnormalities. Neurologists still relied on myelography to evaluate problems of the nerve roots and spinal cord but the development of water soluble contrast which cleared without removal made this procedure much easier for the patient.

Ultrasound imaging of the carotid arteries permitted evaluation of cerebrovascular disease without angiography. By the early 1980's this technology was used at the hospital and in outpatient clinics, including neurology and vascular surgery. Ultrasound was very helpful in demonstrating disease in patients with TIA and stroke. Easy access to this non-invasive technology also opened the door to widespread screening and endarterectomy surgery on asymptomatic patients, although the value of these approaches remained uncertain.

Electroencephalography (EEG) was developed early in the early 20th century. Compact units for hospital and office laboratories were perfected by the Grass Instrument Company in Boston. Dr. George Maltby was trained as a neurosurgeon but had a strong interest in epilepsy and EEG. He came to Portland in 1945 and started the EEG Laboratory at Maine Medical Center (MMC) which he directed until his retirement in1978. EEG technology evolved from tubes to transistors and from paper to computer reading and storage.

The 1970s saw the dramatic growth of medical practices in Portland, aided by the construction of the Park Medical Building across from Deering Oaks Park by physicians who were each interested in expanding their practices as the demands for services increased. These included a neurologist - Bill Leschey, a medical oncologist - Ron Carroll, a rheumatologist - Paulding Phelps, an internist - Jack Davey, two ophthalmologists - Bill Holt and Elizabeth Serrage, and an orthopedic surgeon - Chip Carruthers. This led to the formation of a neurology group that began with Bill Leschey and John Boothby, followed by Richard Sullivan in 1976, Walt Allan in 1978, and John Kelly Sullivan (no relation to Richard) in 1981. This practice model shared overhead and coverage but otherwise had complete independence. This loose model allowed each individual to nurture his own special interests. Bill Leschey had a strong interest in EEG which led him to introduce the allied technologies of brain mapping and evoked potentials. Richard Sullivan was the first neurologist in Maine trained in electromyography (EMG) and neuromuscular disease. Kelly Sullivan was similarity trained and helped increase its availability. Walt Allan was trained as a pediatric neurologist but was comfortable with adult neurology, so he practiced both to help with office and hospital coverage for MMC, Mercy Hospital and the Osteopathic Hospital.

New technologies required investment of time and money from the neurologists and MMC. Two stories illustrate how complications could arise when the economic interests of independent practitioners might conflict with those of the hospital.

> **Maine Magnetic Imaging-** In the early 1980s neurology was experiencing a revolution in neuroimaging. Magnetic Resonance Imaging (MRI) scans provided precise images of the brain and spine - clearly the technology of the future. For MMC to acquire an MRI

scanner for inpatient clinical use a "certificate of need" (CON) from the State would be required. However a CON was not required for an outpatient scanner.

Mercy Hospital was approached by a neurosurgeon from Portsmouth, NH with a proposal to bring an MRI scanner in a truck to Mercy. Upon learning this, a group of physicians including Bill Leschey considered acquiring an MRI scanner for the Portland outpatient community. A large group of physicians (eventually 25 partners) formed Maine Magnetic Imaging to obtain financing and select an MRI machine. Mercy and MMC radiologists were invited to join this venture. However, this would likely make the hospital's application for a CON more difficult. At first the MMC radiologists opposed the idea. The MRI group met with Don McDowell, MMC President, who then suggested to the radiologists that it was in their interest to participate. And so Maine Magnetic Imaging became a very successful and collegial venture in our medical community. Both neurologists and radiologists took courses to learn the physics and interpretation of this new technology, and they shared the reading. If a neurologist read the scans for the day, a radiologist would review all scans with him at 4 pm, and vice versa. This collaborative on the job training worked very well. When the Stark law blocked ownership of imaging facilities by clinicians, control was shifted to hospitals and radiologists. Eventually, in 2005, Maine Neurology and Maine Neurosurgery were able to obtain an MRI scanner for their outpatients and neurologists were again able to become certified to interpret scans.

Cranial ultrasonography of premature infants - Shortly after coming to Portland in 1978, Walt Allan read of the use of ultrasonography to image the neonatal brain through the anterior fontanelle. A brief report in The Lancet suggested that two serious neurological problems in premature infants - intraventricular hemorrhage and post hemorrhagic hydrocephalus - could be diagnosed at the bedside using ultrasound. By coincidence he had seen real-time cardiac echo images of a child with a large cardiac intraventricular clot that was responsible for an embolic stroke. Enthused by the Lancet article he convinced the chief cardiac echocardiogram ("echo") technician to bring the echo machine to the NICU. The first child imaged had a large intraventricular clot that was easily seen. This led to an agreement with Harold Osher,

Chief of Cardiology, to begin imaging all at-risk neonates and to allow Walt Allan to interpret the images. This being a new technology, there was no precedent for interpreting such images. When the Department of Radiology learned that the Department of Cardiology was imaging premature infant brains and a neurologist was providing the interpretation its members felt they should provide this service. Harold Osher felt otherwise and the service continued throughout Walt Allan's career. Interestingly, the expertise acquired by Walt Allan's special interest led to several publications and a partnership between Yale, Brown, and MMC in a major NIH randomized controlled trial to study prevention of intraventricular hemorrhage in premature infants.

In 1987 the Park Medical Building was put up for sale. In order to purchase the condominium in the lower half of the building, 5 neurologists including John Boothby, Richard L. Sullivan, Walter Allan, John Kelly Sullivan, and Stephen Rioux, incorporated to form Maine Neurology, PA. As Maine Neurology grew, its catchment area expanded to include the entire state of Maine and parts of eastern New Hampshire. The group established pediatric neurology clinics in Caribou and Ellsworth and adult neurology clinics in Farmington, Sanford, Norway and Bridgton. The practice diversified by adding physicians with special training. In 1997 Neurosurgical Associates and Maine Neurology co-located to 49 Spring Street in Scarborough where both specialties still reside. In 2002 Maine Neurology doubled the size of its building to accommodate new partners and an MRI suite.

By 2010 Maine Neurology was composed of 12 physicians and 2 nurse practitioners. Subspecialties included: pediatric neurology, electrophysiology, EMG, epilepsy, EEG, stroke, ultrasound, MRI, cognitive neurology, multiple sclerosis and sleep medicine. All physicians were Board Certified neurologists with at least 1 subspecialty board. One physician, John Belden, is certified by 6 specialty and subspecialty boards! Maine Neurology provided MRI imaging and interpretation on site. The group was unique in a number of ways:

- It provided MRI imaging and interpretation;
- It's ultrasound laboratory was certified for carotid and trans-cranial ultrasound procedures;
- It was the only certified EEG laboratory in the state;
- It was the sole group covering both inpatient and outpatient services at MMC;
- It provided neuromuscular disease consultation and EMG services;

- It provided neuro-hospitalist services to MMC;
- The group received statewide referrals for emergency and routine cases, accepting all patients regardless of their insurance status (many neurologists in the state were not accepting Medicaid or "self-pay" patients);
- It provided neurologic teaching for MMC residents and Tufts medical students; and
- The group was involved in several clinical studies.

Maine Neurology was at an important juncture in 2010. Changing economic realities required a decision either to continue as a private practice group and decrease inpatient responsibilities at the hospital, or to join forces with MMC. Ultimately it was decided that the missions of the two organizations were aligned. Maine Neurology merged with MMC, becoming Maine Medical Partners Neurology. This partnership has been very beneficial to all parties and for neurologic care in Maine.

In 2017 in addition to providing the MMC Telestroke Service, Maine Medical Partners Neurology employed neurologists and staff in the following subspecialties:

- 5 pediatric neurologists;
- 4 EMG/neuromuscular disease;
- 3 epileptologists who run a 4-bed epilepsy monitoring unit at MMC;
- 2 in movement disorder;
- 3 in multiple sclerosis;
- 4 full time neuro-hospitalists;
- 4 in neuroimaging;
- 2 in stroke;
- 1 in neuro-oncology;
- 1 in neonatal neurology; and
- 8 nurse practitioners.

The Neuroscience Institute at MMC has developed interdisciplinary programs and research in stroke, epilepsy, movement disorders, neuro-oncology and neonatal neurology.

Since the 1960's there has been a dramatic change in the role of the neurologist, from essentially blind clinical observation to informed diagnosis and treatment. When Dr. Ernie Sachs, Chief of Neurosurgery at Dartmouth Hitchcock, saw the first CT images in 1976 he said that neurologists would no longer be needed. Instead, the number in Portland has increased from 2 in 1976 to 22 today. The list of anticonvulsants available for prescription has grown from 3 to more than 20. Neurologists are able to evaluate medically refractory cases with ambulatory EEG, inpatient video EEG monitoring, high resolution 3T MRI, ictal single-photon emission computerized tomography (SPECT) scanning and intraoperative monitoring leading to appropriate surgical treatment. There are now powerful medicines to treat autoimmune diseases including multiple sclerosis (MS), myasthenia gravis, Guillain-Barre Syndrome, and autoimmune encephalitis. Neurologists have new medicines and Deep Brain Stimulation surgery to treat Parkinson's Disease. Treatment options for brain tumors now include chemotherapy as well as surgery and many forms of radiotherapy. Stroke treatment with TPA and clot extraction has improved recovery from stroke. Neuro-intensive care support has saved many patients with status epilepticus, head injury and CNS infection. Sadly, neurologists are still unable to sufficiently help patients with ALS and Alzheimer's disease.

Neurology has always been a very satisfying vocation. We have evolved from symptomatic and emotional support to a high level of diagnosis and treatment, all to the great benefit of our patients. We hope that further advances will help us as patients in our old age.

NEUROSURGERY

By Donald W. Wilson MD and William F. D'Angelo MD

History of the Division of Neurosurgery at MMC up to 1999

By Donald W. Wilson MD

When I (Donald Wilson) came to Maine in the summer of 1973 there were three neurosurgeons on the staff of Maine Medical Center (MMC), Drs. George Maltby, Robinson Bidwell, and Carl Brinkman. It is my understanding that George was primarily a neurologist by training with a year or two fellowships in neurosurgery with Dr. Gilbert Horrax at the Lahey Clinic in Boston. Dr. Horrax was a disciple of the founder of neurosurgery in the United States, Dr. Harvey Cushing, Chief of Surgery at Peter Bent Brigham Hospital in Boston. I believe George was the first neurosurgeon not only at MMC but also in the state of Maine when he began his practice in 1945. I recently found an article co-authored by him and Dr. Wesley English entitled "Diastematomyelia in Adults" (a rare congenital anomaly) published in the Journal of Neurosurgery in September 1967. I assume Wes was a surgical resident on the neurosurgical service assisting George at the time. George retired in 1978.

Dr. Robinson Bidwell (Bid) was the first physician at MMC to complete a full, formal neurosurgical residency as we know it today having trained at Massachusetts General Hospital (MGH) in Boston. He joined Dr. Maltby in private practice in 1952 and practiced "general" neurological surgery. Bid retired in 1982.

Dr. Carl Brinkman completed a residency in neurosurgery at the University of Michigan in Ann Arbor under the direction of Dr. Edgar Kahn, one of the foremost neurosurgeons in the country. Carl's father, Dr. Harry Brinkman, a general surgeon in Farmington, was a contemporary of Dr. Kahn in their residency years at Michigan. While a resident at University of Michigan Carl wrote a chapter on radionuclear imaging of the brain in the "bible" for all young neurosurgeons at the time, "Correlative Neurosurgery" of which Dr. Kahn was one of the authors.

After completion of his residency Carl joined the staff of MMC in 1964 as an associate of Drs. Maltby and Bidwell. Several years later he decided to leave the group and establish a solo practice. He was "on call" all the time and often had 40-50 inpatients at MMC with the assistance of one surgical resident. Needless to say he needed and was seeking help. This is where and when I came in. In April 1972 while in the U.S. Army in Okinawa, Japan as a neurosurgeon I flew home to Boston to attend a meeting of the American Association of Neurological Surgeons. While there I reviewed a listing of neurosurgeons in the country seeking an associate. I found Carl's name and called him on the telephone that evening. He told me that there were two prerequisites for the job: (1) I had to be young; and (2) I had to love Maine. I informed him that after four years of college, four more of medical school, six years of internship and residency and almost a year in the army I was thirty-three years old. And of course I added that I absolutely loved Maine (which was true). Carl then said "Great, when are you coming up".

I completed my residency at Case Western University Hospitals of Cleveland in June 1971 and after two years in the army joined Carl in August 1973. During the first three or so years we operated together trading various surgical techniques we had acquired over the years. I can remember Carl frequently saying to me "this is the way Eddie (Dr. Kahn) taught me how to do this". One day at a national meeting I had the opportunity to meet Dr. Kahn. After I introduced myself, he exclaimed "you mean you are in practice with Carl?" He obviously had great admiration for Carl as did Carl for him. Carl was an excellent technical neurosurgeon and a wonderful mentor for me. We shared "call" every other night and weekend. My first years in practice with Carl were the most arduous in my career - even compared to my residency experience. Carl introduced the transnasal surgical approach for pituitary tumors at MMC usually operating with an ENT surgeon, Dr. Marvin Adams.

Although I basically performed "general" neurosurgery, I did develop a particular interest and expertise in surgery for far lateral herniated lumbar disks. I recall making a presentation on the subject at a meeting of the Maine Neurosurgical Society which one of my favorite mentors in Cleveland, a guest speaker, found quite interesting. I served as Director of the Division of Neurosurgery at MMC from 1988 to 1993, taking over after Carl Brinkman's term. I retired from practice in December 1998.

During my time at MMC technological advances, particularly in radiology, had a revolutionary effect on neurosurgery. In the 1970's Carl and I would spend half of our day in the Radiology Department performing myelograms, pneumoencephalograms, and cerebral arteriograms. The latter were carried out by percutaneous direct "stick" of the carotid artery or the brachial artery at the elbow (retrobrachial arteriogram). Today these procedures seem extremely antiquated and almost barbaric.

We did have radionuclear brain scans in the early years. Dr. Russell Briggs, a radiologist, assisted in their interpretation. However a far better imaging method has been CT scanning which became available at MMC in 1976. Even though early CT images were crude by later standards, the advance in what we could see inside the brain was tremendous compared to prior techniques. With this modality we were able to envision the entire content of the cranial cavity, namely the brain and particularly the posterior fossa in which lesions such as hematomas were previously virtually impossible to diagnose. Brain neoplasms became much easier to delineate. This made surgical planning more accurate, including the choice of location for the craniotomy.

Fortunately in the late 1970's, cerebral arteriography as performed by Carl and me earlier in the decade using a direct carotid artery puncture was replaced by cerebral arteriography from a transfemoral approach. This advance in technique was introduced with the hiring of Dr. Reed Altemus, a neuroradiologist trained at MGH who arrived at MMC in 1978. The treatment of intracranial aneurysms required the best possible imaging of the arterial circulation of the brain; this was provided by Reed's excellent skill. Early on Carl and I performed surgery for aneurysms with "our eyeballs", later using magnifying "loops" for better visualization. Eventually neurosurgeons in our group introduced the surgical microscope for superior visualization. For many years, particularly before the year 2000, we neurosurgeons applied a titanium clip to its neck to exclude an aneurysm from the parent artery and prevent rerupture after having exposed it via a craniotomy. In a discussion with Jim Wilson I recently learned that now the majority of aneurysms are treated by one of the endovascular neurosurgeons with "coiling" via transfemoral catherization, quite an innovation and a less invasive procedure.

MRI scanning became available in Portland in 1987, first in the basement of our office building on Congress Street and by 1990 at MMC. In addition to providing even more delineated images of the brain it gave the neurosurgeon the more likely nature of a tumor e.g. a benign neoplasm such as a meningioma or a malignant one such as a glioblastoma. MRI angiography (MRA) was a later refinement of MRI which at times has eliminated the need for conventional arteriography which is an invasive procedure. MRI has probably had an even greater impact on the localization and diagnosis of spinal lesions. Myelography has for the most part become a second line diagnostic test used to clarify the few confusing cases not fully diagnosed by MRI. Today a neurosurgeon can sit in his office and on his viewing screen can see and point out to his patient abnormalities such as herniated intervertebral disks, spinal stenosis, or neoplasms without the need for the invasive procedure requiring lumbar puncture.

During my tenure at MMC significant advances were made in the treatment of head trauma - particularly for increased intracranial pressure (ICP) caused by swelling of the injured brain. In the 1980's we began to monitor ICP with the "Richmond Bolt", a metal cylinder placed on the surface of the brain through a small hole drilled in the skull. We put patients into a barbiturate coma along with hyperventilation to reduce the pressure. Later the "Bolt" method was replaced by placement of a catheter in a lateral ventricle to drain cerebrospinal fluid if necessary to lower pressure. I can well remember treating patients with this approach who had wonderful survivals and who I am quite sure would have succumbed previously.

Later additions to the Neurosurgery Division at MMC included Dr. Stephen Klein who joined the MMC staff in 1974 after completing his residency at Emory University and a fellowship in England. Steve had a solo practice and retired around 2005. Dr. Ed Katz joined Drs. Maltby and Bidwell sometime in the 1970's but moved out of Portland a few years later. Dr. Bruce Harris joined Carl and me in 1974 but left in 1977 to work with a neurosurgeon at the Mary Imogene Bassett Hospital in Cooperstown, New York.

Dr. Thomas Mehalic became a member of our group in 1978. He completed his neurosurgery residency at the University of Michigan, spent two years in the air force in Germany and practiced in Pittsburgh a few years before coming to Portland. Tom performed primarily "general" neurosurgery, though later in his career primarily did spine surgery. He served as Director of the Division beginning in 1993, retiring in the early 2000's.

Tom was followed by Dr. William D'Angelo, another graduate of the neurosurgery residency program at Michigan arriving in Portland in 1984. He developed particular expertise in treating patients with trigeminal neuralgia with percutaneous radiofrequency neurolysis for some and microvascular decompression of the trigeminal nerve via posterior fossa craniectomy for others. He is currently functioning as a neurosurgical hospitalist at MMC.

Dr. Lee Thibodeau, a Maine native, became a member of our group in 1988 having finished his neurosurgery residency at Yale. He brought to MMC expertise in the surgical treatment of seizure disorders refractory to control by medication. He was also the first neurosurgeon at MMC to perform spine stabilization procedures with metal plates and screws. He eventually left MMC to form a neurosurgical practice specializing in spine at Mercy Hospital.

Dr. Konrad (Max) Barth joined our group in 1994 after completion of his residency at Presbyterian Medical Center (Columbia) in New York City. He brought to MMC further expertise in spine stabilization surgery.

Dr. Joseph Corbett was the first formally trained pediatric neurosurgeon to come to MMC. Joe completed his neurosurgical residency at the University of Wisconsin; though the earlier years of his training were at the University of Michigan (does this sound like a pipeline beginning with Carl Brinkman?). After completion of a fellowship in Texas, he joined the MMC staff in 1990. Several years later he left to join a neurosurgeon in Vermont.

Dr. James Wilson (no relation to me) became a member of our practice group in 1996. He had spent a year with us as a resident in the University of Vermont program and subsequently completed a fellowship in pediatric neurosurgery at the Hospital for Sick Children in Toronto. In addition to pediatric neurosurgery Jim has been engaged in adult neurosurgery - in particular spinal stabilization procedures.

Sometime after my retirement in 1998 the members of our group became employed by MMC. Since then the practice has expanded to ten neurosurgeons. There have been a number of additions to the expertise offered by neurosurgeons since then but that is another story.

As one can see there were a number of advances made in the 20th century in neurosurgery at MMC. I know that since the year 2000 progress has continued, all of which is of benefit to the people of Maine.

Neurosurgery at MMC from the Late 1990's to the Present

By William F. D'Angelo MD

Taking up the story of the Neurosurgery Division at MMC from where Don Wilson left off, roughly coincident with his retirement in 1998, there has been continued growth in the practice not only in numbers of surgeons but also in the degree of sub specialization. At present, in 2017, there are ten neurosurgeons, covering nearly every aspect of neurosurgical care with the exception of brachial plexus/peripheral nerve surgery. There is a spine deformity program headed by Joe Alexander and a scoliosis program headed by Jim Wilson who also still does the group's pediatric neurosurgery. Phil Anson and Mike Binnette have joined the practice as orthopedic surgeons further adding strength and diversity to the spine program. There are two endovascular neurosurgeons, Rob Ecker and Matt Sanborn who run a robust neurointerventional/ stroke program. Anand Rughani has expertise in movement disorder surgery primarily for Parkinson's disease and is resurrecting Lee Thibodeau's epilepsy surgery program.

Jeff Florman and Anand Rughani do most of the adult brain tumor work. Max Barth and Raj Desai perform the bulk of the complicated multilevel spinal fusions. More recently the practice has developed the position of neurosurgical "hospitalist' to handle all of the neurosurgical emergencies and consults between 6 am and 4 pm daily. This position has been filled by Dr. William D'Angelo since 2014 and became a job-share between Dr. D'Angelo and Dr. Elbert White from Tennessee when he arrived in September 2017.

In August of 2006 after considerable deliberation our neurosurgical practice group, which comprised the entire Division of Neurosurgery at MMC, decided to merge with MMC Practice Partners. This decision largely related to the huge ongoing effort by MMC and its physicians to develop the neurosciences as one of the hospital's key "Centers of Excellence". All involved believe that this has been a success to date. Neurosciences currently constitute the largest clinical line of business at the institution. The neurosurgeons are clearly contributing significantly to this success with their clinical skills and expertise and MMC is seen as an exemplary partner in this large endeavor.

The history of the neuroendovascular program at MMC is of particular interest given how much growth has occurred in this subspecialty in the past decade. Before the arrival of radiologist Eddie Kwan in 1998 endovascular treatment of cerebral aneurysms and vascular malformations required transfer of patients to Boston. Working together with the neurosurgeons Dr. Kwan established a neurointerventional program in Radiology at MMC that at its peak included treatment of about 50 – 60 intracranial cases per year as well as a limited number of extracranial carotid stenting cases. Unfortunately the program was suspended in 2008 when Dr. Kwan left MMC. In 2010 with the arrival of radiologist Chris Baker and neurosurgeon Rob Ecker, the program was reinstituted, and has grown rapidly since that time. In 2015, neurosurgeon Matt Sanborn was added to the team. Currently the number of intracranial aneurysms being treated with endovascular techniques is up to 130 annually. Acute stroke interventions with intracranial thrombectomy have evolved quickly over the past few years to be a viable rescue procedure for many acute stroke patients. The annual volume of these emergency stroke procedures is now over 100 per year and growing. MMC's neuroendovascular program has developed into one of the largest in New England and now includes coiling and stent/coiling for intracranial aneurysms, carotid stenting, acute intracranial thrombectomy, flow diversion for aneurysm, and embolization treatment for vascular malformations, brain tumors, epistaxis and peripheral vascular malformations. Also included in the program are intracranial venous sinus stenting for pseudotumor cerebri and glycerol rhizotomy for trigeminal neuralgia.

Neurosurgery

The neuroendovascular program has also been a key participant in major studies related to the effectiveness of endovascular treatment of cerebrovascular diseases. MMC was the largest New England enrolling site for the SWIFT Prime Study which proved the clinical value of acute thrombectomy after IV tPA treatment of acute stroke. The program has the largest published series ever of revascularization of acute vertebral artery occlusion prior to basilar artery thrombectomy. There is ongoing involvement in multiple national studies: CRESTII, NANO, and STRATIS.

Final Editor's Comments:

Neurosurgery at MMC has grown from a 2 – 3 man "general" practice in the 1950's and 60's to what is currently a ten-physician subspecialty-based practice in 2017. The skills of the physicians involved are remarkable and comparable to the best programs in the country. The division is an integral part of MMC's Neurosciences Center of Excellence, the institution's largest clinical line of business. There is a strong sense of purpose and optimism in the program. There is excitement for what will come in the future, despite the obvious challenges that everyone involved in the practice of medicine is facing. The status of the division is best summed up by a quote from Dr. Bill D'Angelo, a member of the group who is nearing his retirement: "I know it sounds strange, but if I could extend my professional and personal life by 10-20 years, I would do so in a heartbeat. These continue to be exciting and evolving times for neurosurgery here at MMC."

OBSTETRICS AND GYNECOLOGY

By Hector M. Tarraza MD

Caring For Women ---The Maine Medical Center Way

"I was terrified when I went into labor. But my doctor and nurse calmed me down and took great care of me. I will never forget them"
Grateful New Mother

For the first three quarters of the twentieth century, the Department of Obstetrics and Gynecology (Ob/Gyn) at Maine Medical Center (MMC) could have been best described as a vibrant service in a community hospital. The Ob/Gyn physicians in the community were all in private practice. Each had been trained in an out of state residency programs. Many came from either the Boston programs or the University of Michigan. Doctors Warren Baldwin and Stanley Kent were Boston trained physicians who set up private practices in the 1950's near Maine Medical Center. Other private physicians who formed small group practices in Portland in the early days included Doctors Buell Miller, Ken Doil, Harry Bennert, Don McCrann, and Joseph "Skip" Wilkis.

To be able to attract Ob/Gyn clinicians, Maine Medical Center (MMC) needed to develop its own training program. Under the leadership of Dr. Irving Meeker, and working with the community Ob/Gyn's, MMC inaugurated an Ob/Gyn Residency Program in 1975. The first resident to enroll was Doctor David Ernst. The program consisted of a four year program for two residents per year. Doctor Carol Ward became the first female resident. The strength of the program was the dedication of the community physicians whom were all in private practice. Training was carried out by an all-volunteer faculty. During his tenure as Chief of Ob/Gyn at MMC, Dr. Meeker also served as Treasurer for the American College of Obstetrics and Gynecology.

In 1970 the American Board of Obstetrics and Gynecology created three subspecialty areas: gynecologic oncology, maternal fetal medicine, and reproductive endocrinology and infertility. The first Ob/Gyn subspecialist to settle in the Portland area was Doctor Charles Boyce. Doctor Boyce had been practicing at Wayne State University as a gynecologic oncologist. He was one of the 20 original gynecologic oncologists in the United States who founded the Society of Gynecologic Oncology in 1970. In 1986 he succeeded Doctor Irving Meeker as the Chairman of the Department of Ob/Gyn. As a leader Doctor Boyce was charged with recruiting subspecialists for the Department.

The first one was Doctor Hector Tarraza, a Harvard educated gynecologic oncologist who came to Portland 1987. He also recruited Doctor Michael Pinette in 1988, a perinatologist who had grown up in Cape Elizabeth, ME.

As Maine Medical Center began hiring more subspecialists in Ob/Gyn and other disciplines, it needed to create a physician entity to support those practices. The establishment of the Medical Services Organization (MSO) was the predecessor to Maine Medical Partners (MMP). Working as full time employed physicians, the Ob/Gyn subspecialists began to offer their services across the region. The Ob/Gyn subspecialists built a large referral practice. Patients came from throughout Maine as well as from eastern New Hampshire.

With the retirement of Doctor Boyce, Doctor Philip Stubblefield from Boston, MA was recruited to become Department Chair. Doctor Stubblefield was an Ob/Gyn generalist who continued to recruit subspecialists, hire full time academic generalists and develop a clinical research program. The structure of the Department allowed the subspecialists to strengthen its tertiary care role across the state as the residents and academic generalists provided care for the indigent population, and the private community Ob/Gyn's cared for community patients.

Maine Medical Center operated a small indigent clinic on its Bramhall campus for the Ob/Gyn residents. This clinic continued to grow and expand services. It became the MMC Women's Health Center which also serves the large immigrant population in greater Portland. Immigrants from over 40 countries who speak countless number of languages and dialects receive care by Ob/Gyn residents in their continuity clinics. Full time attending physicians supervise all residents and Advance Practice Clinicians (APC) at the MMC Women's Health Center.

The Ob/Gyn full time faculty continued to grow. The residency program also expanded. Initially the program had two residents per year. With the increase in scholarship activity and volume it expanded to three per year and eventually to four per year where it currently stands as of 2017.

Doctor Stubblefield appointed Doctor Daniel Spratt, a reproductive endocrinologist as the Department's Director of Clinical Research. His responsibilities included mentoring residents and attendings to produce high quality research that lead to numerous peer reviewed articles in reputable journals. Clinical research became the other major cornerstone of the Department. Department members such as Doctor Joseph Wax (perinatologist) contributed many articles in premier peer reviewed journals. Doctor Christopher Darus developed a robust gynecology oncology clinical trials program. Patients are now being enrolled in NCI Sponsored national cooperative trials. Doctor

Kalli Varaklis, a medical education expert, brought added knowledge to the medical education literature.

In 1995 Doctor Stubblefield returned to Boston to Chair the Department of Ob/Gyn at Boston University. Doctor Hector Tarraza was appointed as interim – soon to become permanent Chairman - in 1997. During his tenure he hired four Ob/Gyn Residency Program Directors, Doctor Allan Alexander, Doctor Donald "Chip" Wiper, Doctor Kalli Varaklis, and recently Doctor Jason Lachance.

After five years as Residency Program Director, Doctor Alexander retired. Doctor Donald (Chip) Wiper served for five years before taking on the positon as Professor and Chair of the Ob/Gyn Department at Greenville Health System, South Carolina. Doctor Kalli Varaklis completed her Ob/Gyn residency at MMC. After spending several years at Boston University, she returned to MMC and became the first Ob/Gyn resident to serve as Residency Program Director for ten years.

Dr. Kalli Varaklis was recently promoted to serve as the Designated Institutional Officer (DIO) for MMC. In this capacity she oversees all graduate medical education in the Hospital.

These four program directors continue the tradition of academic excellence. Many of the residents conducted outstanding research culminating in the work of Doctor Michael Cerkzes winning the Ob/Gyn Richardson Prize for Most Outstanding Research work by an Ob/Gyn Resident in the United States.

With all of the scholarly activity occurring, over 50% of the residents graduating pursue academic careers and sought highly competitive subspecialty training. It was not uncommon to see a graduating Ob/Gyn resident heading off to Memorial Sloan Kettering Cancer Center, Harvard Massachusetts General Hospital or the Mayo Clinic to enter full time academia.

One of the faculty members became nationally recognized for her cutting edge holistic approach to Women' Health issues. Doctor Christine Northrup published numerous bestsellers and appeared on national talk shows. Her work became an important contribution to how we approach our female patients.

"She had nothing. She was a refugee from Rwanda, single mother to a newborn and were homeless. The nurses, residents and doctors all pitched in to get her a bassinet, diapers, clothes for her baby so that she would have something at the shelter. It was truly an act of compassion by all."

MMC Family Birth Center Nurse

One of the biggest challenges facing the Department of Ob/Gyn in the 1990's was the facility in which it practiced. Despite state of the art medical care being provided by the doctors, nurses and staff, the physical plant was clearly behind the times. Gynecology oncology patients did not have an adequate inpatient facility for them to be cared for. Obstetrical patents were being housed in semi-private rooms with hall bathrooms. High risk obstetrical patients were rooming in triplet rooms with lack of privacy. Gynecologic surgery was not being performed on an outpatient basis because of a lack of facilities.

To meet the needs of expanding services and improved facilities, the hospital embarked on two major capital projects that would greatly impact the Department. The first entitled "Building on a Promise" lead to the construction of the Gibson Pavilion and the Barbara Bush Children's Hospital. The Gibson Pavilion was a modern 43 bed unit built to house the inpatient oncology services. It was here where gyn oncology patients would now be cared for by a dedicated team of professionals. It was the first time that a medical oncology unit would care for gynecologic oncology post-operative patients.

The second major capital project was the "Building on Excellence". A $75,000,000 investment, the premiere cornerstones were the Women and Infants East Tower and the Outpatient Scarborough Surgical Center both of which opened in 2008. The Women and Infants East Tower would house the MMC Family Birth Center. It contained modern private rooms, private bathrooms, with tubs and jacuzzis for the laboring patients and a home like private setting for post-partum patients and their families.

The design of the East Tower was guided by the clinicians, nurses and staff along with patient advocates who were familiar with the requirements for a modern obstetrical facility. It was the first facility built at MMC that was truly patient centered.

The Outpatient Scarborough Surgical Center was built to meet the growing needs of ambulatory surgery at MMC. Gynecologists were the first surgeons to use laparoscopy (minimally invasive surgery) on a large scale. Procedures that had routinely required a 2-3 day hospital stay were now being performed on an outpatient basis. Women were having hysterectomies and going home on the same day. Approximately 65% of gynecologic surgery has shifted from inpatient to outpatient. The new Scarborough Surgical Center provided an excellent facility for patients and staff.

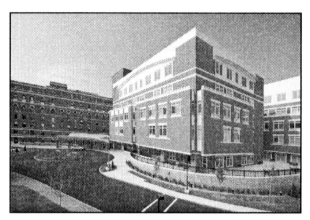

East Tower at MMC – Home to Family Birth Center

"The mother was a high risk patient whose placenta had eroded throughout her pelvis. Four hours of surgery, 20 units of blood transfusion and in the intensive care unit for two days, she did well and went home with her baby on post-operative day number 5. In most institutions in this world, she would have died."

John Pulvino MD, Vice Chairman
of the Department of Ob/Gyn

But bricks and mortar were not the only progress during this time. The Ob/Gyn program had dedicated itself to not only growth, but also to excellence. It developed a state and regional reputation to the point where US News and World Report ranked gynecology at MMC one of the top 50 hospitals in the US (gynecology ranked #41 which is the highest ranking of any department at MMC on any US News and World Report Rankings ever). Many other accolades followed.

New areas of expertise were added. A Division of Female Pelvic Medicine and Reconstructive Surgery (formally Urogynecology) was created and headed by Doctor Mary Brandes. The Reproductive Endocrine and Infertility Division developed a relationship with Boston IVF offering high tech solutions to infertile couples in Maine. Robotic surgery was introduced in gynecologic oncology as well as gynecological surgery.

Community Ob/Gyns came together to form larger private entities. The two largest groups were Generations/Intermed and Coastal Women's Healthcare. All of these physicians remain committed to provide excellent patient care while dedicated to teaching residents and medical students.

By the year 2016, over 2800 deliveries were occurring at the MMC Family Birth Center. More than one in every five infants born in the State of Maine was delivered by MMC staff. A baby was being born within the walls of MMC every 3 ½ hours, 24 hours a day, 7 days a week. Over 12% of all surgeries performed at MMC were Ob/Gyn cases. Ob/Gyn was the fourth busiest service of all of MMC surgical services. 58% of all robotic surgeries at MMC were from the Ob/Gyn Department. The Department of Ob/Gyn received a 5 star rating in maternity care from Leapfrog.

> *"I was told I had Stage IV Ovarian Cancer and there was no hope. The Gyn Oncology Team took great care of me. It has been almost 20 years since and I am grateful."*

> Susan St. Mary MD – Pediatric Nephrologist and Patient

A major initiative in the Department over the past two years has been reducing our surgical site infections (SSI) rates for hysterectomy and C-sections. Using an evidenced based multidisciplinary approach, the Department developed a robust bundle – the pathway to standardize how we care for patients from prehospitalization, to admission, operating room, postoperative care and discharge. Imagine everyone caring for patients with no variation in the approach. SSI bundles led to the Department's achievement of an SSI rate that is currently less than 1%.

As the Department looks toward the future, Maine Medical Center has renewed its commitment through the creation of the Women's Health Service Line. MMC's service lines are committed to three major goals – improving the health of the patient, improving the patient experience navigating the health care system, and optimizing the conditions for doctors, nurses and staff to succeed. The future will see new technologies, new medicines and a focus on preventative health to improve the lives of women. The Department of Ob/Gyn at MMC will be at the forefront of this new era.

> *"I always remind our community and our state that the doctors, nurses and staff at MMC are honored and privileged to care for our patients and families with quality, kindness and compassion…that is the MMC Way!"*

Ophthalmology

By William S. Holt MD

A Free-standing Ophthalmic Surgery Center: Eyecare Medical Group

Personal training and hints of future technology

I graduated from Harvard Medical School in 1967. Vietnam duty slowed things down for me but after discharge I trained in Boston from 1970-75 at the Massachusetts Eye and Ear Infirmary (MEEI). At nearby institutions technologic advances were taking place which would later be incorporated into ophthalmology practice. At MIT in Cambridge prototypes of the first computers were being born. A new type of light energy, "light amplification by the stimulated emission of radiation" (LASER) was being set up on lab benches there. And a few intrepid folk were experimenting with ultrasonic energy to radically change how cataract surgery was done

MEEI was, and remains, a highly regarded ophthalmology center where staid Boston ways prevailed. Even so, we residents could sense and imagine that a dramatically different future lay ahead. Casting about for ways and places to launch my career, Portland seemed perfect. It was large enough to support a progressive ophthalmology practice, had a quality hospital, and offered ready access to the sea and outdoor activities. At New England Ophthalmology Society (NEOS) meetings in Boston I had met and become friends with Dr. Elizabeth Serrage, then practicing ophthalmology in South Portland. She encouraged me to come to Portland. Noticing that there was a need for retinal surgery and laser treatments, I first took a fellowship in retina and then in 1975 returned to my home state of Maine, opening a solo practice on Congress Street in Portland, sharing space kindly made available by Paul Maier MD.

Ophthalmology practices in the 1970's

In 1975 most ophthalmology practices in Portland were office-based, solo affairs. Cataract and all other surgeries were performed on inpatients at Maine Medical Center (MMC) in a single operating room (OR) on the third floor, "P-3". Cataract surgeries were only beginning to be performed with a floor-mounted microscope, the first one in Maine having been introduced by Dr. Maurice van Lonkhuyzen. Cataracts were extracted intact with a cryoprobe through a large incision that was closed with multiple 7-0 silk or nylon sutures. Patients usually stayed in the hospital for three days. Not

155

for long. I knew from training and meetings that cataract surgery was on the cusp of revolutionary changes, including smaller incisions and potentially a device that ultrasonically fragmented cataracts.

Clinically useful argon lasers were developed in the early 1970's and were beginning to be used to treat diabetic retinopathy and to seal around retinal tears. MMC purchased one in 1976 for the eye clinic. I set up the needed diagnostic angiography equipment in my office. Retinal detachments had hitherto been referred to Boston, but because I had spent a fellowship year learning detachment procedures, I decided to offer this surgery in Maine. Detachment surgery is almost always an urgently needed, unscheduled procedure. As referrals developed, our need for detachment surgical times began to be disruptive to MMC's OR schedule. With success in new laser treatments and methods for detachment repair, demand in Portland grew. A full-time retina surgeon, Fred Miller, joined the Portland practice of Drs. Goduti and Frank Read. At that point I shifted away from retina to more emphasis on cataract surgery.

The need for an outpatient eye surgery facility

In 1977 Dr. Serrage and I joined forces and moved into the Park Medical Building on Park Avenue in Portland. Advances were coming in cataract patient treatment that reduced the need for inpatient post-surgery care. One change was the use of soft contact lenses after cataract surgery, replacing unwieldy, thick cataract glasses. The soft lenses improved vision quality however they were difficult for elderly patients to manage.

Another major advance was the introduction of intra-ocular lenses (IOL's), implanted within the eye at the time of surgery. We sought training in Canada and elsewhere. When the first models were approved for use in the U.S., we introduced them into our practice. These early IOL's were technically very challenging to implant using existing techniques. Elsewhere pioneering surgeons were updating older techniques that shelled out the nucleus of a cataract while leaving its capsular membrane intact. Placement of the implant into this 'capsular bag' proved safe. Visual rehabilitation was immediate after the surgery. I did the first 'extracapsular' implant surgery at MMC in 1983. At first we were subject to much criticism by our colleagues. But continuing refinements in technique and success began to lead to increasing patient acceptance and practice growth for us and for other local ophthalmologists. At the same time these better techniques, improved implant designs, and local anesthesia techniques enabled same-day, outpatient cataract surgery. Patients no longer needed to stay overnight, but just a few hours in the hospital ambulatory care unit. With these improvements increased demand followed, and the scheduling capacity of the single eye OR at MMC was exceeded.

Maine Medical Center needed to expand. Application was made for new operating rooms but in an effort to restrain health care costs, the Maine Hospital Cost Containment Commission denied MMC's requests. Dr. Serrage and I approached Mercy Hospital. They did have available surgical time and were willing and able to purchase the necessary equipment. It was challenging to create a fully equipped eye operating room de novo, but we did, and in the process learned a great deal that proved useful later.

Nationally a few intrepid surgeons took advantage of the development of outpatient cataract surgery. They moved out of the hospitals, establishing free-standing surgical centers. They met great resistance from the ophthalmology establishment, regulatory agencies, and hospitals. Dr. Serrage and I visited a few of these pioneering practices, notably a very innovative one built by David McIntyre MD in Belleview, WA, and later, the more established Williamson surgery facility in Baton Rouge, LA. We later used these facilities as models.

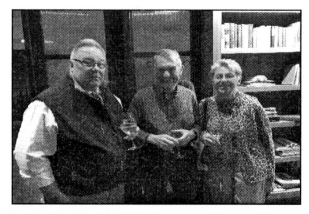

Drs. Cassidy, Holt and Serrage

We began to imagine creating a freestanding eye clinic and surgical center in Portland. Such centers were proving safe, efficient, enabling patient volume and satisfaction, with greatly reduced costs to the system. For example, Medicare paid hospitals about $1350 facility fee for cataract surgery compared with $600 for an outpatient center. We could perform only one cataract surgery per hour at the hospital because of slow room turnover, compared to three per hour in a center with two efficient OR's.

Bruce Cassidy MD whose practice was also expanding, supported the vision of a center. With three ophthalmologists practicing together, we would have sufficient volume to make a new facility viable. With their support and encouragement, I found the nerve to approach Maine Savings Bank with the pronouncement: "Outpatient eye surgery centers are the way of the future. Loan us $3 million, and we will build one." Astonishingly, they agreed! **We were off!** This was 1985/6.

Steps to an ASU

Many challenges followed. In retrospect, it's surprising how much we did in a short time. We had no support - indeed we had resistance - from regulatory authorities, the medical center, and our colleagues. We merged our three practices into the Eye Care and Surgery Center of Maine, LLC ('Eyecare'). Realizing that we required professional practice management we hired a practice manager, Arlene Clifford. She created the needed organizational structure and oversaw the design and construction process. Arlene, as first administrator and each of the CEO's who followed - Donald Cushing, John Wipfler, and currently Clement Berry - have been just right for each different stage of our development. Searching nationwide, we engaged Paul Katz of Minnesota, one of very few architects familiar with eye surgical center requirements. He had been the designer of the Baton Rouge ophthalmology center we used as a model. Paul chose our present location on Sewall St.

Key to our progress was joining the Outpatient Ophthalmic Surgery Society (OOSS), a fledgling national collaboration of surgeons committed to launching such centers. OOSS members learned from each other, facing off against the hospitals, the American Academy of Ophthalmology, and state regulators. It was OOSS's attorney, Michael Romansky, who discovered a loophole in Maine regulations that enabled us to obtain a Certificate of Need from the state. We also benefitted by the support and example of Dr. Jean Labelle at Plastic and Hand Associates who built the first, and at that time the only, surgical center in Maine. Anesthesia management required brief acting agents that induced short-lived relaxation but retained patient ability to obey commands and wore off quickly. We contracted with MMC to accept any complications. Our first anesthetist, Dr. Teddy Eow, led us in meeting these requirements. In our first 10,000 surgeries only one patient had to be referred to MMC, and he was released after a few hours.

Architectural design of ophthalmic surgical centers was necessarily a very innovative process - there were very few to copy. Paul Katz's bold vision was of a first-class practice and surgical facility worthy of being emulated nationally. Construction of the 20,000 square foot facility took more than a year. We moved our practices in and did our first surgeries in October 1987. The surgery section had its own waiting area, two operating rooms and a recovery area. The clinic section contained four separate suites of six exam rooms each, all surrounding a spacious and gracious reception and waiting room. For retinal problems we had an argon and krypton laser center with complete fluorescein angiography capability.

It took several years for the finances to work out. Startup costs, high interest rates in the mid-80's, reduction of Medicare payment rates, and low initial patient volume meant that we did not 'break-even' for several years. Stress from finances and trying to integrate three different solo practices into a cohesive team led us to begin regular planning retreats. A group counselor, Joe Melnick, PhD, facilitated them. These retreats provided focus, averted many potential threats, and may fairly be credited with our success then and later as the group added new surgeons, functions, and equipment.

Growth of the center

Patient acceptance was immediately strong after we opened in 1987. It has never abated. Retina as a sub-specialty has come of age since the 1990's, with vitrectomy, intraocular gases, and sophisticated diagnostic technology. Fortunately, architect Katz had planned for growth. We reconfigured the building and added our first full-time retina person. There are now three retinal specialists at EMG: Dr. Scott Steidl has been joined by Dr. Jackie Nguyen and Dr. Aaron Parme. Similarly, glaucoma as a subspecialty has developed with Ralph Sanchez MD joining us in the mid-'90's, and, at his departure, Drs. Sam Solish and Robert Daly joining and expanding this practice.

A new era in vision correction began in 1995 with federal approval of excimer laser corneal surgery. We joined ASCRS (the American Society for Corneal Refractive Surgery), a newly formed advocacy organization whose publications and meetings have led us, and ophthalmology, through amazing developments that yielded LASIK, a completely new sub-specialty which has made freedom from glasses and contact lenses possible for a great many patients We were among Maine's earliest adopters, with Drs. Serrage, Cassidy, and myself leading the way. We invested heavily in the very expensive delivery systems which required still more space revision. Jordan Sterrer MD, joined to help meet increasing demands for general ophthalmology, LASIK, and cataract care.

Along with LASIK, revolutionary advances in corneal transplants and diagnostics led us to seek a corneal sub-specialist who could keep the group at the forefront of these techniques. Initially Ravi Shah MD and currently Adam Sise MD offer state of the art techniques and enjoy state-wide referrals.

Even as these new techniques and disciplines have been added to ophthalmology and to our group, the mainstay of our group has remained cataract and implant surgery. Continuously evolving, cataract surgery techniques using ultrasonic phacoemulsification, better implant designs and optical accuracy, have dramatically improved patient outcomes. It is fair to say that today's cataract/implant surgery is universally acclaimed as a miracle for quality of life for the elderly.

The Present

With so much added complexity, a few years ago we changed our name to Eyecare Medical Group (EMG) and adopted the motto: "Tomorrow's Eyecare Today". The facility has been greatly expanded in the past two years. EMG now boasts four operating rooms with pre- and post-op areas, with more than 4000 procedures performed annually. An important key to our success has been our insistence on keeping our focus on attending to, and caring for, the patient in the face of computerization of the office, electronic patient records, and ever more constraining government and insurance regulation.

One need only visit EMG today to witness the extraordinary success of our 1987 vision that "Outpatient eye care and surgery is the way of the future". Eight surgeons are supported by over 75 staff members. The annual budget is over $25 million. The Medicare facility payment rate for ASU's like ours remains at about half that required for hospital-based cataract surgery. Our facility has saved the system more than $10 M in this regard alone. EMG has an enviable reputation as one the finest in the country.

As chronicled in this book, during these same years other medical specialty practices in Portland have moved out of the hospital setting as we did, impelled by a vision of reduced patient costs, increased efficiencies, and modern delivery systems. We believe, and research has shown, that centers like ours have brought innovations that have improved patient care delivery and patient satisfaction while providing significant cost savings.

ORTHOPAEDIC SURGERY

By Douglas W. Brown MD

History of Orthopaedic Associates of Portland 1981 - 2010

The idea of creating a multi sub-specialty orthopaedic practice emerged in 1980 from discussions between Don Booth and Chip Crothers, two established Portland orthopaedists, and Doug Brown who was a newly arrived orthopaedist fresh from military service. Booth and Crothers had previously built a successful orthopaedic partnership in Portland. They weren't looking for another partner nor to find a new practice location but they both had orthopaedic sub-specialty interests and training. Both had also done their orthopaedic surgery training at Tufts in Boston. After finishing residency, Booth completed a hand fellowship in Philadelphia and Crothers was a Harris Fellow in hip surgery at Mass General.

Sharing space in the same office building on Park Avenue adjacent to the city's only rheumatologists, Booth and Crothers developed a close working relationship with their rheumatology colleagues and co-sponsored a well-attended weekly teaching conference.

By the time Doug Brown arrived in 1980 with fellowship training and two years of practice experience in the new sub-specialty of sports medicine both Crothers and Booth had well established practices centering around total knee and hip replacements and arthritic hand reconstruction.

More than anything it was their non-competing interests in sub-specialty orthopaedics and their affinity for incorporating academic orthopaedics into the private practice setting that brought Booth, Crothers, and Brown together into a cross-covering arrangement on nights and weekends.

Brown had trained in orthopaedic surgery at the University of Vermont but had fellowship training in Sports Medicine at the Sports Medicine Clinic in Atlanta. Beyond that he had done post doctorate research in biomechanics at UVM and had served for two years as an orthopaedic specialist and team physician at the US Naval Academy in Annapolis, considered then to be one of the premier training positions in sports medicine.

During their first year of working collaboratively, but from different offices, it became increasing evident that all of them had a major need for help with managing the high volume of orthopaedic trauma that came with regular orthopaedic call in Portland.

The demands of managing trauma patients limited everyone's ability to simultaneously maintain and develop a strong commitment to their individual sub-specialty patients and practices.

The answer was to find and recruit an orthopaedic trauma specialist, someone who was fellowship-trained in that new specialty. There was one obvious candidate - Ray White, also a UVM orthopaedic surgery residency graduate and a recent colleague of Brown's. Following residency Ray had journeyed to the University of Mississippi in Jackson to become a junior faculty member in the group headed by Jim Hughes, one of the nation's leaders in the new specialty of orthopaedic trauma surgery. As luck would have it, when they contacted Ray, he indicated he was ready to move away from academic practice to private practice, and from Mississippi to somewhere more desirable – and proximity to skiing was a big factor.

Ray came for an interview and to see Portland in person. Since Burlington, VT - where White had spent 4 years during internship and residency - was very similar to Portland in size and resources, including an excellent teaching hospital, it didn't take long for him to become excited about the move. The only odd thing was that he insisted he wanted to live near a lake rather than the ocean because of his love of water-skiing.

With a house on Highland Lake in his sights, White moved to Portland with his wife Brenda, an excellent pediatrician, and their children in the summer of 1981. His presence ushered in a dramatic change in the standard of orthopaedic trauma care – not only in Portland but throughout the state of Maine. Patients no longer had to routinely endure months of hospitalization, often in traction, for long bone fractures. Instead, applying recently developed techniques of internal fixation, White was able to routinely give patients shorter hospital stays, quicker return to function with fewer complications. He quickly became the "go-to" person for orthopaedic trauma throughout the state. Generously sharing his knowledge and techniques with colleagues, other orthopaedic surgeons were soon able to imitate White's successes.

Coincident with White's arrival, a new practice group was born – "Orthopaedic Associates of Portland." Booth, Brown, Crothers, and White designed a new state-of the-art practice facility occupying the entire top floor of what used to be a shoe factory at 15 Lowell Street. That building had just been converted into first-class space for multiple medical office condominiums. "OA" as the practice was referred to in the community, took the largest space on the 4th floor, sharing the rest of that floor with the first private practice physical therapy practice in Maine.

The idea of combining first-class outpatient physical therapy with orthopaedic surgery practices was a very new concept around the country but one that Brown was familiar with from his experience during his fellowship in Atlanta at the Sports Medicine Clinic, and from the Naval Academy in Annapolis. The integration of supervised physical therapy into the post-op treatment of knee and hip replacement patients at that time was the norm in the hospital setting but routinely continuing it in the out-patient setting was much more novel.

The new private practice PT group "next door" made those transitions simple. The quality and reliability of the recovery of these arthroplasty patients was immediately improved. Soon many orthopaedic surgeons outside the OA group were taking advantage of the private PT group's expertise. The two innovative owners of the PT practice, Brett Eberle, and Frank Gentile, were terrific in developing and guiding the growth of outpatient PT. They too raised the standards of practice of both orthopaedics and PT throughout the state.

While much of the focus of the integrated orthopaedic-physical therapy approach was directed at post-surgical patients an equally impactful focus was on helping athletes and "weekend warriors" recover from a myriad of soft tissue injuries. Appropriate physical therapy greatly enhanced the pace and quality of recovery of everything from sprained ankles to low back injuries in athletes and workers alike.

OA officially opened its doors at the "shoe factory" in December 1981. Other medical groups including some other orthopaedists, an internist, and a group of ophthalmologists occupied the rest of the space. One orthopaedic surgeon who did not actually join OA but agreed to share office space with the group deserves special mention. Larry Crane had been the "dean" of orthopaedic surgeons in Portland for many years prior to 1981. He was an extraordinary innovator, having brought one of the earliest arthroscopes to Portland from Japan in the mid-1970's.

In the 1960s Dr. Crane had been the first champion of total hip arthroplasty in Maine, having journeyed to England to train with Sir John Charnley. When his interest in arthroscopy developed in the late 70's he began to host a series of annual arthroscopic surgery training courses which attracted all the leading innovators from all over the world. His impact on the orthopaedic community in the US was huge. He was later honored as the President of the Arthroscopy Association of North America. While Dr. Crane felt he was too near the end of his orthopaedic career to join a new group he was welcomed by Booth, Brown, Crothers and White into an informal association with OA, where he remained until he retired about 8 years later.

OA also employed a full-time practice administrator, Debbie Alpern, who proved to be a highly effective executive and ushered them through the initial formation of the group, the move into new facilities at Lowell Street, and the gradual expansion of the group for the next 5 years. 1982 was the first full year of practice at Lowell Street. Very soon, the need for additional orthopaedic subspecialists to round out the group became evident. The following year Phil Anson, a new graduate of the orthopaedic surgery residency at the University of Rochester, expressed his interest in joining the group to help with both trauma and sports medicine. He agreed to do additional fellowship training in orthopaedic trauma surgery in England and Switzerland and returned in the summer of 1984 to officially join the group bringing the number of surgeons to five.

At about that time physician assistants were starting to be utilized in some orthopaedic surgery practices around the country. The concept of physician assistants (PA) began in the military with many of the early ones being former military "corpsmen." High quality PA programs quickly developed at places like Yale and Duke and other leading medical teaching institutions. The OA group sensed the value of PAs. By 1984 the group had hired several to work one-on-one with the orthopaedic surgeons making rounds, assisting at surgery, and in the office. These were highly collaborative and closely supervised relationships. They were also immeasurably valuable to patients and physicians alike, and obviously enhanced the quality and continuity of care. Mike Sheldon from Yale, was the first. He worked closely with Dr. Brown. Chris Hillman soon followed from Duke as did Alan Hull and Claudia Shedd.

OA quickly became a very successful orthopaedic group practice. The elements that most contributed to that success were the specialty training and commitment of the surgeons, the collaborative and cooperative organization of the physicians and staff led by Debbie Alpern, the carefully designed facilities which greatly enhanced the efficiency and quality of the practice processes, and the integration with physical therapy, and physician assistants. Everyone sensed the differences OA brought to Portland - patients most of all.

Extensive discussions ensued about expansion, and after a vacant parcel of land became available on Sewall Street, about a mile from Maine Medical Center, those discussions became much more serious. The group engaged George Therrien Architects to design a building "from the inside out" specifically for the purpose of practicing orthopaedic surgery with both physical therapy and out-patient surgery facilities, as well as room for expansion.

At that time, the OA group felt that there was no reason the group could not successfully expand to mimic the best groups of multiple specialists found at the leading orthopaedic training programs. In fact the group at UVM which Brown and White were very familiar with became the primary model to imitate.

A big issue of concern with building a new practice facility was cost - in an environment where reimbursement was being reduced. To build the kind of facility that the OA physicians envisioned was going to involve millions of dollars. They felt confident they could be successful from the orthopaedic standpoint but they needed to be sure they could afford it.

By 1986 Debbie Alpern felt she needed to reduce her time commitments in order to devote more time to her family so OA turned to a well-respected nurse administrator, Sandra Putnam. She came on board and quickly established herself as an essential component in the planning and administration. Planning with the architects progressed through 1986 at which time OA purchased the land on Sewall Street.

Initially, OA considered building a combined facility with the rheumatologists but it became apparent as the discussions progressed that the groups' needs were quite different. Therefore Rheumatology Associates proceeded with the purchase of a parcel of land on Sewall Street adjacent to that of OA that incorporated a design better suited to their needs.

Late in 1986 the architects had produced a nearly complete set of drawings. But before OA could feel comfortable with the surgery center component of the plans, they brought in a consultant who specialized in the design of out-patient surgery facilities to review them. That meeting generated a great deal of concern because it appeared that the space and requirements for the surgery center had been underestimated and under designed. It became critical to re-think that whole portion of the building or risk owning a facility that was inadequate the moment it was built. After a great deal of soul-searching and further consultation with the Portland architects and others the OA partners decided to put the project on hold for a year to carefully re-evaluate everything.

In September 1987 Linc Avery joined the group as the third sports medicine specialist. He had been actively recruited during the previous year following his residency at Strong Memorial Hospital in Rochester, NY. At the same time Don Endrizzi approached OA about joining the group. Not only was Don an exceptionally well-trained orthopaedic surgeon who had just finished residency at Columbia in New York, but he was also exceptionally well-connected to Portland. His wife was Peggy Pennoyer, daughter of prominent Portland physicians: surgeon Doug Pennoyer and allergist Doris Pennoyer.

Despite lots of discussion to convince Dr. Endrizzi that OA would be a perfect venue for him he decided to join another group. OA had envisioned him as their shoulder expert because his experience at Columbia under renowned shoulder specialist Charles Neer was second to none. Dr. Endrizzi ended up changing his mind in January of 1988 at which time OA gladly welcomed him as surgeon number seven.

At this point, it became obvious that OA needed to re-activate its plans for building a facility on Sewall Street. The original architectural design plans were basically very sound. Changing the surgery center to make it larger and more functional would eliminate most of the previous design concerns. In addition the reimbursement trend began to appear as though everyone could live with it. However, the project needed more land so OA added to the parcel they had already purchased and the decision was made to push forward.

A major problem then developed with PT. Brett Eberle and Frank Gentile would have been perfect to run the new PT center but the political climate in Washington began to change such that any physician-owned PT facility might be subject to prohibitive regulation. Gentile and Eberle were reluctant to take those risks while OA was not prepared to abandon the integrated PT approach that had been so beneficial. The OA physicians decided to risk the possible regulatory backlash from Washington and hired new PT providers.

In August 1988, OA broke ground on the Sewall Street project which was completed by November of the following year. It was a spectacular building of almost 40,000 square feet with beautifully designed work-flow in the patient care areas, a large PT facility, a two-lane lap and therapy pool, extensive "Nautilus" exercise equipment, and two operating rooms designed for arthroscopic surgery as well as the other orthopaedic procedures that were becoming more frequently done in out-patient surgery centers. There were also two x-ray suites and large spaces for future growth, meetings, and staff dining.

The building quickly became referred to as the Taj Mahal, a term which was sometimes tinged with envy by other members of the medical community who by tradition had been practicing in facilities which were far more restricted in size and far less purposely adapted to the functions of a medical practice. While facilities like the Sewall Street became relatively common in the next 20 years, in 1988 OA Centers for Orthopaedics was highly unique. Soon, physicians and administrators from all over the country would come to visit.

Within a few months of moving into the Sewall Street facilities another superbly-trained Columbia orthopaedist, Mike Becker, agreed to join the group. Becker had just finished a respected fellowship in New York with John Insall, one of the giants in knee arthroplasty with a special knee implant design of his own. Also in January 1990 the group welcomed Bill Heinz, a Board Certified internist from Indianapolis who had just completed one of the country's first and most innovative "primary care sports medicine specialist" training programs. Dr. Brown knew the people who trained Bill at Methodist Hospital in Indianapolis who wanted Bill to stay and work with them however he recognized the Portland opportunity as unique. He would be working collaboratively with 3 sports medicine trained orthopaedic surgeons in a brand-new facility which included a true state of the art PT facility.

The new outpatient surgery facility, known internally as the Orthopaedic Surgery Center (OSC), began operations in early 1990. It was a huge success from a patient standpoint and for surgeons and staff as well. Almost everyone welcomed the opportunity to have surgery in a facility designed from the ground up to support the specific surgeries which would be done there, and with staff who were doing the same things day after day, enabling them to be highly expert. Patients and staff both benefitted from the efficiencies and precision of this specialization.

OA physicians recognized from the beginning they would not be comfortable with anything but the highest quality staff and facilities if they were to undertake the responsibility of owning and running an innovative out-patient facility. They wanted absolutely no problems from a risk and quality-control standpoint. That led to joining forces with the large hospital-based anesthesia group then known as APA (Anesthesia Professional Associates). The sub-set of anesthesiologists from that group who agreed to work on a rotating basis at OSC were absolutely the best anesthesiologists in Maine. Very quickly their skill and experience in managing out-patient anesthesia grew as did their satisfaction at working in the OSC environment. Patients were confidently and routinely told that the anesthesiologist who would be giving their anesthesia had very likely provided anesthesia in the hospital for patients having open-heart surgery the day before or the day after.

No discussion of the success and quality of the OSC would be complete without mentioning Linda Ruterbories. Linda was a young but very gifted OR nurse who earned a reputation for leadership and expertise at Mercy hospital prior to coming to work at the OSC. At first she worked as one of the staff OR nurses at OSC but very quickly it became evident she was the person who should be running the entire operation. She made that switch and for the next 25 years guided the facility through multiple expansions, while at the same time earning an advanced degree as a nurse practitioner. She turned the OSC into a highly respected prototype of excellence in outpatient design and operations.

In 1992 OA was fortunate enough to attract another superbly trained orthopaedic surgeon to help Ray White in the orthopaedic trauma area. George Babikian was already a Board Certified general surgeon before he became certified as an orthopaedic surgeon. He was an extremely gifted surgeon and, just as importantly, a very innovative and insightful practice manager. George not only paired beautifully with Ray to expand the orthopaedic trauma portion of our practice but he helped in numerous ways over subsequent years to align and insightfully grow the practice.

In the same year OA recruited John Chance as a hand surgeon to work with Don Booth. John was another Columbia-trained orthopaedist with the added value of a hand fellowship with master hand surgeons Larry Schneider and James Hunter in Philadelphia. With the addition of Babikian and Chance the group achieved expansion to a total of 11 physicians – ten sub-specialty orthopaedic surgeons plus one sub-specialty trained internist.

Tragedy struck the group suddenly in the spring of 1993. Don Booth's son Andrew, a very capable sailor, was tragically killed in a freak accident while sailing solo off St. Thomas in the US Virgin Islands. The boat was found sailing in circles. The entire practice was badly shaken by the news. Dr. Booth took an extended period of time off and everyone rallied to help manage his patients. Later that same year Dr. Crothers suffered a heart attack which led to heart surgery followed by a six-month leave of absence. Dr. Babikian stepped up to take over his hip surgery practice. This set the stage for the future when Dr. Babikian was to become one of Maine's premier hip replacement surgeons himself.

Dr. Booth returned to practice for a short time in late 1994 but found the transition too difficult and decided to retire. That left the hand practice managed by Dr. Chance. Also in that year OA hired Mats Agren, another University of Vermont orthopaedic graduate and a fellowship-trained spine surgeon.

By 1995 the OSC was functioning extremely well with volumes that suggested the need for future expansion. The controlled environment of the surgery facility facilitated completion of an influential study of multi-modal pain management in outpatient ACL (anterior cruciate ligament of the knee) reconstructions which ultimately ended up influencing how ACL patients were managed at many other institutions around the country.

1995 and 1996 saw OA expand by five physicians – and contract by one. Dr. Crothers made the difficult decision to retire early because of health issues, giving up his hip practice in the summer of 1995 to Brian McGrory who arrived in August from the Mayo Clinic having also completed a prestigious fellowship in hip surgery with Bill Harris at

Mass General in Boston, the same mentor that Dr. Crothers had trained under years earlier. Crothers' total hip arthroplasty practice had grown over the previous 15 years to the point where patients came from all over the state for his expertise and experience. He also had been heavily involved with consulting work for some of the major hip implant manufacturers and was well-recognized nationally for his contributions to the study of hip replacement surgery.

In January 1996 Mike Totta, a physiatrist with special interest in interventional injection techniques for managing back and neck pain arrived to complement the work that Mats Agren was doing in the spine area. Also in January of that year John Herzog and Peter Guay decided to merge their private practices into OA. Both were osteopathic orthopaedic physicians who had been practicing together in Portland. With the closure of the Osteopathic Hospital of Maine and its merger into the ever-expanding Maine Medical Center sphere of influence it became apparent that more integration between the osteopathic and allopathic communities was clearly the way of the future. OAP decided to be part of that and brought Herzog and Guay aboard.

Bill Dexter also joined OA in late 1996 as a part-time primary care sports medicine physician, primarily to work with Bill Heinz to develop a fellowship in primary care sports medicine co-located at OAP and the Maine Medical Center (MMC) primary care department. Dexter had previously trained in MMC's primary care program and following that at a fellowship in sports medicine in Michigan. His strong personal athletic background at Dartmouth made him a perfect match for his interest in creating a sports medicine fellowship training program in Portland.

Bill Heinz and Bill Dexter's contributions to that primary care sports medicine fellowship program over the next 20 years were enormous both in terms of the quality of the training the fellows received and in the number of well-trained primary care sports medicine physicians who ended up practicing in the Greater Portland area and elsewhere in Maine.

Unfortunately 1996 also brought another loss to OA. Dr. Anson decided to leave to practice independently in Portland. That same year Dr. Babikian began to focus more and more of his energy on hip replacement surgery. Over the ensuing 15 years he became one of the most innovative hip arthroplasty surgeons in the northeast, perfecting "minimally invasive" approaches which opened the door to immediate weight-bearing without risk of dislocation and same-day, out-patient hip replacement surgery. This was as much of a revolution in hip surgery as arthroscopy had been for the knee. Dr. Babikian was clearly one of the country's pioneers.

OA's loss of Crothers and Anson in 1995 and1996, combined with the addition of the five others, left the group with 12 orthopaedic surgeons, one primary care physician, and five PAs.

Things remained relatively stable at OAP through the beginning of 1999 when Dr. Tom Murray, a fellowship-trained sports medicine and shoulder specialist, decided to shift to OAP from another orthopaedic group in Portland. Murray brought substantial expertise in the new field of arthroscopic shoulder surgery, being generally recognized as an extremely proficient arthroscopic shoulder specialist. He was a great compliment to Dr. Endrizzi's widely recognized broad-based shoulder expertise. Although initially Dr. Murray emphasized his shoulder expertise he had equal proficiency in all aspects of sports medicine, including knee surgery, consistent with his fellowship training in sports medicine in southern California following his residency in Hartford, CT.

Eight months before Dr. Murray arrived, Eric Hoffman, a Duke-trained orthopaedic surgeon originally from Seattle but influenced by his wife's strong family connections in Scarborough left a position in Manchester, NH which he had held for a few years after residency to join OAP. Because he had not completed a fellowship in any sub-specialty Dr. Hoffman initially filled a position as a general orthopaedic surgeon, before eventually narrowing his interest to sports medicine. As his experience grew in that specialty, Dr. Hoffman eventually received sub-specialty certification in orthopaedic sports medicine – the functional and academic equivalent of having completed a fellowship in that specialty.

Unfortunately Dr. Agren decided to leave OA in the summer of 1998 to pursue private practice in spine surgery elsewhere in Portland. However, Jim Findlay who was an experienced osteopathic primary care physician with impressive experience in spine diagnosis and manual therapy joined OAP's spine team in the summer of 1999.

By the end of 1999, in its 18th year of existence, OAP consisted of 13 orthopaedic surgeons, a full-time primary care sports medicine physician, a physiatrist and a primary care osteopathic physician both specializing in spine problems.

Dirk Asherman, another surgeon with a strong Portland connection, having grown up in Falmouth and educated at Bowdoin before medical school and residency at Dartmouth, joined OAP in 2000 after completing a foot and ankle fellowship in Texas. Dirk had a strong interest in OAP and decided on the foot and ankle specialty to complement OAP's existing resources. Asherman also had a strong interest in sports medicine, having been an outstanding soccer player at Bowdoin and Falmouth High.

Dr. Herzog retired from active practice and left OAP in the summer of 2001. Shortly after that in January 2002, Dr. Andy Burgess left his academic teaching practice in Baltimore to join forces with Ray White and George Babikian thereby augmenting Maine Medical Center's growing orthopaedic trauma service. Dr. Burgess was extremely well established and experienced in orthopaedic trauma having taught at the famous Maryland Shock Trauma Service at Johns Hopkins in Baltimore. His reputation was widely recognized in academic circles and his position as an educator in Baltimore was solid. He had maintained a summer home in Rockport for many years and he decided in mid- to late- career that his quality of life might be better if he could combine his expertise with Ray White's at OAP and Maine Medical Center to expand the orthopaedic trauma center services there. At about this same time MMC received certification as the major Level I trauma center in Maine so bringing Andy Burgess on board was a logical and impressive move. Although Dr. Burgess was certainly a powerful and positive addition to OAP – and to Maine Med's Trauma Service - the fit was not a perfect one so Dr. Burgess decided to leave a little over a year later, in the fall of 2003.

At about that same time, Dr. Sacha Matthews joined OAP as a hand specialist working alongside John Chance. Like Dr. Chance, Matthews was a Columbia University orthopaedic residency alumnus. He had followed his residency with a fellowship in hand surgery with Martin Posner in New York. Mathews immediately developed a high-quality hand surgery practice and a reputation for depth of knowledge and expertise in hand problems.

The seven years from 2003 to 2009 brought OAP to its peak in size, expertise, and development as a sub-specialty group. In primary care sports medicine Scott Marr and Lucien Ouellette, both highly regarded fellowship graduates from the MMC primary care program, joined OAP in 2004 and 2007 respectively. Steve Kelley, a fellowship trained joint replacement specialist from the University of Vermont came on board in the summer of 2006. Soon after that Matt Camuso, a superbly-trained orthopaedic trauma specialist, joined the group following a distinguished and impressive Navy orthopaedic career. With Dr. Camuso's military surgical training and experience, Dr. White's master surgeon status, and Dr. Babikian's participating whenever possible, OAP's orthopaedic trauma service achieved new heights. Nowhere in Maine – and most of New England was there a more impressive and capable team.

During the same time period the OSC became sufficiently busy that expansion in the number of ORs seemed absolutely necessary. Once again OAP partners went to the architects to design two more specialty ORs and much larger pre-op and post-anesthesia recovery areas. With the possibility of 24-hour-stay orthopaedic procedures such as total knee and total hip replacements in mind, the architects also designed enough space into the facility to allow that function should the partners determine to move in that direction in the future. There would be many regulatory hurdles to overcome for a 24-hour stay facility yet the partners wanted to design in the option. While maintaining the original 2-room OSC facility at full capacity the architects and builders were able to pull off a full renovation over the course of about 12 months. The new 4-room facility opened in 2004. It was a remarkable construction feat resulting in an even more remarkable new state-of-the-art facility.

The expanded OSC wasn't the only facility improvement which the OAP partners undertook at that time. In close collaboration with the radiology group, a new 1-Tesla MRI was incorporated into the expansion plans. The new MRI facility opened its doors at the same time as the upgraded OSC in 2004. This was a major improvement for patients and physicians alike, greatly increasing the efficiency and scheduling for patients and physicians. By focusing the MRI protocols on just a few musculo-skeletal exams it was possible to increase the quality of the individual studies while lowering the costs. The OSC and the MRI were designed to offer patients and insurers demonstrably lower unit costs for procedures done there compared to hospital-based surgeries and MRIs.

The sports medicine team received three welcome additions in 2007. First was Ben Huffard, a Yale medical school graduate and Hospital for Special Surgery trained orthopaedic surgeon. Dr. Huffard then completed a fellowship with renowned sports medicine specialist Richard Steadman in Vail, CO before signing on at OAP. Ben's wife had grown up in Cape Elizabeth so the move to Portland was a natural choice for the Huffards.

Two more primary care sports medicine physicians, Mike Pleacher and Jeff Bean, joined OA in 2009. Dr. Pleacher re-located to Maine from the University of New Mexico sports medicine department where he had gone following completion of his fellowship in sports medicine at MMC and OAP. His experience at New Mexico was a perfect fit for his being located in OAP's new Brunswick practice facility and for assuming the role of team physician for Bowdoin College. Dr. Bean had also completed a primary care sports medicine fellowship and shifted his practice from Saco to OAP's Windham facility.

Unfortunately, Dr. Huffard's arrival in 2007 was almost simultaneous with Linc Avery's decision to leave OAP to pursue his own solo sports medicine practice in Portland. As one of the core OAP surgeons Avery had helped influence and guide OA's development for many years. He had also built an impressive reputation for excellence as a sports medicine expert for many years. His departure was a big loss which unfortunately ended up being a prelude to even bigger losses for OAP.

In 2009 MMC persuaded Drs. Camuso and White to change their practices to become full-time employees of the hospital. While a logical and strategically sound decision for MMC which was looking to consolidate and better control its comprehensive trauma services, the loss to OAP of an extremely important component of its comprehensive orthopaedic profile was severe – and one that could never be reversed even if OAP could somehow convince new trauma orthopaedic specialists to come to Portland. A year later Drs. Babikian, McGrory, Becker, Endrizzi, and Guay made similar moves to MMC to create a new joint arthroplasty division. Those five departures represented the loss of irreplaceable assets for OAP. In effect 2009 and 2010 saw OAP gutted of about 30% of its six major practice components – trauma and joint arthroplasty – with only sports medicine, hand, foot and ankle, and spine remaining.

After the departure of the core group of 7 senior orthopaedic surgeons in 2009 and 2010, Orthopaedic Associates of Portland's 29-year history effectively came to an end. At its heyday in 2009, OAP had consisted of 22 physicians -16 orthopaedic surgeons and six physicians in various primary musculo-skeletal care roles.

The still impressive physical facilities on Sewall Street and the strategically located satellite offices north, south and west of Portland all remained after 2010 but the large, comprehensive team of expert sub-specialty orthopaedic surgeons dramatically and inalterably shifted as did the balance of power in the orthopaedic community - from private practice towards hospital-controlled and from entrepreneurial and independent to corporate and institutionalized.

It is important to point out that most of medicine outside of OAP also dramatically changed over the same 29-year period. Everything evolved - from government regulation to insurance company policies to the eventual dominance of hospital-controlled medical practices. When OAP started in 1981 only 30% of physicians worked in hospital-based practices. By 2010 that number had risen to 70%.

At OAP, the departure of the core group of orthopaedic surgeons dramatically and permanently altered the founding principle of OAP as a multi-specialty group practice. The loss of seven specialist surgeons with a combined experience of over 115 years represented far more than the loss of seven individuals. Master surgeons like Ray White, George Babikian, Don Endrizzi, Brian McGrory and Matt Camuso, each at the peaks of his career, were not replaceable. Each had helped define and shape OAP's culture over many years. They also represented 80% of OAP's in-patient practitioners. All were architects of OAP's growth and development.

The dramatic consolidation of providers into hospital-based systems of care delivery occurred not just in orthopaedics and not just in Portland, Maine but throughout the country. While many politicians and citizens might applaud the shifts to more "organized" and "integrated" medical care, only the future will tell whether these fundamental shifts will deliver the higher quality, lower cost care that its proponents so confidently predict. Ironically what OAP demonstrated more than anything over a 29-year period was that high quality, efficient, patient-centered care was possible through the efforts of a group of dedicated, innovative, and entrepreneurial independent physicians who were ahead of their time when they started the project in 1981.

After 2010 OAP was transformed into a mainly outpatient-surgery-based, hand and sports medicine group with a meaningful presence in foot surgery and spine. Over the course of the ensuing seven years from 2010 to 2017, the number of its primary care sports medicine physicians increased, another knee arthroplasty surgeon (Dr. Kelly) left to practice elsewhere, and Drs. Totta and Binette who were both spine-focused also left to join the Maine Medical Center group. This effectively ended OA's presence in spine and joint replacement. Totta and Binette brought the number of OAP alumni physicians at MMC to 10 if you include Dr. Avery who eventually left his individual practice to become hospital-employed. The more narrowly focused OAP of 2017 continues to provide high-quality, specialized orthopaedic care through its state-of-the-art Sewall Street facility in Portland and three satellite facilities in Windham, Saco, and Brunswick.

Over the course of the 29 years between 1980 and 2010 OAP elevated the standards of orthopaedic care in Maine. Coordination and teamwork among orthopaedic subspecialists allowed each surgeon to deepen his expertise, offering patients a level of care comparable to that of acclaimed academic medical centers. The integration of physical therapy, comprehensive imaging, and an outpatient surgery center gave patients the opportunity for efficient, comprehensive, one-stop, high-quality orthopaedic care at demonstrably lower cost. That was the defining goal of OAP and the source of pride for everyone associated with the practice throughout its history.

Pathology

By Michael A. Jones MD

Introduction

In many ways, the evolution of pathology services at Maine Medical Center can be divided into two eras, pre-regionalization and post regionalization.

The pre-regionalization era characterizes services prior to the early 1990s and reflects the traditional practice of anatomic and clinical pathology based on a single hospital and dependent on a single hospital's patient volume, albeit the largest in the state of Maine. In this model, which was the predominant model practiced in the United States, pathology services were carried out by generalist pathologists who focused only on the needs of the hospital at which they worked and subspecialization in pathology was in its infancy. The pathologists in Portland throughout this period were employees of the Maine Medical Center (MMC), forming its Department of Pathology, and depending on the hospital for all Departmental resources. This inhibited their ability to take the lead in determining their direction. Hospital employment in that era impeded many of the entrepreneurial and growth initiatives that would come later. Importantly, pathologist compensation at MMC in this period was pegged to the low end of academic compensation nationally yet the Department was by no means academic in the traditional sense and didn't offer the aspiring academic pathologist an upward path or the promise of the benefits of a truly academic career. Thus pathology was caught in a dilemma, unable to attract aspiring academic pathologists on the one hand and similarly unable to attract entrepreneurial, driven private practice pathologists due to the low compensation. In retrospect, pathologists in this period (up until the mid-1980s) were compensated at rates 20-30% less than what pathology assistants would be paid only 15-18 years later. In addition, the science of pathology was yet to be affected by the explosion in molecular genetic information and technologies that would transform it in the 1990s. As such the practice of pathology was largely carried out with the traditional light microscope and standard hematoxylin and eosin histochemistry stained tissue sections with almost no ancillary technologies available to improve diagnosis. In this era, the practice was also largely inpatient driven with most of the laboratory services and generation of specimens coming from the inpatient environment.

The post regionalization era coincided with the confluence of several critical events that would forever change the trajectory of pathology services. By the late 1980s and early 1990s, molecular technologies were being introduced that exploded the base of knowledge and complexity of pathologic diagnosis and started to drive substantial subspecialization in the discipline. Significant pressure was developing on the Department to find ways to recruit recently trained physicians who had taken fellowships in specific areas required to support the clinical services that were similarly undergoing increasing subspecialization. In addition new, entrepreneurial leadership was needed and ultimately came in the person of Dr. Michael Jones who was recruited to Maine Medical Center in the late 1980s. It became clear that a new practice model was needed in order to expand the geographic base of pathology services and achieve the volumes needed to support new, subspecialized professional talent. This model would come when the pathologists moved from hospital employment to private practice, a move which, under the leadership of Dr. Jones and others, would lead to rapid expansion, unprecedented growth in the scope and depth of services and ultimately the formation of Spectrum Medical Group. These factors all ushered in the era of regionalized pathology services.

Historical Perspective

A key figure in the early years of pathology at Maine Medical Center was Joe Porter. Dr. Porter was a revered and magnetic figure who served as the first formal MMC Chief of Pathology. He was also responsible for initiating the pathology residency which existed at the Medical Center until being disbanded in the early 1960s. Under Dr. Porter's guidance the Department grew from a few generalists to seven physicians primarily by adding graduates of the residency program including Joe Stocks and Lou Taxiarchias. The MMC pathology residency program was eventually terminated in the early 1960s due to lack of adequate volume and resources to properly train residents. Joe Stocks became Chief of Pathology in the 1960s.

In this era, the pathologists received general pathology training but tended to focus in specific areas through "on the job training" while continuing to practice the full spectrum of pathology services. This period in pathology featured very limited techniques by which to interrogate tissue and blood specimens. In fact, other than the few specimen types that required electron microscopic examination, the light microscope reigned supreme. Other than light microscopy - based on the hematoxylin and eosin stain - and electron microscopy, the only other technique was histochemistry in which certain chemicals were used to stain for various substances such as iron, amyloid and microorganisms.

In the 1970s, MMC developed more academic aspirations. In the Pathology Department this culminated in the recruitment of John Batsakis in 1979. Dr. Batsakis had trained at the University of Michigan and taken a faculty position at the same institution where he quickly developed a national reputation as a head and neck pathologist. He was the first pathologist recruited to MMC bringing a national reputation and a track record of publication. Dr. Batsakis recruited Ron Nishiyama to join him in Portland. Dr. Nishiyama had a national reputation in endocrine pathology, particularly thyroid pathology. The recruitment of these two physicians was a watershed moment in that they brought a broader more national perspective with them. Dr. Batsakis was a prolific writer and was putting together what would be the first text book on head and neck pathology. Ironically, he was also a chain smoker and would sit in his office smoking and writing endlessly on yellow legal pads. He added significant structure to the Department, creating two divisions, anatomic and clinical pathology. The former dealing with surgical pathology, cytology and autopsy pathology and the latter focused on the clinical laboratory. While the arrival of Dr. Batsakis potentially signaled a new commitment to academic pathology, the MMC was not a fit and did not deliver enough of an academic environment to keep him satisfied. He left after only 3 years to become the Chairman of Pathology at the MD Anderson Cancer Institute in Houston, Texas where he remained until his retirement. Dr. Batsakis recruited Rich Porensky who had looked at a position at Maine Medical Center two years earlier when Dr. Stocks was Chief. At that time the funding for the position fell through and he practiced in Pennsylvania for two years until he moved to Maine in 1979. Rich would prove to be a mainstay in pathology and ultimately would be one of the few early physicians to move into private practice and ultimately Spectrum Medical Group. In addition to Drs. Batsakis and Nishiyama, Rich joined a group that included Joe Fanning, Joe Stocks, Bob Luke (who's wife Barbara was a radiologist) and Ron Howard (who would leave shortly thereafter to pursue a PhD).

While Dr. Batsakis did not stay at Maine Medical Center for very long, his fellow Michigan faculty member, Ron Nishiyama, did and so the impact of Dr Batsakis's recruitment lived on in the form of Dr. Nishiyama who continued to have a major and lasting impact on the Department. His departure did however create the need for a new Chief and likely raised significant questions about the real academic potential of the Department particularly in light of the absence of a training program. The search for a new Department Chief would prove to take several years during which time Joe Fanning assumed the role of Interim Chief.

Ultimately, Allen (Lou) Pusch, a pathologist from the Chicago area who had focused largely on clinical (laboratory) pathology, assumed the Chief position in the mid 1980s

177

with Dr. Nishiyama as the Director of Anatomic Pathology and Joe Fanning as the Director of the Clinical Laboratory.

At this point, the Department was still a traditional hospital-based service, with the clinical laboratory focused primarily on inpatient testing and limited outpatient or outreach services. The surgical pathology service was similarly inpatient focused. All of the pathologists continued to be employed by the Medical Center and as such were disinterested in growing volumes or extending services more broadly. All other non-MMC pathologists in Maine were in private practice but had little to no interest in building a larger group. Ancillary diagnostic techniques such as immunohistochemistry and molecular diagnostics were still in the future so pathology continued to be practiced largely as it had for decades.

The 1980s were relatively stable with little entrepreneurial activity. Dr. Eric Mann from Erie Pennsylvania was hired. Eric's father had been a dermatologist in the Penobscot Bay area where Eric had grown up. Surgical pathology volumes were in the 10-14,000 range and cytology exams were less than 10,000 per year. In 1986, Dr. Nishiyama recruited Stuart Flynn, a pathologist who he had known as a medical student at the University of Michigan. Dr. Flynn was accomplished, energetic and very well-trained as he had done a fellowship at Stanford University, one of the top such programs in the country. However, much like the fate of Dr. Batsakis, Dr. Flynn was not happy with the modest level of academic commitment within the Department and left after only one year. In spite of his brief tenure, Dr. Flynn was able to initiate an immunohistochemistry lab, a critical ancillary diagnostic testing capability that was revolutionizing anatomic pathology across the country.

The impact of immunohistochemistry would be profound and continues to the current day. Dr. Flynn left Maine Medical Center for Yale University and the Yale-New Haven Hospital in 1986 where he joined the faculty. At that time Yale had recruited Dr. Juan Rosai, one of the preeminent pathologists in the world and as luck would have it became friends with Dr. Michael Jones, who had completed a pathology residency at the University of Vermont and started a fellowship in Surgical Pathology at Yale in 1987. Dr. Flynn used his relationship with Dr. Nishiyama to pave the way for Dr. Jones to get on Maine Medical Center's radar. Halfway through his fellowship, Dr. Jones was recruited to Maine to take over for Lou Taxiarchis who had announced his intention to retire. Dr. Taxiarchis provided support to the fledgling gynecologic oncology service, at that point comprised largely of Charlie Boyce who had only recently recruited Hector Tarazza. Dr. Jones was hired by Maine Medical Center in the summer of 1988 but spent the first few months of his employment doing an abbreviated fellowship in gynecologic and urologic pathology at Massachusetts General Hospital, ultimately starting work at MMC in the late fall of 1988.

Regionalization of Pathology Services

In the early 1990s major changes were underway in the practice of laboratory medicine and pathology. Hospital laboratories, which to this point had focused on delivering inpatient laboratory testing and were largely seen as cost centers, began expanding into the outpatient market by developing infrastructure elements that allowed them to compete with the for-profit commercial laboratories. The key investments included better, more sophisticated information systems and courier services to cover the outpatient market as well as a pricing structure that could be competitive. Meanwhile, professional pathology services were coming under greater and greater pressure to develop more subspecialty expertise primarily because it needed to support clinical medicine disciplines that were becoming more subspecialized. The depth and breadth of clinical medical knowledge was growing too large for a generalist practice to keep up with.

Arriving at Maine Medical Center with Dr. Jones in the late 1980s was Ted Bailey, a pathologist who had specialized in microbiology and laboratory medicine. He came to Maine from the Centers for Disease Control. More importantly, Dr. Bailey shared an interest with Dr. Jones to create a more entrepreneurial pathology group that could grow regionally, cover a broader geography and therefore get large enough to generate specimen volumes that would support more subspecialization and improve the quality and depth of professional pathology services. They felt that getting out from underneath the hospital employed model was critical to achieving these goals.

At that time, Maine Medical Center, reflecting a desire to expand laboratory services into the outpatient market and turn the lab from a cost center to a profit center, had recently acquired a small non-hospital based lab with the intention of expanding outpatient testing and potentially moving certain services out of the hospital. The challenge however was that the pathologists were still employed and were not incented to have volumes and work load increase as it made no difference in compensation. Salaried compensation in pathology at that time was loosely pegged to academic salaries but the Department had essentially no educational or academic mission since the residency program had disbanded 20 years before and little to no research was being done. It was the worst of both worlds, academic based compensation models but private practice level productivity expectations. The Department had recently experienced two major failures in its inability to provide a sufficiently academic environment and enough professional growth opportunities to retain Drs. Batsakis and Flynn, both of whom had left abruptly and went on to high achieving academic careers. In addition, significant regional expansion and growth would likely require merger with smaller local pathology groups that were already private practices and had no interest in becoming employed by MMC.

Maine Medical Center's early foray into outpatient laboratory services quickly became NorDx Laboratories which was structured as an entity independent from the hospital organized under the MaineHealth umbrella. NorDx became the nidus of a larger plan to form a regional laboratory with the goal of merging labs from Brighton Medical Center, Mercy Hospital, Maine Medical Center and Southern Maine Medical Center. It was felt that considerable savings could be achieved in a consolidation and since the regional laboratory would not be under the hospital profit cap, could generate additional revenues. Ironically, this vision of laboratory services mirrored many of the goals being sought by a few of the Maine Medical Center pathologists, primarily Drs Jones, Bailey and Porensky. They felt that, free from the limitations of hospital employment, a new, independent pathology group would be incented to grow the volume to move away from the generalist model, recruit new, young talent and improve the quality and breadth of pathology services. The reality of achieving this vision however would come at significant personal time and cost as the move into private practice was still opposed by the hospital. Many of the older, existing pathology physicians, while not actively opposing the move, were very concerned about the unknowns of starting a new practice. The time required to move into private practice would prove too long for Dr. Bailey who left to become Chief of Pathology at a large hospital in Indianapolis, leaving a group of Lou Pusch, Ron Nishiyama, Joe Fanning, Eric Mann, Rich Porensky, Joe Stocks and Michael Jones. Dr. Nishiyama took over as Chief of the Department in the early 1990s and threw his support behind the initiative to move out of the hospital. By this time NorDx Labs had started to grow its volume and it was clear that to align incentives toward growth, the physicians needed a new practice vehicle.

The regional lab initiative meanwhile was gaining momentum and meetings between the pathologists at Mercy Hospital, Brighton Medical Center, Southern Maine Medical Center and Maine Medical Center were taking place. The desire to form a professional pathology group in parallel to the regional laboratory finally provided the opportunity for the pathology group to separate from MMC and form Maine Pathology Associates, with Dr. Michael Jones as its first business director. Ironically, Mercy Hospital and Southern Maine Medical Center would ultimately pull out of the regional lab initiative leaving only Maine Medical Center and Brighton Medical Center in it. Dr. Art Vanderburgh who had practiced alone at Brighton for many years and was moving quickly towards the end of his career, joined Maine Pathology Associates early on and stayed at Brighton providing services. Dr. Vanderburgh had also recruited Bob Cawley, a recently trained pathologist from Temple University.

Once Maine Pathology Associates was formed the pathology group entered a phase of rapid, unprecedented growth that would continue for the next 20 years and see the recruitment of many young, highly trained pathologists who brought a host of new subspecialties to MMC and the southern Maine area. The long time senior pathologist at Southern Maine Medical Center retired and his young partner, Dr. Sharade Pailoor joined Maine Pathology Associates. The 1990s also saw the retirements of Drs. Stocks, Nishiyama and Pusch while Dr. Fanning moved up the coast to Penobscot Bay Medical Center. Dr. Mann had left Maine Medical Center employment to join Dr. Bob Wilhoite at Mercy Hospital which meant that, of the original employed MMC group, only Drs. Porensky and Jones spent significant parts of their careers in the new private practice group. Dr. Jones had taken over as Chief of Pathology at Maine Medical Center in January of 1997 upon Dr. Nishiyama's retirement. It was Maine Medical Center's desire that there be alignment between the Pathology Department and NorDx regional laboratory (now organized under MaineHealth rather than Maine Medical Center) so Dr. Jones, as the new Department Chief, was made Medical Director of NorDx.

The early and mid 1990s were a time of rapid change for Pathology. As Maine Pathology Associates was forming, many of the original employed pathology group were moving on or retiring. As such, recruitment of new physicians was rapid. Doug Dressel arrived in the late 1990s bringing the first subspecialty certification in cytology. Doug also received additional training in renal pathology at the Brigham and Women's Hospital in Boston and became the group's first trained medical renal pathologist. Tim Hayes joined after a fellowship in laboratory coagulation from the University of Vermont. The recruitment of Dr. Hayes was an important step forward as it represented the first pathologist focused solely in laboratory medicine (clinical pathology), a move which brought much needed depth and expertise to clinical pathology services across the board, not just limited to coagulation. Tim also quickly became a transfusion medicine expert and really brought the first ever significant efforts at blood utilization to MMC. Tony Mattia, an anatomic pathologist trained at Massachusetts General Hospital also arrived in the late 1990s. Dr. Mattia had subspecialized in gastrointestinal (GI) pathology, again being the first such pathologist with specific GI training to practice in Maine. Dr. Rob Christman joined the Department from a fellowship in hematopathology at Temple University becoming the first pathologist at Maine Medical Center to be Board Certified in Hematopathology in addition to anatomic and clinical pathology. A long-neglected area in pathology at Maine Medical Center was dermatopathology.

Dermatopathology had been a long-established subspecialty certified area within anatomic pathology that largely focused on outpatient skin biopsies, that had never had a presence within the Pathology Department. Dr. Jones initially recruited Danielle Bouffard a recent trainee in dermatopathology at Mass General Hospital. Dr. Bouffard was from Montreal and ultimately found Portland too pedestrian for her liking so she moved back to be in academics in Montreal. The lack of a dermatopathology presence was quickly felt however and luckily was quickly filled by Chris Dowling who had grown up in Cape Elizabeth and whose father was a Portland orthopedic surgeon. Local roots proved helpful and Chris really became the first dermatopathologist to establish a long presence in the specialty for Maine Pathology Associates. It was the arrival of all this young, recently trained talent that started to rapidly fulfill the promise of a new private practice group's impact on improving the depth and breadth of pathology expertise in Maine.

The late 1990s and early 2000s continued to see rapid expansion and growth in pathology. After only three years as Maine Pathology Associates, Dr. Jones and his partners joined colleagues in Anesthesia, Radiology and Radiation Therapy (all of whom had long track records as private practice groups) in forming Spectrum Medical Group (described in more detail in the Spectrum Medical Group chapter in this book) which in addition to the Maine Medical Center also included radiology and anesthesia practices at Eastern Maine Medical Center and St. Joseph's Hospital in Bangor.

Fueling the rapid expansion of pathology was in part a national trend that saw the decline of the small, one to three-person pathology practices. As the medical knowledge base in pathology grew exponentially and was accompanied by the need to subspecialize, it became harder and harder for small generalist practices to keep up and many pathologists saw the benefit of becoming part of a larger practice not only to avail themselves of the subspecialists in the group but also to avail themselves of more sophisticated business infrastructures that could deal with the ever-growing administrative burdens of running a practice.

With the Spectrum business infrastructure now behind it, the pathology practice rapidly expanded to include numerous small and mid-sized hospitals in Maine and New Hampshire. The group acquired the Mercy Hospital contract when Robert Wilhoite retired. While viewed negatively at the time by Maine Medical Center administration, the arrangement allowed Mercy patients access to a much broader and deeper level of expertise that benefited the Portland community at large and continues to this day. Small, rural hospitals also benefited from the expertise. Ciellette Karn was recruited as another general and hematopathologist and after serving briefly at MMC, became the Chief of Pathology at Mercy Hospital where she was later joined by Ron Guibord, another certified cytopathologist who had come from Berkshire Medical Center. Memorial Hospital in North Conway New Hampshire and Huggins Hospital in Wolfeborough, New Hampshire came on board as did Miles and Boothbay Hospitals in Mid Coast, Maine. Additional MaineHealth network hospitals to contract with Spectrum for pathology services included St. Mary's in Lewiston, Franklin Memorial in Farmington, Waldo Hospital in Belfast and Henrietta Goodall (now Southern MaineHealthcare) in Sanford, Maine. While many of the hospitals that contracted with Spectrum Pathology were MaineHealth members or affiliates, the benefits of a large, diversified and subspecialized set of services were sought well beyond the MaineHealth network. These sites ultimately included Exeter Hospital in Exeter, New Hampshire, Wentworth-Douglass Hospital in Dover, New Hampshire and York Hospital in York, Maine. Growth occurred not just with successful bids to acquire open hospital contracts but also through merger with other groups. Ramesh Gaindh, and Ola Melhus merged with Spectrum in the 2000s and brought with them the contracts for Mid Coast Hospital and Stephens Hospital.

All of this exponential growth could never have happened in the employed environment that had characterized the MMC Department of Pathology for most of its existence. This rapid expansion required the recruitment of many pathologists. As pathology regionalized and developed more subspecialty expertise, the discipline was undergoing a revolution as molecular medicine started to blossom. Rapid advances in the basic science community allowed the interrogation of cancer and other diseases at the genetic level that pushed our basic understanding of disease, particularly cancer, into an entirely new arena. The onslaught of molecular genetic information would ultimately seep into diagnostic pathology forever changing it and continuing to push the need to subspecialize further as disease complexity grew to new levels. Spectrum Pathology now provides coordinated, regional services from as far north as Waldo Hospital in Belfast, Maine all the way down to Exeter Hospital in Dover New Hampshire. The story of pathology's growth in Portland from a small, generalist, seven-person group based at and employed by Maine Medical Center, to a 17-member regionalized and subspecialized group providing standard of care diagnostic services, is one that reflects a complex mix of physician leadership, entrepreneurial spirit, the ever-changing medical environment, timing and luck.

PEDIATRIC ONCOLOGY

By Stephen R. Blattner MD, MBA and Julie A. Russem MPH

Prologue

Bringing pediatric hematology and oncology services to Maine was a labor of love and an expression of idealism on the part of many people. Sprinklings of serendipity and even naiveté were also present. If the latter had been appreciated at the time, the ultimate results might never have happened.

Between 1981 and 1993 pediatric cancer care in Portland evolved as a unique academic-community comprehensive children's cancer treatment program. What is now a firmly established component of the Barbara Bush Children's Hospital originated from the private medical practices of Drs. Stephen and Francine Blattner launched in 1981. Having recently completed portions of their residencies in pediatrics and psychiatry at Maine Medical Center (1977-1979) they undertook a "green pasture" startup. With the addition of Julie Russem, MPH in 1983 as a critical founding partner the effort developed strong community support, culminating in the formation of the Maine Children's Cancer Program (MCCP) in 1986. By 1994 MCCP had become a prototype for MaineHealth's emerging suite of pediatric subspecialty programs and services.

Mirroring the largely unscripted path of this journey, this chapter follows a thematic rather than a strictly chronologic approach.

The Maine Pediatric Practice and Cancer Care Environment in the Early 1980's

Pediatric practice in Maine was traditional - but poised for change in the late 1970's. General pediatricians in the early 1970's delivered most of what is now considered primary care while also managing complex conditions such as asthma, diabetes, seizure disorders, gastrointestinal conditions, prematurity, developmental disorders, and others that were at the time considered well within the purview of generalists. General pediatricians were at times supported by adult specialists in pulmonary medicine, endocrinology, neurology, etc. as fellowship trained pediatric subspecialists were few and far between. Pediatrics as a specialty was itself entrepreneurial in Maine as care for children had been traditionally provided by allopathic and osteopathic general practitioners (GP). The few general pediatricians in practice served as "consultants" to the GPs for complex conditions and sick newborns.

The small number of pediatric subspecialists in the Portland community in the late 1970's practiced a hybrid of general pediatrics and subspecialty medicine – mostly as members of general pediatric groups. They delivered pediatric primary care, sharing call with their partners, while also serving as consultants and/or principal caregivers within their subspecialties. Elsewhere around the state, older general pediatricians were curiosities, peppered in solo or small group primary care practices. Specialty children's health care was truly a "new idea" to those communities. While Eastern Maine Medical Center (EMMC) in Bangor was an early pioneer in the retention of hospital supported pediatricians and pediatric subspecialists, the approach in Portland was - by custom - "market based". Neither Maine Medical Center (MMC) nor Mercy Hospital employed primary or subspecialty pediatricians in the 1970's other than one or two neonatologists. MMC provided modest financial support to help maintain two pediatric surgeons and thereby the viability of that critical pediatric service.

The Portland general pediatrics environment was considered to be "saturated" in the late 1970's and early 1980's. Younger recently trained and Board Certified general pediatricians found other places to practice, scrapping their way to viability in communities such as Skowhegan, Augusta-Waterville, Presque Isle, Fort Kent, Farmington, Lewiston-Auburn. Meanwhile, pediatric subspecialty training was becoming increasingly appealing and available to new trainees, some from Maine, who wanted to blend their desire to provide direct care and pursue more academically oriented careers with their passion for living in Maine.

During the 1970's changes were also taking place in the approach to the care of children with cancer. Nationally, the established "single institution" model for childhood cancer trials conducted only at the very largest centers (e.g. Dana Farber Cancer Institute in Boston, Sloan-Kettering in New York, St. Jude's in Memphis, Children's Hospital of Philadelphia) was giving way to collaborative clinical trials within regional and national cooperative groups (e.g. the Children's Cancer Study Group, CALGB, SWOG). This had the effect of expanding access to investigational clinical protocols to smaller academic pediatric centers that wished to accrue cancer patients, treat them closer to their homes, and share treatment data with a larger community of investigators. As a result of this broadened availability of standardized, research-based care, the overall cure rate for childhood cancers as a group rose from under 30% to nearly 60% by the early 1980's.

Children treated for cancer at major pediatric centers in the late 1970's also experienced enhanced quality of life due to palliative and programmatic innovations, regardless of the ultimate outcome of their treatment. Collectively, these accomplishments were attributable to a comprehensive approach to the childhood cancer experience that combined the provision of clinical research based multidisciplinary medical treatment with integrated psychosocial and practical support services within a pediatric academic medical center environment where passionate and highly trained subspecialists cared for this high-risk population.

Prior to 1981, the 40-50 children from Maine diagnosed with cancer annually had nearly universally received their diagnosis and treatment in Boston - principally at the Dana Farber Cancer Institute/Children's Hospital (DFCI/CH). Some pediatric cancer care for patients in the Bangor region was provided by a veteran pediatric oncologist at EMMC. In Portland, teens with "adult" type cancers such as Hodgkin's disease were frequently treated by adult cancer specialists, with or without consultation from pediatricians in Maine or specialists at the Boston centers. Some younger children received selected portions of their lower acuity care from these physicians who were committed to easing travel for families. Children with solid tumors, if referred to MMC, were treated by the pediatric surgeons in consultation with distant centers in Boston or elsewhere.

While children with cancer during this era may have received treatment consistent with trials conducted at major centers, formal participation in pediatric collaborative group clinical trials was non-existent. Other than inpatient playrooms and limited bereavement services, modern psychosocial programming for children with cancer were not available. The DFCI/CH did provide comprehensive services through the Jimmy Fund to Maine children – but only when they were referred to Boston for care. At this time the Jimmy Fund considered Maine to be within its primary catchment and fundraising area. The choice for families was therefore to receive some care closer to home, without the benefit of comprehensive services and clinical research participation or to receive the "full package" but be uprooted to Boston. There was no plan to change the status quo.

The absence of a university medical center in Maine to provide comprehensive services for children with cancer in the late 1970's and early 1980's created space for an entrepreneurial Portland based pediatric cancer program.

Opportunity/Model

Having completed two years in MMC residencies and liquidated their initial "Maine footprint" consisting of a small house in the then undeveloped town of Freeport, Steve and Fran Blattner furthered their academic and clinical training, in pediatric hematology-oncology and child psychiatry respectively, at the University of Rochester's

Strong Memorial Hospital ("Strong"). At Strong they were exposed – both from the pediatric and psychiatric perspective - to a new model of pediatric care that was highly integrated with liaison psychosocial/behavioral health. They spent six months formally working together in a customized pediatric liaison fellowship, becoming co-designers and facilitators of a unique hematology-oncology parent support group. With these combined new skill sets they decided to return to Portland, Maine – recognizing that its high quality medical center, relatively underdeveloped pediatric specialty environment, and potentially mutable referral patterns presented the opportunity to launch a practice providing resources that could benefit infants, children and teenagers and their families who were experiencing pediatric cancer and blood disorders.

Pediatric and adolescent medicine services at university medical centers in the 1980's preceded the adult medical care world in developing comprehensive models of care that included clinical research based medical care integrated with psychosocial and practical support services and programs extending from the hospital into the community and home. As patient survival increased both overall and for specific cancers, energy shifted from a focus on "death and dying" to "life and living" for pediatric oncology patients and their families. While offering the important bereavement support that was unfortunately still needed in this field, the opportunity to design and deliver services that supported "usual and normal" childhood activities – participation in school, sports, extra-curricular and social pursuits, and healthy family interactions – was attractive to optimistic, recently trained professionals wishing to make a difference for this population.

The unique opportunity in Maine was to build a pediatric oncology program that encompassed the triad of medical treatment, clinical research participation and psychosocial programming from a non-university base. From the outset, Dr. Stephen Blattner's private practice of pediatric hematology oncology was a mini-programmatic experiment that mimicked the academic model. It was unique nationally as a private practice based statewide center for pediatric cancer.

Startup, Healers, and Therapeutic Spaces

Modern pediatric oncology in Portland therefore began with a solo pediatric oncology private practice, enrolling patients in clinical research protocols from DFCI and providing an increasingly full range of psychosocial support services. The practice remained solo until the nonprofit Maine Children's Cancer Program (MCCP) was developed in 1986 to fund non-reimbursable research and support programs. This community supported institutional base was critical to attracting second (1986), third (1988) and fourth (1993) pediatric oncologists.

The first outpatient pediatric oncology nurses, Ann Baiocchi, RN and Gay Petersen, RN and later Cindy Stevens, RN and Cathy Cestaro, RN were recruited from the ranks of Maine Medical Center's best neonatal intensive care center (NICC) nurses. Established by a general pediatrician turned neonatology entrepreneur, Dr. John Serrage, the NICC at MMC was a respected environment where high touch, high tech, high stress, yet family centered care for critically ill babies was provided. By 1993 the outpatient pediatric oncology nursing staff had grown to a team of gifted caregivers, nearly all recruited from the same setting. These skilled, compassionate, unflappable RNs in upbeat, bright clothing served simultaneously as orchestrators of outpatient care and education, designers and providers of the practice's earliest school and outreach activities, clinical research coordinators, and critical personal and phone lifelines for patients and families requiring guidance, information, and day to day psychosocial support during and after treatment.

Inpatient care was delivered on the pediatric unit at Maine Medical Center (then located in P2CD). There were no inpatient dedicated pediatric oncology nurses at the time. Expertise in the care and support of newly diagnosed and acutely hospitalized pediatric cancer patients was learned on the job. Outpatient nurses from the private practice gained adjunct status at the hospital and served as early models of advanced practice nurses – teaching inpatient nurses about modern pediatric cancer programming, visiting inpatient children and families to provide disease and treatment specific education, and more or less inventing what is now called "care coordination" across the inpatient-outpatient continuum. As the practice's physician staff grew it assigned one physician to the hospital at all times while the other physician(s) tended to the ambulatory setting. This "hospital doctor" role for pediatric oncology patients in Portland, instituted in 1986, was itself an innovation. The "hospitalist" discipline, dedicated solely to inpatient care, was not recognized until about 1996.

Treatment for childhood cancer is a family experience. It was fitting that Drs. Steve and Fran Blattner, themselves starting a young family, searched for an office space to begin practice and together work with patients and families. It was clear even in the startup period that two professional offices within a common suite that included several treatment rooms and a lab would be required. Both oncology and behavioral health services would be needed to support childhood cancer patients as well as their parents and siblings. While Dr. Francine Blattner's child psychiatry practice had independent access for patients, joint psychosocial care was delivered from the beginning by designing her office in a larger "living room" style open suite also accessible from the cancer treatment space. This permitted families and staff to conference with each other and with both physicians when appropriate. With growth more in-house mental health support was required. MCCP experimented with various models that included sharing a social worker with MMC and employing its own child psychologist, Joe Fitzpatrick, PsyD. Over time MCCP determined the best fit to be a dedicated social work program as its primary mental health resource. Liz (Gibbons) Murray LCSW, hired as the first full time MCCP social worker in 1992, continues to provide professional assessment and support for children and families.

The original Portland practice location was in a carriage house converted by two orthopedists, Drs. Steve Monaghan and Larry Leonard, at 19 West Street. That office as well as two subsequent in-town locations at 685 Congress Street (1986-1992) and above what is now the Hannaford supermarket at 295 Forest Avenue (1993-1997) featured paradoxical environments. Children and adolescents underwent uncomfortable and at times terrifying bone marrow aspirations, spinal fluid sampling, and chemotherapy while also surrounded by massive toy repositories, studios for patient produced art, and galleries for the display of art work and candid photos of happy kids who came for care. Warm and welcoming design, bright colors, child and teen friendly spaces and activities created environments where children felt safe and loved while also being subjected to uncomfortable procedures, treatments, and conversations.

These were the days before safe, easy, oral or parenteral ambulatory sedation and anesthesia were available to mitigate discomfort and anxiety from chemotherapy and painful procedures. Cooperation was gained and anxiety relieved largely through the milieu itself - the safety and comfort communicated to children by the design, décor and compassionate staff present in the treatment space - all of which supported their comfort and psychological well-being.

The move from West Street to Congress Street in 1986 provided a larger space completely outfitted to the needs of patients and families. An empty storefront was creatively renovated and redesigned as a fun and functional outpatient treatment center. The central feature was the huge waiting area playroom with long carpeted steps and a toy filled platform for endless play. Kids often stayed long after their treatment was finished, a testament to their claiming the healing space as a haven. "Fisher-Price colors" on the doors invited entry into the treatment rooms with walls filled with patients' and siblings' art. Comfortable futons with bright colored covers were available for children receiving day long infusions. This was truly an early iteration of the "ambulatory infusion center" which has become the mainstay of contemporary adult and pediatric cancer care.

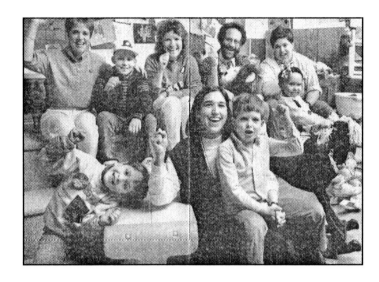

The move to Back Cove in 1993 further expanded the program space to accommodate growing staff and yet more user-friendly design elements. Primary colors and futons and play areas were central as was the evolving sense that the space was in part owned by the patients who were in treatment, recently off treatment or long-term survivors. Technology had advanced all the way to the presence of VCRs and color TVs in every treatment room and a shareable rolling cart Nintendo – each a welcome replacement for black and white TVs and Walkman cassette players which at the previous office had been the major form of personal distraction and entertainment for kids and adolescents.

As the practice moved from one location to the next, large bulletin boards filled with patient photos and art work were carefully transported to new walls – a powerful message imprinted from early patients to those who came later. These constituted the permanent archives of Maine's children with cancer - who in most circumstances progressed from illness to health. Photos of patients wearing personalized "off treatment" T-shirts were treasured as a remembrance of the challenging path traveled together. When the clinical outcome was poor and death resulted, the many joyful and poignant moments of the journey were nonetheless documented, celebrated, and preserved.

Of course, the most healing space for children is at home. Despite the complexity of direct and supportive care required for this patient population, the goal of providing it closest to home was always a programmatic aspiration. From early on, the practice prioritized outreach education and training initially funded by the Dana Foundation. The Comprehensive Pediatric Oncology Outreach Services Program was established in 1987 through grant support from The Maine Division of Maternal and Child

Health and the Maine Elks Association. This creative endeavor focused on training and supporting primary care physicians of patients from Augusta to Presque Isle and Fort Kent to deliver first line selected elements of care in their own communities. In addition, staff – sometimes fearful for their own lives flying in the winter to Aroostook County on the ancient prop and turbo-prop aircraft of then extant Bar Harbor Airlines - conducted clinics around the state. As high-tech home care capabilities and providers became available in Maine in the 1980's, the practice pioneered home based active therapy and palliation, in partnership with infusion pharmacies and community health agencies, long before these approaches became mainstream for cancer patients.

Proto-Entrepreneurs and Entrepreneurs

In order to bring pediatric oncology care to Maine, a broad community, entrepreneurial approach was essential. Multiple motivated and willing sponsors were required - each committed to a local care solution for this special population with complex medical and psychosocial needs.

Dr. Blattner brought a robust clinical and support program vision informed by his training at Strong. He was joined later by like-minded associates who served the practice for many years. Dr. Susan Light (for one year) followed by the permanent addition of Drs. Gary Allegretta, Lewis Cohen, and Craig Hurwitz brought enhanced clinical depth, expertise, and innovation. They worked tirelessly to deliver intense, complex, and compassionate care. As referral patterns shifted and therapeutics became more aggressive, larger numbers of sicker children came into the pediatric oncology care system. Expanding the program to support more patients and families with newly available approaches was increasingly necessary. This required dedicated structure, leadership and operational management.

In 1983 Julie Russem, MPH was a young woman already passionate for developing programmatic and psychosocial support services for children with cancer and their families. She moved to Maine after serendipitously "cold calling" Dr. Blattner, having learned from other New England program leaders that "there was a guy in Maine trying to start a new pediatric cancer program." Ms. Russem had recently earned her MPH at Yale University, writing a Master's thesis that analyzed the experience of children with cancer dying at home. Seeking to apply her skills to developing an innovative childhood cancer program in a relatively underdeveloped environment, Julie was attracted to the Maine vision, to which she brought organizational creativity, fresh ideas, and an irrepressible passion to package the emerging program elements into a vibrant and durable community resource. A close partnership with Dr. Blattner rapidly developed as did deep bonds with patients and families.

In August of 1983 Ms. Russem and Dr. Blattner collaborated to write a prototype grant proposal to seek funding for support services under a new entity, the Childhood Cancer Support Program (CCSP). Julie was Program Coordinator. Over the next three years the CCSP evolved to become the Maine Children's Cancer Program (MCCP), established in January 1986. Dr. Blattner, a co-Founder, served as MCCP's first Board President and Chief Executive/Medical Director. Julie Russem, also a co-Founder, became MCCP's Program Director and served as Vice President of the Board.

Dr. George Hallett, Chair of Pediatrics at MMC during the early and middle years of the pediatric oncology program's development was critically supportive of building this resource for Maine's children with cancer. Although the model for pediatric practice development at the time was strictly private practice, Dr. Hallett realized that the expanded services being developed such as outreach training for physicians across the state, school based services, and participation in clinical research required additional, non-practice generated funding. He was a ceaseless advocate and networker, connecting the pediatric oncology practice to community philanthropists and funding sources and advocating for reversing referral patterns from Maine communities away from Boston and back to Maine. It was due to Dr. Hallett's tireless efforts that initial funding for the CCSP was secured.

When Dr. Blattner left Rochester in 1981 and headed to Maine to begin the entrepreneurial effort in pediatric oncology, he realized – perhaps a bit late in the game – that a strong affiliation with Maine's historical referral and research base at the DFCI/CH would be essential and perhaps was not to be assumed. A major developmental serendipity was his ability to successfully and rapidly secure close and warm relationships with Drs. Stephen Sallan and Howard Weinstein leaders of the pediatric oncology program at the DFCI/Jimmy Fund Clinic and internationally known leaders in pediatric oncology. After a drop-in visit to their office in Boston while literally en route from Rochester NY to Portland in a moving truck, Drs. Sallan and Weinstein rapidly moved to secure the endorsement of their boss, the iconic academic hematologist Dr. David Nathan, to take the brave step of supporting a new and untested practicioner in "Jimmy Fund territory" who would contribute patients to DFCI's institutional clinical trials. This crucial step ensured that patients treated in Portland would be formally registered on DFCI protocols and thus could truly receive state of the art research based cancer care in Maine. It also opened the opportunity which endures today for Portland based pediatric oncologists to serve on research teams with peers at DFCI. Dr. Blattner initially served as co-investigator on DFCI childhood leukemia and brain tumor trials thus establishing the Maine practice as a legitimate partner to its much better-established research base. Gay Peterson RN served as MCCP's first Research Nurse Coordinator, onboarding and educating patients and families about clinical trials. Melanie (Leavitt) Feinberg served as the first Clinical Research Assistant, organizing and managing data and trials operations. DFCI served as a backup for referral pathology, consultation regarding complex treatment planning, as well as the center for the occasional out-referral for management of unique problems that required deeper subspecialty pediatric resources or technologies than were available in Portland. As DFCI analyzed data from its highly successful and widely published childhood acute lymphoblastic leukemia trials, subsequently published as a series in 1994, MCCP's patient population was indistinguishable from any of the academic center participants in treatment outcomes and complication rates.

Pediatricians in the Portland area proved supportive from the outset. They were willing to change historically comfortable referral patterns, trusting that local care would prove to be equally effective to that received at distant centers. Members of the Portland generalist and subspecialist pediatric community at that time, including Drs. Dan Miller, Marty Barron, Everett Orbeton, Sarah Cope, Ed Matthews, Dick McFaul, John Goodrich, Jim Haddow, Jack Mann, Walt Allan, Susan St. Mary (Williams), Sumner Berkovich, Tom Brewster and many others provided a fertile environment of referrals, encouragement, and internal promotion. Portland's pediatric surgeons, Drs. Albert Dibbins, Michael Curci, and later Dr. Allen Browne, themselves entrepreneurs in providing highly specialized, academic medical center level pediatric surgical care rapidly agreed to co-management of their pediatric solid tumor patients with pediatric oncology.

Elsewhere, around the state, general pediatricians and general/family physicians were willing to refer patients to Portland and then move out of their practice comfort zone to assist in the local provision of selected elements of care, assuming responsibility for ensuring pediatric cancer patients both received maximal care close to home and were promptly transported to Portland when local capabilities were exceeded. These included Drs. David Poleski (Presque Isle) and Michael Hofmann (Skowhegan) both from the same MMC pediatric residency cohort as Dr. Blattner as well as Drs. Norman Seder (Fort Kent), Mead Hayward (Caribou), Lilian Snyczer and her husband Abner Taub (Fort Kent), Terrence Sheehan (Augusta), David Walter and Gil Grimes (Lewiston-Auburn), Houghton White and Dana Goldsmith (Rockland), Burtt Richardson (Winthrop) among many others.

Physician leaders at MMC were crucial to creating the hospital based clinical resources required to diagnose and treat gravely ill children with cancer. Without them, it would have been impossible to treat children requiring inpatient care at the time of diagnosis or when experiencing complications of disease or treatment.

Dr. Paul Cox, head of MMC's critical care program, committed resources to adapting adult oriented critical care services to support a new and potentially extremely ill patient population without which the provision of complete care during periods of life-threatening complications would not have been possible. He eventually sponsored Dr. Sandra Bagwell from his staff to obtain formal pediatric intensive care training. With the blessing of their Chief, Dr. Jake Hannemann, Drs. Stuart Gilbert, Jeffrey Young, and Chris Seitz adapted MMC's Department of Radiation Oncology services and environment to better accommodate treatment of children. This care involved significant changes – there were complex technical considerations, a new need to provide/coordinate sedation and anesthesia, and an imperative to closely collaborate with colleagues at DFCI in Boston to maintain protocol standardization With the active support of Dr. John Gibbons, then Chair of Radiology, Dr. Charles Grimes innovated and advocated for an outstanding level of service and responsivity from the Department of Radiology at MMC – a key diagnostic service required for the care of pediatric cancer patients. Drs. Phil Villandry and Kate Sewall committed the Anesthesia Department to developing pediatric protocols for the provision of sedation and anesthesia for young children undergoing radiation treatments and painful procedures. Drs. Joseph Stocks and Robert Luke facilitated changes in laboratory and pathology protocols to accommodate collection of research samples, developing "micro" techniques for pediatric blood sampling, and obtaining rapid reference pathology opinions from DFCI for pediatric leukemia profiling and solid tumor staging. Each of these hospital physician leaders participated in local innovation to support the broader effort to successfully support pediatric oncology. Later, Drs. E.J. Lovett and Ken Ault and their colleagues at the Foundation for Blood Research (FBR) and subsequently the Maine Medical Center Research Institute (MMCRI) developed local capabilities in diagnostic and research techniques critical to the characterization of childhood cancers.

Patients and Families

Patients came to the Portland based Maine Children's Cancer Program from throughout Maine and adjoining New Hampshire. Newborns through adolescents and their families found care and compassion from a dedicated staff aimed at curing childhood cancer and providing psychosocial and practical support regardless of the outcome of the child's disease. As treatments for some cancers became more aggressive and sophisticated, at times requiring care at distant centers (e.g. Boston, Minneapolis, Seattle) for bone marrow transplants which were then still relatively experimental, the Portland based program remained the focus of support for families who valued the intimate relationships and assistance in understanding and planning care that developed during challenging times.

A joyful spirit of love and fun existed simultaneously with the fear and dread implicit in a childhood cancer diagnosis. Staff and the playful environment set the tone and patients of all ages and their families came to welcome these potentially challenging visits. Uncomfortable and frightening venipunctures were minimized by the wider use of indwelling central venous catheters and later implantable ports. Conscious sedation was increasingly an option for painful procedures such as lumbar punctures and bone marrow aspirations. Patients came to view office visits more as fun outings with a requisite post-procedure pause at the "Balloon Box" stocked with donated toys to be taken home. Teenagers were allowed as much independence as possible and involved in decisions and discussions to enhance their influence over what often felt like an "out of control" experience. Visits to the outpatient care setting became an opportunity to check in with favorite staff who had become their away from home supplemental support system. MCCP developed school transition services that brought staff to educate teachers, students, and administrators about the disease, treatment, side effects, and educational impact. The School Visit Program was delivered to schools throughout Maine in order to maximize effective school re-entry and support accommodations for children who had been long hospitalized, perhaps disfigured or limited by disease, treatment, or side effects.

The addition of social work staff directly impacted the establishment of therapeutic relationships at all phases of treatment. In addition, medical, nursing and administrative staff all played an important role in developing and maintaining a milieu that enhanced positive experiences amidst the drama of childhood cancer. MCCP's physicians and staff were significantly involved in the initial launch of Camp Sunshine in 1984 and provided clinical support and backup for several years thereafter.

The pediatric oncology patient population receiving Portland based care increased each year, with new patients increasingly approaching the estimated 40-50 pediatric total cancer diagnoses expected for Maine in any year. The majority of children survived their diseases to became long term follow up patients of the practice for surveillance or management of late effects of treatment - the unfortunate accompaniment to curative cancer treatment. When children did not survive, continuing family support services were provided.

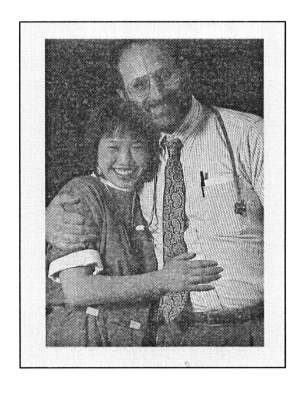

Community Support and Philanthropy

As outlined above, non-clinical pediatric cancer programming, research, and support services for patients and families were initially funded by a private medical practice. An early philanthropic vehicle, the Rainbow Fund, was created to receive small memorial contributions to assist in funding support services. In 1985 these funds were used by the nascent Childhood Cancer Support Program (CCSP) to launch a 501(c)(3) parents' organization named IMPACT (Involving Maine's Parents and Children Today) Against Childhood Cancer. This organization provided peer to peer support, sponsored family activities, published a newsletter and engaged in fundraising. IMPACT demonstrated the value and power of parent involvement in both defining and meeting the needs of the pediatric cancer population while helping to create and fund resources. From a Cabbage Patch doll raffle to a "Mug-A Thon" to a 10k Walk (1988-present), IMPACT contributed crucial early energy and financial support for services that positively impacted families until it was absorbed into MCCP in 1990.

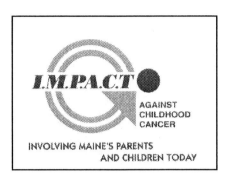

Program growth and activities rapidly outstripped the scale and scope of the initial grassroots fundraising efforts plus the resources that could be provided solely from the private pediatric oncology practice. The staff required to coordinate and deliver pediatric cancer support services was significant, increasingly co-sponsored by the CCSP, generously supported by the Visiting Board of the Children's Hospital and the Maine Elks Association due in large part to the advocacy of Dr. George Hallett.

The Maine Children's Cancer Program was incorporated as a Maine charitable, tax-exempt, nonprofit, 501(c)(3) organization in January of 1986 as the final iteration of these efforts. Its mission was to maintain clinical services and to capture and deploy strong community support for childhood cancer clinical research and supportive programming. MCCP was from the outset governed by a community board of directors. MCCP's co-founders, Stephen Blattner MD and Julie Russem MPH, were full time Chief Executive/Medical Director and Program Director respectively, responsible for administration, planning and implementation of clinical research based medical care and a range of psychosocial and practical support services for children and families. Medical, nursing, and social work staff coordinated care throughout the state while providing outpatient evaluation and treatment at MCCP's community based outpatient facilities in Portland. Medical and social work staff also treated patients when hospitalized at MMC. MCCP's success and durability was and remains a direct result of substantial individual and organizational philanthropy. Fundraising from community generosity plus grant funding were ongoing, ultimately underwriting the approximately 50% of MCCP's $1,200,000 budget not compensated by clinical care revenues in 1993.

When the initial Board of the Maine Children's Cancer Program was formed in January 1986, Stephen Blattner and Julie Russem as well as parents were among the Founding Board members. John Bay soon became the first community volunteer President.

Parents of children under treatment, post-treatment, and of deceased children remained a critical Board presence. Fundraising efforts included participation by parents who were best able to tell the story of receiving cutting edge care in Maine from a comprehensive program and enthusiastic in their support of MCCP. Solicitations for significant support began and culminated in the Davis Family Foundation's three-year grant of $300,000 This generous support continued for an additional four years ultimately totaling $750,000.

The Board expanded over the years, driving MCCP's success in corporate, individual and community fundraising. The 10 K WALK, initially an annual event at Back Cove, Portland, expanded from Portland to other communities. Creative events such as DINE (Dinners to Insure MCCP Never Ends) were organized around the state. Brochures with smiling kids and targeted mailings raised both visibility (friend raisers) and funds. Informational luncheons and tours of the outpatient facility increased awareness and support as did colorful canisters placed at retailers around the state. Mr. Bagel sponsored an annual tennis tournament, Shaw's organized golf tournaments, the Black Point Inn hosted parties and a long-term relationship was established with the newly arrived Sea Dogs baseball team. It was a tireless, coordinated and successful effort of the Board, staff and often families and it translated to the provision of clinical research activities and psychosocial services not covered by medical reimbursement. By 1993, MCCP was a thriving organization with a challenging and ongoing need to raise funds in the local and statewide community.

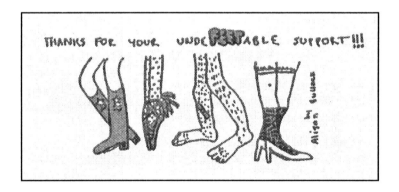

Transforming

In May 1988, two years after its founding, MCCP reorganized from a side by side relationship with Dr. Blattner's medical practice to a single entity that included the direct delivery of medical care services, thus becoming a truly comprehensive children's cancer program in the model of a university medical center. Prior to this reorganization, the medical practice had been responsible for employing medical and nursing staff, fractionally funded for the non-revenue-generating support and research services they provided for MCCP. In 1988 all practice personnel became employees of the nonprofit MCCP. Community support continued to increase, funding program elements not covered by medical reimbursement. That year Stephen Blattner and Julie Russem were nominated by MCCP families and awarded a shared Jefferson Award, a national public service award given locally, for founding the Maine Children's Cancer Program.

The Maine Children's Cancer Program benefited greatly from its dedicated Board which worked energetically to provide the necessary financial support to maintain a comprehensive program. Early Board members from the community included Marian Albee, Bill Dunnett, Gordon Erickson, Lee Jones, Bob MacLaughlin, Kathy Hillman-Reed, Chris Rogers, Roger Sicard, and Barbara Turitz, several of whom provided decades of leadership and support. By 1993, MCCP had become an integral part of the health care delivery system in Maine. But success had its challenges. While successful in raising the $600,000 annually from grants and/or philanthropy required to maintain a full suite of services, the MCCP Board realized that sustaining that level of community funding over time would be difficult and distracting. Options included creation of a substantial endowment or partnering with a larger organization and using the greater part of the Board's energy to advocate for staff and program development. In late 1993 Dr. Blattner, Ms. Russem and the MCCP Board concluded that a financial partnership with Maine Medical Center was the most prudent course to ensure uninterrupted provision of services for a growing patient population and an ever-evolving service mix. On December 16, 1993, the Boards of Directors of the Maine Medical Center and the Maine Children's Cancer Program voted to integrate the two organizations as of January 1994. This guaranteed the durability of comprehensive care for Maine's children with cancer and their families.

Epilogue

Today the Maine Children's Cancer Program is thriving. Headquartered at the Scarborough MaineHealth campus, MCCP is a vibrant part of the MaineHealth family of subspecialty pediatric services. Its dedicated team of pediatric oncologists, nursing, clinical research, social work, and administrative staff deliver care and programmatic services to children with cancer and their families based on the original vision. MCCP's Board remains active in program advocacy and fundraising. Transformative community programs such as the School Visit Program continue. The early support of the Maine Elks Association has been sustained as an Elks Major Project. For more than 30 years the Maine Elks statewide membership has enthusiastically contributed over four million dollars to benefit MCCP's programming.

The Maine Children's Cancer Program had its roots in the entrepreneurial efforts of individuals who were committed to serving the complex medical and psychosocial needs of Maine's children with cancer and their families. MCCP is now a durable component of Maine's health care delivery system. Today the overall long-term survival rate for childhood cancers has increased to nearly 85%. The MCCP logo was drawn in pen and ink depicting five exuberant jumping kids of different ages in various stages of treatment. The image illustrates the goal of MCCP – preserving childhood and enhancing the quality of the cancer journey for children and for families, regardless of disease outcome. The MCCP logo accurately reflects the experience of hundreds of Maine families.

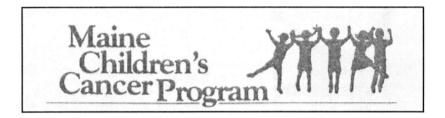

Editor's Addendum

Dr. Blattner and Julie Russem have described the psychosocial care emphasis of the Maine Children's Cancer Program, but I believe the following vignette will illustrate to the reader the effect it had not only on the patient and their family but also on the community.

An eighth grader in the Cape Elizabeth Middle School was a family friend. She was diagnosed with acute lymphoblastic leukemia and was treated with multi-drug chemotherapy accompanied by consolidation low dose radiotherapy to the brain, which was the standard of treatment in the 1980's.

What made this young girl's treatment so memorable is that the Maine Children's Cancer Program made a special effort to keep children in school and to involve the teachers and fellow students in their experience of care and recovery. The nurses from the MCCP went to the school and gave an in-service to the teachers and discussed the plan of treatment and the expected side effects and how to handle them. They stressed how effective the current management was and that she had an excellent long-term prognosis. These nurses then stepped into the classroom to 'teach' her classmates about leukemia. They created a very real picture for those children, including her treatment and the real hope that she would be cured as a result of her treatment. Students came to understand that their classmate would feel nauseous, tired, have a decreased appetite and lose her hair. Lots of questions were asked and answered in that classroom with the hope that their support would make her treatment and recovery just a bit easier.

The patient went through her treatments with tremendous support from her school and friends. She did very well and returned to a full active life very quickly after completion of her therapy. I attended her graduation ceremony from Cape Elizabeth High School four years later and was moved when her classmates gave her a special award for the courage and spirit she demonstrated in defeating her leukemia. There was then a prolonged standing ovation as she came forward to accept her award. I don't think there was a dry eye in the building.

The great lesson of this story is that a terrible tragedy can become an important teaching moment not only for the school but also for the whole community. Her classmates, who think they are invincible and will live forever learned that good health is precious and should not be taken for granted and a genuine word of encouragement and support can make a huge difference for those who are suffering.

Stuart Gilbert MD

PEDIATRIC SURGERY

By Michael R. Curci MD, Allen F. Browne MD and Albert W. Dibbins MD

The Development of Pediatric Surgery at the Maine Medical Center

Pediatric surgery developed as a specialty at the Maine Medical Center (MMC) during the formative years of 1970-2000. This was a transition period in the US, and certainly in New England. Pediatric surgery was beginning to be recognized as a distinct specialty by surgeons. Newborns and young pediatric patients had historically been regarded as "small adults," with similar physiology to mature persons. They had not been considered to require different management or technical skills. The limited recognition of a need for specialized pediatric training is evidenced by the small number of fellowship training programs at the time (only twelve in North America in 1972). Except for a handful of pediatric surgeons who were salaried at academic institutions, the basis for their compensation was private, fee-for-service practice with poor support from insurance companies, state Medicaid or hospitals. Board Certification in Pediatric Surgery was established in 1975. There was no "grandfather" clause, so everyone was expected to take the written exam – full professors and new graduates of the training programs alike.

The local barriers to the establishment of pediatric surgery in the Portland community were several. Everyone, with the exception of Dr. George Hallett, Chief of Pediatrics at MMC, was in private practice. There was no departmental or hospital support. The general surgeons weren't sure they needed this new surgical specialty. There was also a New England philosophy about infants and children with serious defects, expressed by Dr. Ike Webber, the first Board Certified general surgeon in Maine, that "bad apples should be thrown back". The need for a pediatric surgeon was thought to be dubious since correction of pediatric anomalies did not produce good results and the quality of life for survivors would be limited. Pediatric tumors were rare and even more rarely cured, and surgeries such as pyloromyotomies, hernia repairs, appendectomies, etc. could be performed by general surgeons. Medicaid and insurance payers did not understand the complexity of the care needed for pediatric surgical problems and, therefore limited their reimbursements to what would be paid for similar procedures on adults. A gastroschisis (a congenital malformation in which the abdomen remains open) was just another "hernia repair" - not recognizing the need for extended ventilation support and intravenous nutrition over a four to six-week postoperative period and prolonged follow-up for malabsorption, gastroesophageal reflux, incisional hernias and late bowel obstructions.

Prior to the arrival of the first fellowship-trained pediatric surgeon in Maine, the general surgical staff provided all of the surgical care. Dr. Allen Browne was a surgical intern in 1971 and 1972. He remembers rounding with Dr. Richard Dillihunt on a newborn that Dr. Dillihunt had explored. He had found multiple small bowel atresias and had closed for lack of anything else to do. A pediatric surgical attending, Dr. Angelo Eraklis from Boston Children's, was in the hospital giving Pediatric Grand Rounds and a consultation was arranged. The consultant described excising the atretic areas and long-term intravenous nutritional support via central venous access while the remaining bowel adapted. These were all new concepts to the state of Maine, so the child was transferred to Boston Children's Hospital.

The Maine Medical Center was recognized nationally in 1974 as a result of a precedent-setting legal opinion in the Maine Superior Court. The case of MMC and Martin Barron, Jr. vs Marie and Robert Houle involved a full term newborn child with esophageal atresia, a tracheoesophageal fistula, an absent left eye, and a rudimentary left ear. The parents requested NO surgical intervention or intravenous support. The landmark decision by the court in favor of treatment for the infant changed the management of children with disabilities and has been a frequently recognized decision:

> "In the court's opinion, the issue before the court is not the prospective quality of the life to be preserved, but the medical feasibility of the proposed treatment compared with the almost certain risk of death should treatment be withheld. Being satisfied that corrective surgery is medically necessary and medically feasible, the court finds that the defendants herein have no right to withhold such treatment and that to do so constitutes neglect in the legal sense. Therefore, the court will authorize the guardian ad litem to consent to the surgical correction of the tracheal esophageal fistula and such other normal life-supportive measures as may be medically required in the immediate future".

The patient eventually died from complications secondary to pneumonia, but a community hospital in rural northern New England was now recognized nationally.

The first fellowship-trained pediatric surgeon in Portland was Martin Bell who arrived in 1973 but stayed only briefly before leaving early in 1974. Following his departure, Albert Dibbins arrived in August 1974. He had received his pediatric surgery fellowship training at the Pittsburgh Children's Hospital and had spent several years there as a staff member. His practice start date was September. His move into his new home was interrupted when he received a telephone call from the pediatrician Jan Wnek. A term newborn with esophageal atresia and a tracheoesophageal fistula had just been born. He was asked if he would be available. Not having ever been in the MMC OR, he did not know its location or any of the personnel, but he agreed and went to the hospital to care for the infant. As the case proceeded, Phil Villandry, the anesthesiologist, stuck his head over the ether screen and asked if Dr. Dibbins really knew what he was doing. The patient did well and established the benefit of this new specialty. Dr. Dibbins went on to become a legend in Maine for his care of infants and children, his availability, and his dedication to teaching. He was known by the nurses on the pediatric floor for somehow showing up just in time when a pediatric patient became sick and the seeming ever-presence of his Volkswagen beetle outside the hospital.

Michael Curci arrived in July 1976, having just completed his pediatric surgery fellowship training at the Pittsburgh Children's Hospital. This began a 24-year professional relationship with Albert Dibbins during a period of extensive change in both surgery and pediatrics at MMC. In 1976 the only specialty-trained pediatric physicians were Ed Mathews and the newly arrived Dick McFaul in cardiology, Dan Miller in genetics, and Sumner Berkovich in infectious disease. Over the next 25 years, new pediatric subspecialists arrived in both pediatrics and surgery. These important additions are discussed in other chapters.

During this time period, working an every-other-night schedule, the pediatric surgeons became responsible for all the patients requiring specialty coverage and acute care that the community pediatricians were not comfortable managing, and for whom there were no pediatric subspecialists. The pediatric surgical service established central lines and long-term TPN for the infants and children; they established pediatric critical care and pediatric trauma care for the State of Maine. Although Marjorie Boyd cared for selected leukemia patients, the pediatric surgeons managed solid pediatric tumors. When Stephen Blattner returned from his pediatric hematology-oncology fellowship in 1981, he established pediatric oncology for the care of both "solid" and "liquid" pediatric cancers. Prior to Dr. Blattner's arrival the pediatric surgical service partnered with Boston Children's Hospital, who advised them on protocol management which fortunately was less complicated than it is today.

John Serrage and Madonna Browne initially provided critical care for neonates, until Doug Dransfield arrived in 1980 as the first fellowship-trained neonatologist. The NICU was located in a very small, crowded unit with limited nursing experience. This changed rapidly under Dr. Dransfield's hands-on care and the surgeon's "kind" but sometimes intimidating style. The demands were clearly outlined and consistent, which provided the basis for more sophisticated nursing care.

Both medical and surgical GI diseases were managed by the pediatric surgical service, associated with a steep learning curve. Ph probe testing became available in the early '90s under their leadership. The Department of Pediatrics provided the equipment so that this could be utilized for pediatric patients and limited adult patients. This "burden" became overwhelming until adult GI physicians invested training time to provide the service for adults. The pediatric surgical service also established upper and lower flexible endoscopy for children in the early '90s. Pediatric GI disease remained in pediatric surgery's domain until Ken Lombard arrived in 1993.

In the 1980's additional needed services were provided by radiology. John Gibbons encouraged Charlie Grimes, a radiology resident, to pursue additional training in pediatric radiology at the Boston Children's Hospital. After Grimes completed his fellowship, he returned and provided the needed support for the adult radiologists, who were very committed but at times uncomfortable with the new management skills required for the pediatric surgical patients. The pediatric surgical service was also very fortunate to have Kate Sewell in the Department of Anesthesia, since she was the first member of that department who had additional training in pediatric anesthesia. Many of the successes achieved by the pediatric surgeons would not have occurred without her presence.

Acute care, trauma and burns took up a great deal of time. Acute care for both medical and surgical inpatients was initially covered by the pediatric surgical service. This provided supervised training for the pediatric residents. The pediatric surgical service was integrated with one of the adult surgical services in terms of resident coverage, resulting in variable house staff coverage. The pediatric surgeons were required to be "chief residents" again in order to provide consistent, quality care. After this, full-time attending coverage became a model for all services.

Transfer options for major burns were few in New England, as the Boston Shriners burn unit had limited bed availability. In the '80s, with the support of the Chief of Surgery, Dick Britton, a burn unit was created at MMC. Extensive burns required daily dressing changes with sedation. This created the need for a tank room with monitoring capabilities. Besides performing the daily management, the pediatric surgeons also handled the extensive skin grafting needed by children with burns.

During the years 1976-1990, Dr. Dibbins and Dr. Curci continued to maintain an every-other-night on-call service and handle additional requests for services not provided by other specialists. This burden was aggravated by poor reimbursement by the insurance companies and the Maine State Medicaid program. For a private practice, this was not viable. Two changes occurred that provided limited economic support. The first was that Dr. Curci became an advocate and made multiple trips to Augusta to explain the health care needs of the pediatric patients in Maine. He emphasized that the pediatric surgical services were available not just for the Portland community but for the whole state. The Portland based pediatric surgeons were being asked to provide complex services for the larger population without adequate reimbursement (our service was 40-50% Medicaid). After multiple discussions, the administration in Augusta agreed to provide additional financial support. The second change was the introduction of limited support from the hospital in the form of providing malpractice insurance.

As pediatric surgeons we enjoyed a unique personal relationship with our patients. Maine has a large geographic area with a poor population who have difficult transportation issues. To accommodate these patients, we established a clinic at EMMC until a pediatric surgeon was retained at that institution.

A more unconventional approach was to make follow up visits to patients at outlying facilities during otherwise recreational trips made by the surgeons in Maine. As an example, a 2-year-old female from Fort Kent underwent a skin coverage procedure for a giant omphalocele during the newborn period. She developed a large ventral hernia extending to her knees. This required multiple corrective operations and frequent follow-up. During Dr. Curci's fishing trips to Baxter State Park, he would arrange to see her at a local "facility". Initially this was at the dumpster behind the McDonalds in Millinocket but eventually privileges at the local hospital were arranged in order to use their ER. Similar trips to Saddleback to ski provided him time to see patients at the group home in Strong, Maine for evaluation of major neurological disabilities.

The pediatric surgical service took on an additional responsibility in 1988, when Dr. Dibbins became the General Surgical Residency Program Director. Allen Browne arrived in 1990 as the third pediatric surgeon, providing additional coverage and an every-third-night on-call schedule. Dr. Browne also became the Director of Undergraduate Surgical Education. Dr. Dibbins remained as the program director until his retirement in 2000 and was replaced by Dr. Curci until Curci's own retirement in 2008. Dr. Browne remained Director of Undergraduate Surgical Education until 2002. During this period, the hospital reimbursement for the program director and the directorship of undergraduate surgical education was returned to the practice as the means to sustain three in-practice pediatric surgeons. The hospital also provided the pediatric surgical service with a pediatric surgical nurse practitioner.

The pediatric surgical service helped establish advanced, minimally invasive surgical procedures. It cared for international patients by cooperating with Partners for Health in Maine, and with Veterans for Peace. It offered international health care experiences through trips to the Albert Schweitzer Hospital in Haiti. It was involved in research for children with colonic dysmotility with the pediatric GI service and Harlan Winter at Massachusetts General. It sponsored an international conference on colonic dysmotility with participants from Ireland and Switzerland. It also established the Maine Pediatric Trauma Program.

In 1998, the Barbara Bush Children's Hospital was created. Dr. Curci was very involved in its development, as well as in the establishment of the Ronald MacDonald House in Portland. Hospital-based practice became a reality in 2008, expanding the service to four pediatric surgeons assisted by two nurse practitioners. This ensured the continuation of a quality pediatric surgical program that was respected and equal to any other pediatric surgical service in New England.

These changes, and the creation of the Barbara Bush Children's Hospital in 1998, could not have been imagined when pediatric surgery first arrived in the 1970s. Although there is a certain nostalgia for the "old days", with their more hands-on care approach, this will hopefully be remembered as part of the legacy passed on to the new generation of pediatric surgical care providers.

PEDIATRICS

By J. Daniel Miller MD

The year was 1967 and going into the Maine Medical Center (MMC) for an internship interview was a bit like stepping back into the Dark Ages. The city of Portland was nothing like the destination spot it has become today. The Old Port area of the city was comprised mostly of abandoned buildings and young house officers upon arrival at their new home were warned to stay out of that dangerous area especially after dark. Coming from larger metropolitan areas and medical school most new house officers found the rental housing market very grim.

Once inside the Maine Medical Center and once getting a sense of the medical community the outlook completely changed. At that time, as was the case for most of the country, a rotating internship was mandatory. The standard at MMC was for the intern to serve three months on the medical service, three on surgery two on pediatrics, two in the emergency room and two months on elective including OB/GYN and orthopedics. The house staff was small and consisted of 12 rotating interns and 6 surgery residents along with 2 pediatric residents, 2 radiology residents and 2 family practice residents who covered the unfilled 2 positions as medical residents. There was at that time only one part-time employed medical position, that person being Dr. M. Bacastow, the Medical Education Director.

The MMC facility in 1968 was old fashioned to say the least. The Richards Wing was being built at the time giving hope for a better place to train and work. The oldest part of the hospital consisted of large wards on three floors. The hospital beds were closely packed and the only sense of privacy was a thin curtain that could be pulled around the bed. The interns and residents took care of the people on these floors and they were loosely supervised by private attending physicians who were there briefly in the mornings. The house staff was supportive of each other and much of the teaching that was done was from senior resident to junior to intern. After one year of a rotating internship at MMC most young doctors felt they could handle anything.

The medical staff in 1968 was made up entirely of private practicing physicians who would spend two to four weeks a year serving as attending physicians on the various services. There was a wonderful sense of collegiality among the doctors in the community and there were several events every year when the entire medical staff and house staff and spouses would get together socially and most young physicians had the feeling they were in an extended family.

The hospital in 1968 was for the most part run by the medical staff. The President of the Medical Staff was the person in charge and there was only one hospital administrator, who in 1968 was Phil Reiman. One promising fact about the medical staff in the late 1960s was that there were some very capable visionaries who were leaders of their various departments. Two of those physicians who influenced many young pediatricians were George Hallett and Ed Matthews.

From the viewpoint of the house staff the MMC was being run on a shoestring as the annual income of an intern was $3,500. At $65 per week this came down to an hourly wage of about eighty cents. The one enticing factor economically was the free food that was served on linen table cloths by some of the nicest kitchen staff in the world. The average intern gained 10-20 pounds in the year and the most common answer to how many lamb chops would you like was seven.

George W. Hallett MD was Chief of Pediatrics at Maine Medical Center from 1968 until 1986. He and Al Aronson MD were hired by MMC as the first full-time department chiefs. George had been trained at Columbia University and Babies Hospital in New York and at Children's Hospital in Philadelphia. He left a successful pediatric practice in Portland to become hospital employed.

Edward C. Matthews MD had been trained at McGill University and had done his fellowship in pediatric cardiology at Cincinnati Children's Hospital. Ed was the first pediatric sub-specialist in Maine. He ran a busy pediatric private practice and at the same time took care of infants and children with complex congenital heart disease. He was instrumental in starting the first pediatric group practice in Maine in 1972 with Drs. Marty Barron, Sumner Berkovich and John Serrage who called themselves the Pediatric Center with offices on Vaughan Street in Portland.

In 1968 the pediatricians in Portland included Drs. Francis Fox, Everett Orbeton, Sarah Cope, and Ralph Heifitz along with Drs. Barron, Matthews and Phil Good. Phil was winding down his practice at that time but he had been the person most responsible for starting the MMC residency in pediatrics in the early 1960s. All of these people were involved when George Hallett set out to revive the program in 1968.

Most of the credit for turning around the MMC Pediatric program belongs to Doctors Hallett and Matthews. These two men, who had previously been in competing private general pediatrics practices, shared a vision of what would become a very important part of Maine Medical Center in the future. George Hallett, who became President of the New England Pediatric Society, had close ties with some of the major academic leaders in the early 1970s. Several people who wrote or edited the major pediatric textbooks in that era were frequent visitors and lecturers for the Portland pediatric community. Dr.

Hallett re-energized the residency program which to this day has attracted well trained candidates from all over the country. Many of those candidates came to Maine partly because of the attractive life-style that Portland provided. It was common in the 1970s and 1980s for young physicians to do a residency in pediatrics at MMC and then go away for specialty training and then return to Maine along with their new expertise.

Dr. Matthews remained in private practice doing both pediatrics and pediatric cardiology. It is remarkable that Ed Matthews in 1968 was performing cardiac procedures on tiny infants in a catheterization lab that he had set up in a way that had not been seen before in Maine. Ed was an excellent pediatric cardiologist who did all the work by himself at the same time carrying on a busy pediatric practice. It was because of exposure to this brilliant sub-specialist that many young house officers had a glimpse of MMC and Portland as a future hub of pediatrics.

The 1970s were years of great advances in the newly formed field of neonatology. Dr. John Serrage retired from private pediatric practice and became part-time Chief of Neonatology at MMC. He was also instrumental in setting up a statewide program to serve sick neonates in Maine. Hyaline membrane disease associated with prematurity was a dreadful condition for pediatricians to treat as many of the respiratory assistance devices had not yet been invented to serve infants. Under the encouragement of Dr. Hallett new procedures were attempted for the first time in Maine. What was to become a hugely successful Neonatal Intensive Care Unit (NICU) at MMC had its roots in a little room off the fourth floor nursery where the use of positive pressure ventilation in a premature infant took place for the first time in Maine.

During the 1970s a national change toward specialization occurred in medicine. The MMC terminated the rotating internship and it was replaced by straight residencies. At MMC the pediatric residency became a three year program.

Because the emphasis of this project is to explore the physicians who made significant impacts on the Portland medical community, the views that were expressed in a previous history of pediatrics in Maine, "A View From The Sun Parlor," will change to a focus on the impact makers. The development of what in a quarter century would become one of the top twenty ranked children's hospitals in the United States really got off the ground in the late 1970s and early 1980s. A number of physicians deserve special mention as their contributions laid a solid foundation for the rapid ascent of pediatric sub-specialties that occurred in Portland during the 1980s and beyond.

Several of the important physicians are separately contributing their accounting of events in other chapters of this book. One of the most important individuals who helped transform the pediatric community in the early-1970s was Dr. Albert Dibbins.

Al quickly established himself as a highly competent pediatric surgeon and one of the best teachers on the pediatric floor of MMC. Even more important was the way he cared for his patients. It was an impressive accomplishment for Dr. Dibbins to come here as a solo pediatric surgeon with little financial help from the hospital at a time when most of his patients were on Medicaid, a notoriously poor payer. Al Dibbins deserves credit for being one of the founding fathers of the future children's hospital. In 1976 with the expansion of pediatric surgery to include more complex cases Portland was fortunate to have a "clone" of Dr. Dibbins with the arrival of Dr. Michael Curci. For more than three decades Portland has been blessed with the absolute best in pediatric surgeons. These two men were compassionate artists in their field who made themselves available to the Portland medical community 24/7 and helped start a program that has expanded and prospered.

Maine Medical Center and pediatrics were gradually changing as the 1980s approached. What had previously been a good community hospital was evolving into a tertiary care center and a major teaching hospital. The adult services in MMC had expanded at a prodigious rate while the children's services remained underdeveloped. Entering the 1980s the Department of Pediatrics still had only one full-time employed physician – the Chief. Most of the graduates of the pediatric residency program went into general pediatrics and settled in Maine. Some of the graduates went away for fellowships and brought their sub specialties back to MMC. In the early 1980's a glaring deficiency in the pediatric community was the sub-specialty of hematology-oncology. Dr. Stephen Blattner singlehandedly solved the problem for the pediatric community. Prior to that time all children with leukemia or cancer or other complex blood disorders were referred to Boston. Dr. Blattner completed his pediatric residency at MMC and moved to the University of Rochester's Strong Memorial Hospital to complete a fellowship in pediatric hematology-oncology. He came back to Portland and began giving around the clock care to seriously ill pediatric patients with leukemia, cancer, and rare hematologic disorders and had outstanding success rates. He was instrumental in starting the Maine Children's Cancer Program – at that time funded largely by voluntary contributions. Dr. Blattner deserves great credit for pursuing such a work-intensive program that went on to become one of the pillars of the future children's hospital.

It is difficult to imagine during these times when neonatology has become such a successful sub-specialty of pediatrics that through most of the 1970s there was no such thing as a NICU. In 1979-1980 Dr. Hallett recognized the need for moving towards a NICU. With MMC assistance several neonatologists were hired to lead the newly formed NICU. Dr. John Serrage, having retired from general pediatric practice was the first. Dr. Doug Dransfield, a graduate of Columbia University with neonatology training at Children's Hospital of Philadelphia eventually came to MMC to become full-time Chief of Neonatology. Doug immediately established himself as a "hands-on" neonatologist. In addition to being an extremely caring physician he was one of the finest neonatal teachers. His teaching style emphasized basic physiology and the new graduates of the MMC pediatric residency left the program with a strong sense of competence in neonatology.

During the 1980's the Portland medical community experienced a transformation from a community based medical staff into a tertiary care center. MMC was at the center of this change. The entire medical community was essentially private practice based with physicians doing voluntary teaching and supervision of the house staff at MMC.

Several pediatricians deserve special credit for the contributions they provided to the greater Portland children's services. Dr. Keith Megathlin came to town after completing a fellowship in pediatric allergy and immunology. Most of the general pediatricians in the 1980s took care of many children who suffered from asthma. Dr. Megathlin brought a new level of expertise to the management of these very sick children. He started a private practice of pediatric allergy and became one of the leaders of the pediatric community, still all private practice based. Until 1986 there was still only one full time pediatric physician at MMC other than the neonatologists, that being George Hallett, the Chief of Pediatrics.

Two other pediatric specialists who brought major change to the medical care of children in southern Maine are Dr. Walter Allan and Dr. Richard McFaul. In 1980 Walt Allan arrived on the pediatric scene in Portland as the first pediatric neurologist. Walt graduated from Northwestern and did post-graduate training at Barnes Hospital and Washington University in St. Louis, Missouri. Before he came to Portland, pediatricians managed most seizure disorders with occasional help from the adult neurologists. With the arrival of Dr. Allan, the care in pediatric neurology flourished. Walter Allan will add his words to this book in the chapter on neurology, but there is no question that he was one of the pillars in the future children's hospital.

Dr. Richard McFaul came to Portland after finishing a pediatric cardiology fellowship at the Mayo Clinic. He was recruited by the Pediatric Center physicians to be of help to Ed Matthews who was being swamped by pediatrics and sick cardiac patients. Dick McFaul was instrumental in elevating pediatric cardiology in Portland and in fact he and Ed Matthews split away from pediatrics and started Pediatric Cardiology Associates an organization that remains a solid part of the medical community today. There were many other young pediatricians who played a major part in the development of Portland into a major tertiary care center but these physicians along with a few others were the leaders of a movement to advance the care of children in Portland. At a time when adult medicine was expanding rapidly with strong centralized hospital support, the pediatric unit remained small. A small working committee organized and met weekly to push for programs that had not been provided for children. This committee that included Drs. Blattner, Allan, Megathlin, McFaul, Allen, Browne and Dan Miller pushed for more specialty support. The greatest need was for the community to have a pediatric intensivist. Other glaring weaknesses included the lack of pediatric gastroenterology, endocrinology, infectious disease and nephrology.

When the search committee was formed to look for a new Chief of Pediatrics to succeed the retiring Dr. Hallett, there was finally an emphasis placed on seeking the input of the pediatric community. After a prolonged search for a new Chief of Pediatrics, Dr. Paul Dyment, was chosen to head the Department at MMC. Paul had built a substantial pediatric department at the Cleveland Clinic. He was the son of a physician and had a strong sense of medical history so the pediatric community hoped he would build the department into a children's hospital. Dr. Dyment's tenure as chief was relatively short-lived before he moved on to Tulane University. In early 1991 several leaders of the pediatric community organized to formulate a game plan for the future. Dr. Stephen Blattner helped form a committee that later became known as the Pediatric Planning Committee consisting of Drs. Allan, Miller, Browne and Blattner. This committee met every other week during the winter of 1990 and produced a long list of requests to present to MMC administrators.

As the purpose of this composition is to focus on the physicians who helped establish MMC and Portland as a major health center, two pediatricians deserve special attention. Dr. Stephen Blattner had a vision of a new direction for the Pediatric Department at MMC. Although he appeared to be a rebel to some people, he had a clear vision of where pediatrics within MMC was headed in the 1990s. Dr. Keith Megathlin was another quiet strong leader in the pediatric community. His calm leadership led to a complete shift in the direction of MMC pediatrics. In 1991 a committee under his direction notified the Chief of Pediatrics that the majority of the pediatric community was not satisfied with his performance. Dr. Megathlin handled the awkward task with utmost diplomacy and helped carry the Pediatric Department during an extremely difficult era.

Portland's pediatric community which had consisted of eight pediatricians in 1968 had grown to thirty general pediatricians and more than fifteen pediatric subspecialists in 1991. It is remarkable that in 1991 there was still only one full-time pediatrician in the

Department of Pediatrics at MMC. It had become clear that before a new chief of the department was chosen many of the issues that had not been previously addressed by MMC administration needed to be resolved.

Many meetings and conferences took place in the Portland pediatric community in 1991. As a result of those evaluations it was felt to be important to have the hospital commit to a new direction for children's services before a new Chief of Pediatrics was chosen. Once again a search committee was formed and chaired by Dr. John Tooker from pulmonary and intensive care. This time there was ample pediatric representation on the committee and through communications with MMC CEO Don McDowell there was general agreement that the hospital would support the needs identified by the pediatric community. After a prolonged search with some major candidates from the top pediatric hospitals the committee chose Dr. Paul Stern to lead the department. Paul had been Acting Chief of Pediatrics at Dartmouth and had just supervised the building of a new children's hospital in that community so most of the pediatricians in Greater Portland hoped that he could help advance MMC to accomplish something similar in Maine.

As the new chief arrived at MMC the hospital saw a rapid evolution in pediatric services. Dr. Loraine McElwain was hired as the first pediatric hospitalist and held the title of inpatient chief. It was under her direction that the pediatric hospitalist program was developed as an essential part of a future children's hospital. During the next few years with the help of Paul Stern and the listening ears of Don McDowell, new additions to MMC included Dr. Jerrold Olshan in pediatric endocrinology, Dr. Kenneth Lombard in pediatric gastroenterology, Dr. Carol McCarthy in pediatric infectious disease, Dr. Anne Marie Cairns in pediatric pulmonology, Dr. Eric Gunnoe in critical care, Dr. Matthew Hand in pediatric nephrology, Dr. John Bancroft in gastroenterology and Dr. Reed Quinn in cardio thoracic surgery. The pieces were falling in place for a new children's hospital within MMC.

As we are now about to celebrate the twentieth anniversary of the Barbara Bush Children's Hospital it is important to appreciate the transformations that took place laying the foundation for this important institution. Much of the turmoil in the pediatric community in 1990-1991 resulted in meetings and correspondence between pediatricians and MMC hospital administration. Essentially the pediatric community wanted some more full-time in- hospital pediatric specialists. The greatest need at that time was for a pediatric hospitalist in addition to one or more pediatric intensivists. The planning committees also requested support for pediatric endocrine, infectious disease, nephrology, hematology-oncology and gastroenterology.

The timing was excellent because MMC administration had evolved in a parallel track to the physician community. The first full-time physician-President of MMC was Dr. Doug Walker a retired pediatrician connected to Johns Hopkins Hospital who became President of MMC in 1974. He was followed by Edward Andrews MD who served as President of MMC after arriving from Vermont. Under Ed Andrews' administration the MMC grew and prospered and essentially became a tertiary care center.

For the pediatric community it was the next President and CEO of MMC, Don McDowell who was instrumental in listening to and helping to answer the needs of pediatricians. It was he along with the Chairman of the Board of Trustees, Owen Wells who were the people who most assisted in the evolution that led to the formation of Barbara Bush Children's Hospital.

The 1990's were years of transformation of the Portland medical community. One area where the result was most dramatic was in the field of pediatrics. The foundation of change had been built by a group of private practicing pediatricians who realized they needed more and better care for their patients and the community. Hospitals across the country had been enjoying financial success and Maine Medical Center like other institutions began to explore purchasing physician practices. In the early 1990s pediatric practices were facing tremendous pressures from rising costs especially in the area of immunizations.

In 1991-1992 meetings were held among the various practice groups to consider merging with Maine Medical Center. After several years of negotiations MMC agreed to purchase the practices of twelve pediatricians in Greater Portland. This group of pediatricians, including Drs. Barron, Fowler, Britton, Browne, Miller, York, Osborne, Blumenthal, Savadove, Brewster Faucette, and Stomatos, became the MMC owned Greater Portland Pediatric Associates (GPPA). This was the first group of physicians to be purchased by MMC. It marked the beginning of a quarter of a century of forming a multi-specialty group that has grown into MMC Partners employing more than 400 physicians. The 1990s was also the time of competition as the organizations of Intermed and Martin's Point were starting and growing.

The evolution to a children's hospital occurred quite rapidly between 1991 and 1996. The events that took place were accurately described in the book "A Hospital For Maine". One of the facts that was not adequately explored was the commitment of Don McDowell. He was the first person to fully comprehend the needs and desires of the pediatric community. He became convinced that the community would not settle for anything less than a children's hospital. One step in that commitment was his decision to add a pediatrician to the Board of Trustees of MMC.

In 1988 George H.W. Bush was elected President of the United States. First Lady Barbara Bush was well known for her interests in children and literacy. When in the mid-1990s the MMC was adding physician strength to the full-time Department of Pediatrics, the thoughts of an MMC Children's Hospital were entertained by Don McDowell and the Board of Trustees of MMC. It was largely through the efforts of Don McDowell and Owen Wells that the Barbara Bush Children's Hospital became an entity. Inspired by a generous gift of $3 M dollars from Elizabeth Noyce who served on the Board of Trustees of MMC at the time, Barbara Bush agreed to have her name be used for the hospital. In 1995 the concept of a Barbara Bush Children's Hospital was born and in 1998 the institution came into existence.

The "hospital within a hospital" concept was successful in other parts of the country and the BBCH within MMC has become a beacon for pediatric care in northern New England. This short pediatric story is only a reminder that hard-working caring physicians helped build an institution that continues to provide the highest level of pediatric care and remains a partner of a supportive community. BBCH is a highly respected children's hospital that dates back to many caring pediatricians who worked in partnership with their community over many years to build a place that will continue to shine for years to come. The pediatric expertise of today is a far cry from those dark days in 1967.

Plastic Surgery

By Therese K. White MD

Plastic and Hand Surgical Associates

I have the honor of archiving the story of Plastic and Hand Surgical Associates. The founders were my mentors. I have had the great privilege of returning after my fellowship to join this practice. Its influence on my career and that of so many other now practicing general surgeons and plastic and reconstructive surgeons in this country cannot be over estimated. Their vision and commitment to grow a private practice in plastic and reconstructive surgery to serve the state of Maine with the highest standard of quality and ethics is a story worth telling.

Plastic surgery is comparatively new among the recognized surgical subspecialties. The society was established in 1931. Much of the work in the early days was being done at the larger academic centers. Smaller, more rural medical communities often did not have a single trained reconstructive surgeon.

Jean Labelle, a French Canadian with a larger than life personality and a work ethic to match, relocated his young family to southern Maine in 1971. He was the son of a pharmacist and spent his youth working in the family drug store and the Canadian mines. He completed college and medical school in Canada. He then completed his general surgery training in Detroit and returned to Montreal to complete a fellowship in plastic and reconstructive surgery.

When Jean completed his training and arrived in Portland there was only one trained plastic surgeon in the community. Bert Olmstead by all accounts was a quiet gentleman and was doing beautiful work. Some of his hand drawn surgical sketches and glass photography of patient images remain at the office today documenting his talent.

Jean however was anything but quiet and reserved. He was the epitome of surgical enthusiasm. He was ambitious. He loved to operate and he loved to teach. He arrived in Portland when physicians had autonomy. This would prove to be essential as his vision of plastic surgery in the community became reality.

When Jean arrived in Portland, Maine Medical Center (MMC) had a thriving general surgery residency. With Jean's enthusiasm and drive to educate, he became the surgical resident equivalent of the pied piper. All surgical residents spent time rotating through the "subspecialties". Plastic surgery was one of these rotations and Jean reveled in his teaching role. As the surgical residents joined him in the emergency room, office and operating room his enthusiasm for the specialty was infectious. As he continued to make himself available - essentially without limit - to the emergency room staff, the medical staff and his surgical colleagues, his expertise and results expanded the medical and surgical communities understanding of the role of a trained reconstructive surgeon in the modern medical era. He was also inspiring many training surgeons who had no significant prior exposure to the specialty to consider further training in reconstructive surgery.

Jean worked hard and created alliances with his colleagues. Plastic surgery was a specialty exploding with new techniques. There were major new developments in wound care, burn care and hand surgery. It was the era of developing reconstructive flaps that would enable limb salvage and wound coverage. Cleft lip and palate techniques were being improved. Jean's practice was growing and he began looking for partners. He looked no further than the residents he was training. I remember speaking with him about how the partnership grew. He looked for talent. He looked for residents with technical talent but he also looked for residents with work ethic and moral character.

The first colleague to join was Bob Waterhouse. Bob came to Maine Medical Center from Philadelphia. Completing college at Middlebury and medical school at Jefferson he had spent childhood summers in Maine. He arrived in Maine for his general surgery training with his childhood sweetheart and with a young and growing family. In addition to being an excellent surgical resident Bob had a gift for mediating and negotiating. This would serve the developing partnership well in the years to come. Bob had been interested in a career in orthopedics but with Jean's encouragement and persuasion, he changed course and went to McGill for plastic surgery residency, returning to Maine to join Jean in 1978.

Dick Flaherty, another surgical resident and contemporary of Bob's also came under Jean's influence. Dick was from New England, born in the Boston suburbs. He completed college at Boston College and Georgetown medical school. He arrived in Maine with his young family in 1974 for a 5-year general surgical residency. Dick also possessed all of the qualities that predicted success including technical talent, confidence and integrity. He was principled and disciplined. He arrived in Maine considering a subspecialty surgery career and under Jean's influence, was drawn to reconstructive surgery and secured a plastic surgery fellowship in Rochester New York. While at Rochester, Dick gained a wealth of experience and techniques that would complement Jean and Bob's skill set. In addition to a solid general plastic surgery experience, Rochester provided excellent experience in head and neck reconstruction. With a skill set that would expand and complement what Jean and Bob were offering,

Dick returned to Portland in 1981. These three pillars would develop and grow the practice we now know as Plastic and Hand Surgical Associates.

Plastic and Hand Surgical Associates was incorporated in 1976. Jean Labelle, Bob Waterhouse and Dick Flaherty were forward thinking. Their expanding practice needed office space. In 1976 they purchased land and constructed an office building in South Portland. Although only a few miles from Maine Medical Center and Mercy Hospital this was seen as a peculiar location choice. All medical offices were in close proximity to the hospitals at that time. But the new 295 interstate allowed efficient travel between office and hospitals and land in South Portland was available more reasonably priced. This decision would also allow for future expansion.

Bert Olmstead remained on excellent terms with the new and aspiring practice partners. Although he did not officially join the group he rented space in the new office building and practiced there until he retired in 1987. The new office had character. The front was built with an A frame. The waiting room had a stone fireplace and high vaulted ceiling for a welcoming atmosphere. It was unlike any other medical building in the community. The culture of the group was maturing. Plastic and Hand Surgical Associates was collaborating with the medical community on many fronts. The emergency room, the trauma service, orthopedics, cardiac services all began to utilize the growing reconstructive team to collaborate for wound issues. The practice continued to thrive.

The rules that ultimately would govern the success were seemingly simple. There was total transparency among the partners. Partners had equal responsibility for call, an agreed upon method of delegating overhead expenses and equal voice in all major decisions that would affect the practice. A weekly partners meeting was established. Every Thursday morning the partners would meet at 6:30 to discuss the management of the practice. Although I was not present in those years, knowing the dynamics with these three men, the meeting scripts were undoubtedly ambitious. They were committed to their community, committed to their careers and to their families. The formula was successful. And the practice continued to grow.

In another memorable conversation with Jean Labelle, I recall his theory on asking new partners to join the practice. "If there is a talented surgeon there is room..... never let a talented one go because it is not the right time to hire." And so when John Attwood arrived as a surgical resident he was an obvious recruit for Jean and the others. John was raised in Vermont. He attended College at St. Michael's and medical school at Dartmouth. John was a true New Englander. He was soft spoken by nature. His compassionate bedside manner was striking. He also had the required elements. He was technically gifted and a team player. Jean saw his talents and knew he would be a perfect addition for the Plastic and Hand team. After completing the 5-year general surgery residency at Maine Medical Center, John secured a fellowship in plastic surgery at the prestigious Massachusetts General Hospital.

Microsurgery techniques were being perfected and new reconstructive procedures were being developed. Burn care, cleft lip and palate techniques were also improving. Cosmetic surgery was also becoming more accepted even in the conservative New England culture. The team wanted John to return and bring with him these new techniques. And so, choosing from multiple opportunities, in 1986 John Attwood returned to Portland to join the Plastic and Hand team.

A year following John Attwood, another promising resident arrived in the general surgery program at Maine Medical Center. David Fitz, having graduated from Harvard College and from medical school in Cincinnati, arrived in Maine with a spirited enthusiasm. He was an innovator and challenger of the norm. With his unbridled spirit he added to the enthusiasm and he too was seen as a complement to the team. When he completed his five years of general surgery he went to Pittsburgh, another prestigious reconstructive program, where he too was trained in the latest techniques. David wanted to return to what was developing into an unmatchable team. Like the four partners who were already in the group, David knew that practicing in Portland was a unique opportunity. The quality of medicine was equal to that of the academic centers but there was a quality of life and freedom in private practice that didn't readily exist in academic medicine. The partners recognized that David would be an asset. So in 1987 David returned and he and John Attwood would bring modern microsurgery to Maine Medical Center. They would also bring many new reconstructive techniques and continue to elevate the skill set of the group.

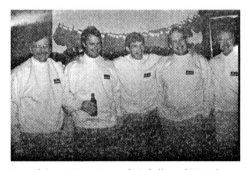

Drs. Flaherty, Fitz, Attwood, Labelle and Waterhouse

In late 1980's surgical services were thriving and expanding at a rate that was outpacing the medical center's capacity. Elective cases, those medically indicated but not emergent, were being cancelled on a more and more frequent basis. Often cases were cancelled the afternoon prior to a planned and scheduled surgery. This was disruptive to patients and to the practice. Efficiency was being destroyed and the ability to provide predictable, scheduled elective surgery was suffering. In a visionary way that was unprecedented the partners decided to build a free standing surgical center.

This would be the first non-hospital affiliated, fully accredited surgical center in Maine. By all reports MMC was fully supportive of the concept. There was no dissent from the partners, so they leveraged their personal assets, and broke ground in 1986. The surgical center was completed in June of 1987. The anesthesia staff from Maine Medical Center, also an independent provider group, had agreed to staff the surgery center. The first case was the excision of a wrist ganglion performed by Dr. Labelle with Dr. Hank Adams providing anesthesia. The surgery center was up and running! It was fully accredited with the highest standards for a free standing surgical facility. It was licensed by the state of Maine, certified by Medicare, accredited by AAASF (American Association for Accreditation of Ambulatory Surgery Facilities), and AAAHC (Accreditation Association for Ambulatory Health Care, Inc.).

In the first year of operation of Western Avenue Day Surgery Center, 289 cases were done. The following year the number grew to 732. The quality of care exceeded that at the hospitals for the outpatient procedures as the team was subspecialty trained. The surgeons could staff and outfit the facility for the specific needs of the practice. They did not need permission from an administration for new equipment. They were able to choose their own staff and assistants. The efficiency was unprecedented.

The Thursday morning meetings continued to glue the group together. Decisions were made to benefit the practice and strengthen the group. As the practice expanded so did the services provided. X-ray equipment allowed on site x rays. Hand therapists were employed to provide collaborative occupational therapy services on site as well.

With the Western Avenue Day Surgery Center up and running the partners continued to be innovators. They presented to the New England Plastic Surgery Society the first known series of outpatient breast reduction procedures. Formerly requiring inpatient stays, the society was skeptical in its response – to what is now a standard practice throughout the country, Plastic and Hand had again set the bar. With excellent anesthesia, efficient surgeries, and one-on-one recovery care, the patients had an excellent experience. The satisfaction surveys were a testament that this was a major advance.

Although the practice had developed a successful and growing private surgical facility, its partnership with the hospitals remained strong. Four of the five partners had done their 5 years of general surgical training at Maine Medical Center. Their fellow physicians were colleagues and friends. There was a true commitment not only to the medical community but to the community as a whole. The surgeons understood that their service to the community as a whole was part of their mission. They remained integrally dedicated to the success of the medical community. All were on the teaching staff for the residents and medical students. Resident and student rotations on the plastic surgery service were common place. John Attwood served as the Division Director for the plastic surgery service at Maine Medical Center. He frequented the student lecture rotation. Bob Waterhouse worked with the hospital administration and served as President of the Medical Staff from 1992-1994. Dick Flaherty was Chief of Surgery at Mercy hospital. The practice covered emergency call and inpatient consults. In these days none of these services were compensated but were an expected responsibility as a member of the medical community.

It was in this time frame that I was first exposed to plastic surgery and the Plastic and Hand team. I was a surgical resident and had assigned rotations on the service. My first rotation was as a second year resident. My plans to pursue a career in neurosurgery quickly came into question. The plastic surgery team was the most dynamic group of surgeons that I had yet to encounter. The breadth of the surgeries they performed was mind boggling to a junior resident. Trauma reconstruction, oncology reconstruction, cranio-facial reconstructions, congenital reconstruction, hand surgery and cosmetic procedures - they were all doing all of these! They were passionate about their work and all were enthusiastic to share their time with those of us who were learning. As so many of my fellow residents in general surgery, a plastic surgery fellowship became a goal.

In my fellowship years I saw from the outside the strength and vision of the Plastic and Hand team. They were great surgeons, but as I came to understand what made them successful as a group was something quite unique among surgeons. Their individual egos were dwarfed by a commitment to the success of the group. They understood their success relied on the success of the entire team. They organized teaching conferences for the residents. Case conferences were scheduled after office hours to review difficult cases at the end of the day at the office as a team. They were collaborative, enjoyed working together, they implicitly trusted each other, and most importantly they respected each other. The more senior partners worked as hard, took as much call and did as much charity work as the newer partners. They remained entirely transparent with each other with all of the financial decisions of the practice. With their commitment to their local community and peers, unlike many plastic surgeons, they maintained the respect of their colleagues. Their example in those first 20 years was exemplary and they became known throughout our plastic surgical society as a uniquely talented team.

Plastic and Hand Surgical Associates is now celebrating its 40th year as a practice. Much has changed in the health care community over the third and forth decades of the practice. Under the continued strong leadership of the original partners, the practice has continued to expand and thrive. In 1996 in collaboration with Spectrum pathology division, on site pathology services became available at Western Avenue Day Surgery Center so skin cancer care with evaluation of surgical margins at the time of excision became available. Previously this had only been available in the hospital setting. The office and surgery center underwent major renovations in 2002, providing more recovery room bays and additional administrative area. By 2012 over 40,000 cases had been safely performed. The first esthetician was hired in 1999 and the first physician directed skin care practice, Skin Solutions was launched in 2001.

I had the great honor of being invited back to Maine to join the team in 1996. I proudly helped establish a relationship with the Lahey Clinic plastic surgery fellowship. Plastic and Hand has since become an integral part of the Lahey plastic surgery fellowship program. The fellows continue to enjoy their time with us as much as we enjoy collaborating with new ambitious colleagues. Their time with us remains one of their strongest clinical rotations.

We have continued to collaborate with the hospitals, both Maine Medical Center and Mercy Hospital. We continue to cover their emergency rooms and inpatient consults. We have helped to establish the breast centers at both institutions offering reconstructive services to breast cancer patients. Our commitment to the greater community remains strong.

This year the last of the founding partners retired. They have left us with a great tradition and an incredible opportunity. In an environment when many of our colleagues have merged with larger groups, sold their practices and become employed, our group remains collaborative, committed to the service of our local community but also strongly committed to maintaining our independence. Our Thursday morning meetings continue. We believe we can provide the most efficient and cost-effective quality care with this model. We are grateful for the visionary work of our founders who have made all of this possible. We look forward to carrying on the tradition of providing excellence in our specialty in collaboration with the greater medical community.

PSYCHIATRY

By Carlyle B. Voss MD & Girard E. Robinson MD

History: MMC Dept. of Psychiatry

Psychiatry has undergone dramatic changes since the 1960's. During that period many psychiatric disorders were labeled "neuroses" which were thought to be the product of unconscious feelings and impulses unacceptable to the patient's conscious mind. Treatment (psychoanalysis) would bring these unconscious impulses and feelings into consciousness and the symptoms (depression, phobias, obsessive compulsive thoughts and behaviors, etc.) would be cured. It was a hopeful and appealing concept but was not based on any scientific studies. Sigmund Freud and others developed these concepts which dominated much of psychiatric theory, training and treatment, especially in America.

In the 1970's and going forward these psychoanalytic concepts were largely superseded by the expectation that psychiatric concepts should be scientifically based as much as existing knowledge would permit. Other theories and treatment began to include behavioral and cognitive approaches.

Medication that impacted mood and thought processes went from a few drugs with, at best, modest effectiveness to some that had dramatic beneficial effects. For the first time there was a medication, Thorazine, that relieved and controlled psychosis. Tricyclic antidepressants worked for many. Lithium, an element, could stabilize people with manic depressive disorder. It was finally approved in the USA in 1971 although had been available in other countries for years.

A major change in how diagnoses were made took place. The Diagnostic and Statistical Manual (DSM III) was published in 1980, replacing DSM II which had been heavily based on psychoanalytic theory. Diagnoses in DSM III and subsequent iterations (currently DSM V) are based insofar as possible on reproducible scientific studies. Revisions by teams of leaders in psychiatry are undertaken when new knowledge warrants reexamination of diagnostic criteria.

There have been tremendous advances in our ability to study activity in the living brain with SPECT scanning, functional MRI scanning, and other techniques. These have confirmed that (surprise) the brain is an organ that functions on physical principles. Psychiatric disorders are not the product of being possessed by demons or the devil which was (and still is for some) the explanation for psychoses, obsessive compulsive symptoms, mania, depression, etc.

It has been an exciting time to be in this challenging, wonderful specialty. It has also been a privilege to be at Maine Medical Center (MMC) as it has evolved in the last 40-50 years and to interact with the skilled and compassionate physicians in the other specialties. The collegial and professional interactions among us has been stimulating and gratifying.

In the 1960's psychiatric care in the Portland area was provided by psychiatrists in private practice. They provided some services at MMC for patients in the hospital and emergency room but there was no formal department of psychiatry at MMC although some attempts had been made to develop one.

The People

Alan Elkins MD was recruited in 1969 to develop MMC's Department of Psychiatry. When he arrived there was a small adult outpatient service. Psychiatric inpatients were treated in scattered beds in the medical/surgical units. Alan was the person whose vision and energy founded the Department. He valued equal treatment and access regardless of ability of patients to pay. He emphasized adherence to traditional medical values in the treatment of psychiatric patients. Under his leadership the inpatient unit, Pavilion 6 (P6), was developed. He obtained approval from the Residency Review Committee (RRC) for a psychiatric residency with 3 slots in each of the four years. A child psychiatry fellowship was developed.

Alan was very involved with MMC administration. He also had important connections with psychiatry nationally. He was an examiner for the American Board of Psychiatry and Neurology, later bringing in Drs. McNeil and Voss as examiners as well.

Carl Jackson MD, a fourth year resident at the New York State Psychiatric Institute did an elective rotation at MMC and then stayed on as the Inpatient Director.

Adair Heath MD, a child psychiatrist was recruited. He trained at Albert Einstein in New York and became Director of Child and Adolescent Psychiatry.

Lyle Voss MD was recruited upon finishing his residency at the New York State Psychiatric Institute to be the Director of Outpatient Psychiatry. Over 31 years at MMC Lyle had several responsibilities in the Department. He was Inpatient Director and Interim Chief and was Director of Forensic Psychiatry for training residents.

A number of graduates of the psychiatric residency and child fellowship became attending physicians in the Department, including:

- Walter Christie MD who finished his residency as Chief Resident at MMC after completing two years at the University of Michigan. At different times he was the Inpatient Director, Outpatient Director, and Assistant Chief;

- George McNeil MD who was Training Director for over 35 years. During his tenure the residency grew and became a strong program;

- Steve Soreff MD who was the head of Consultation and Liaison for many years;

- Ted McCarthy MD who was the head of Consultation after Steve; and

- Andy Hinkens MD who was the Training Director of Child Psychiatry and also provided clinical care.

Psychiatrists were also recruited from outside of MMC. These include:

- Doug Robbins MD who became the Chief of Child Psychiatry after Adair Heath left;

- William McFarlane MD who was appointed Chief of Psychiatry in 1992. Bill led a nationally recognized research project for early intervention in adolescents and young adults with signs and symptoms of psychotic disorder;

- Cindy Boyak MD who was recruited in 1991. She was Director of Outpatient Psychiatry and was President of the Medical Staff from 2014 – 2016; and

- Girard Robinson MD who was recruited upon graduation from his residency at Cornell-Weil in New York in 1988. He was Inpatient Director before being promoted to Chief of Psychiatry after the merger of the Department with Jackson Brook Hospital (now Spring Harbor Hospital.) Jerry has led the Department to new heights, growing and strengthening the residency and greatly expanding psychiatric services from York to Rockport.

There were many other professionals who contributed much to the development of the Department of Psychiatry including psychiatrists practicing in the community, nurses, social workers, occupational therapists and psychologists.

The Department

The last 17 years have brought significant growth and change to the mental health system under the MaineHealth umbrella. A number of key events have shaped the evolution of the MMC Department of Psychiatry and what is now Maine Behavioral Healthcare (MBH).

As noted above, the Department of Psychiatry at MMC began as a clinical service in the 1960's. The psychiatric residency began in 1970. The residency expanded from 3 to 5 residents per year in 2004 and the child psychiatry fellowship expanded from 2 to 3 fellows per year in 2007. There is now a total of 26 residents and fellows.

In 1999 a private for profit psychiatric hospital, Jackson Brook Institute (JBI) in South Portland, fell into bankruptcy. MMC purchased the license to the 100-bed facility. JBI thus became a non-profit, free standing, teaching, psychiatric hospital, Spring Harbor Hospital (SHH). SHH has been overseen by a community representative Board of Trustees and initially operated as a subsidiary of MMC. In 2001 SHH became an independent entity and a full member of MaineHealth (MH), the parent health system. At that time SHH was contracted by MMC to provide management oversight of the Department of Psychiatry and the Chief of Psychiatry at MMC and the Medical Director of SHH became a single position with the expectation that this would provide leadership toward a unified local mental health system between the two separate employers. As a full member of MH, SHH was positioned to become the principal support of mental health services for the other member hospitals of MH. This led to several management agreements by which SHH provided oversight of local hospital psychiatric services such as at Southern Maine Medical Center. It also provided the platform to launch system wide behavioral health integration services for hospital owned primary care practices.

This growth subsequently led to the vision for a more region wide mental healthcare system which would bring together hospital and community based care programs. In 2008 Maine Mental Health Partners was formed as the original confederation of this region wide network. The network consisted of well-established behavioral healthcare organizations in Maine. These included Spring Harbor Hospital and four community mental health agencies (Community Counseling Center, Counseling Services, Inc., Mid-Coast Mental Health Center, and Spring Harbor Community Services). This was a passive parent model that ultimately led to the creation of more unified organizational structure. Maine Behavioral Healthcare was founded in 2014 by the merger of these organizations. By most measures, Maine Behavioral Healthcare is Maine's largest behavioral healthcare organization with 1,150 employees

(850 FTEs), 45 physicians and serving over 20,000 clients and patients with 30-plus clinical programs at more than 30 service locations in southern, western, and mid-coast Maine. Maine Behavioral Healthcare also manages behavioral health services for several of MaineHealth's member facilities including as noted previously Maine Medical Center (20 additional psychiatrists), Pen Bay Medical Center and Southern MaineHealthcare. The latter two are served by MBH employed psychiatrists. Other services include inpatient psychiatry, crisis services, case management, outpatient psychiatry, tele-psychiatry, substance abuse services, trauma services, primary care integration, behavioral health homes, residential services and several other important programs such as Peer Support Services, Elder Services, Employee Assistance Program, and Trauma Intervention Programs. The Chief Medical Officer now encompasses the roles of Senior Vice President of Medical and Clinical Affairs for MBH and Chief of Psychiatry at MMC.

Undergraduate Medical Education (UME)

Undergraduate medical education within Maine Behavioral Healthcare and the Maine Medical Center Department of Psychiatry is primarily focused on the education and training needs of Tufts School of Medicine (TUSM) Maine Track students.

Partnership with TUSM began in 2005. This partnership initiated a substantial change in the academic landscape for Maine Medical Center and other affiliates. The Tufts Maine Track, a Maine focused division of TUSM, has its own admissions committee through which between 35 to 40 students with ties to Maine are admitted each year. They spend the two pre-clinical years at TUSM in Boston, followed by two clinical years at Maine Track clinical teaching sites. In addition to Maine Medical Center, these sights now include several more rural sites for those students in the Longitudinal Integrated Curriculum, an innovative longitudinal, patient focused approach to medical student education. The Maine Medical Center Department of Psychiatry has six to eight medical students who also rotate through Spring Harbor Hospital.

Graduate Medical Education

The Department of Psychiatry has operated a psychiatry residency training program since the 1970, most of that time under the leadership of Dr. George McNeil and more recently of Dr. Daniel Price. The child psychiatry fellowship at MMC began in 1971, most recently led by Dr. Sandra Fritsch and Dr. Erin Belfort. Since 2000 Spring Harbor Hospital has been an important addition to inpatient resident clinical experiences.

Dr. William Brennan has been an important and consistent clinical educator at SHH over the last 17 years. This increase of training opportunities and community need allowed for the expansion in 2004 of the general psychiatry training program from three to five residents per year and from two to three child fellows per year in 2007. The Department's training programs now have a total of 26 residents and fellows.

Over the course of the past 10 years the residency program has become highly regarded and more competitive. This year the program is on track to have over 300 applicants from American medical school graduates and several hundred more from foreign medical schools for the five residency slots. The residency has consistently received positive evaluations from the RRC and from the trainees through an annual program review process.

Research

Research within the Department of Psychiatry and MBH took an important step with the appointment of Susan Santangelo ScD as the Director of the Center for Psychiatric Research in 2013. Dr. Santangelo has expertise in epidemiology and genetics with particular expertise in the genetics of autism. Her partnership with Dr. Matthew Siegel has resulted in a robust research program on autism including the multisite Autism Developmental Disorders Research Inpatient Collaborative (ADDRIC). Prior to the arrival of Dr. Santangelo research in the Department of Psychiatry had been initiated by Dr. William McFarlane, the Department Chair from 1990-2001. As noted above, Dr. McFarlane became best known for his pioneering work on the early identification and treatment for young people at risk for developing psychotic disorders.

Future Directions

In addition to education and research, the overall clinical direction of the Department at MMC and Maine Behavioral Healthcare (MBH) includes the deliberate strategy to be more integrated with the general medical system and medical subspecialties. The vast majority of MaineHealth primary care practices have MBH clinicians integrated into their practices. There are several fledgling projects to enhance psychiatric expertise and availability to specialty medicine such as obstetrics, oncology, neurology, transplant medicine, pediatrics and pediatric subspecialties. Drs. Cindy Boyack, Steve Stout, Leora Rabin, Dena Whitesell, Maya Buhlman, James Wolak, Doug Robbins, Robert McCarley, and Patrick Maidman, among others have all played important roles in expanding the vision and scope for psychiatric services within Maine Medical Center and the larger health system.

Pulmonary and Critical Care Medicine: 1970-1990

By George Bokinsky MD

The two decades included in this story were periods of major growth in the scientific knowledge and practice of medicine both globally and at the Maine Medical Center (MMC). Three important leaders of pulmonary medicine and critical care medicine in this formative period are no longer living to tell their stories leaving it to those of us fortunate to have worked with them to describe their achievements. In this regard the author is grateful to colleagues, staff members, and family of those founders for perspectives and insights. The two decades of this chronology will be subdivided into five-year segments related to the time of arrival at the MMC principals and the changes that occurred during those half decades. Of course, all change is a continuum of gradual process but this story seeks to match progress with the individuals and groups involved.

Pulmonary medicine, as we know it today, began with the arrival of Edgar Caldwell MD from the University of Vermont in 1971 bringing with him funding for advancing the pulmonary function laboratory from simple spirometry to a sophisticated pulmonary function laboratory. The change from analog to digital data processing required computer expertise. The laboratory hired the first systems analysts to provide the necessary support for the process which soon enabled remote site testing and transfer of data for interpretation. Systems to precisely measure airflow and simultaneously display airflow and the volume of expired air advanced the diagnosis of airways disease. Body plethysmography and gas dilutions techniques allowed determination of static lung volumes and served to separate restrictive from obstructive lung diseases. Diffusion capacity for carbon monoxide (DLCO) became a key measure in the differentiation of emphysema from other forms of airflow obstruction such as asthma and chronic bronchitis.

The laboratory also acquired state gas mass spectrography equipment. The first oxygen saturation monitor at the MMC was much closer in size to a desktop computer than the current models used throughout the hospital that have become part of the bedside vital signs taken on all patients. These early accomplishments set the stage for future developments to be described later.

During Dr. Caldwell's tenure respiratory therapy and blood gas analysis became part of the Division of Pulmonary Medicine. Mr. Cliff Hoover, RPFT was working as a respiratory therapist at the time of Dr. Caldwell's arrival at the MMC. He describes a conversation that he had with Dr. Caldwell in which he asked Dr. Caldwell why he chose to practice at the MMC. Dr. Caldwell replied that, among other factors, he was impressed with respiratory care already in place as developed in the 1960's under the capable leadership of Robert Miller, RRT. Mr. Miller was a respected leader in respiratory care with the MMC providing services in intermittent positive pressure breathing (IPPB) as well as ventilation support in the intensive care unit. Other leaders of respiratory care services to follow Mr. Miller include George Ellis RRT and Kathryn Harris RRT. Each made substantial contributions to the extension of respiratory therapy into the critical care units, the blood gas laboratory, hemodynamic monitoring sections, pulmonary rehabilitation, and patient education. Epidemiological research into asthma and chronic lung disease in Maine began during this time by Dr. Caldwell with support of the Maine Lung Association and the Department of Respiratory Therapy.

Critical care medicine transitioned from the domain of anesthesiology to that of pulmonary medicine beginning in 1973 with the arrival of Paul Milton Cox MD after his completion of a pulmonary medicine fellowship at Colorado University Medical Center (CUMC). The Pulmonary Medicine Fellowship at CUMC under Thomas Petty MD featured research into the management of adult respiratory distress syndrome using volume cycled ventilation with positive end expiratory pressure (PEEP). Pulmonary fellows learned how to assemble the ventilators, intubate the patient, draw and analyze the arterial blood gas sample, and manage the ventilator as that was their duty during nights on call.

These hands-on skills coupled with his analytical engineering mind made Dr. Cox an ideal leader in critical care medicine at the MMC. Working well with administration, nursing leadership, and respiratory therapy he developed a single Special Care Unit (SCU) with staff skilled to support medical, surgical, and pediatric patients using well considered protocols that could be modified as knowledge was advanced. Recognizing that skilled technical staff was essential to the success of the operation, Dr. Cox was instrumental in the creation of a respiratory therapy curriculum at the Southern Maine Technical College (SMTC). He would continue as the medical director of that program for 20 years.

By 1974, Drs. Cox and Caldwell had obtained initial approval for a one-year program that would ensure the training of physicians skilled in pulmonary medicine through an American Thoracic Society funded pulmonary fellowship. John Tooker MD arrived the next year to become the first of many to begin their careers in pulmonary medicine

at MMC. The fellowship would increase to two years, increase in numbers of fellows, and in 1987, add a third year in critical care medicine to begin in 1988.

1975 saw the arrival at the MMC of J. Mark Kjeldgaard MD upon completion of his research fellowship in pulmonary medicine at the University of Rochester in Rochester, New York. He joined Dr. Caldwell in the Division of Pulmonary Medicine bringing additional skills in pulmonary physiology and testing of value to the fellowship program and in teaching of medical students and residents. Dr. Kjeldgaard also recognized a need to support the neonatologists at the MMC in the ventilator management of premature infants with respiratory distress syndrome. He returned to the Colorado University Medical Center where he had completed his residency in internal medicine and served as Chief Resident to acquire those skills which he applied with his pulmonary medicine colleagues until increased numbers of neonatologists in the NICU solved a temporary staffing problem. Dr. Kjeldgaard also had interest in asthma and pediatric lung disease, serving as a consultant and attending clinician before the arrival of fellowship prepared pediatric pulmonologists to fill that need. Dr. Kjeldgaard established pediatric clinic within the Division of Pulmonary Medicine outpatient clinic partially staffed by Dr. Daniel Shannon who traveled from Boston to Portland one day a month.

1977 saw two new members added to the Division of Pulmonary and Critical Care Medicine. Dr. John Tooker had graduated from the Colorado University School of Medicine in 1970 before serving as an intern at Bellevue Hospital and resident in internal medicine at New York University Medical Center and Colorado University Medical Center. He served in the US Navy as a medical officer directing the intensive care unit at the base. Having done one year of fellowship at MMC, Dr. Tooker had completed his second year of pulmonary fellowship at the University of Washington in Seattle, Washington where he had worked in the intensive care unit and conducted research in pulmonary vascular disease and the use of pulmonary artery balloon-tipped catheters. Dr. Tooker was recruited by Dr. Cox in the Special Care Unit to expand the educational program for students, residents from multiple disciplines, and pulmonary fellows. Working with the Department of Nursing, a nursing outreach education program to rural hospitals was created.

George Bokinsky MD arrived in 1977 upon completing a research fellowship at the University of California, San Diego and serving as associate investigator at the Veterans Administration Hospital where he received training in exercise physiology, pulmonary rehabilitation, surgical treatment of chronic pulmonary thromboembolic disease, pulmonary pathology, and in the new area of testing for obstructive sleep apnea. He had graduated from the Medical College of Virginia in 1970 and completed internship and residency in Internal Medicine at the Colorado University Medical Center in Denver before serving in the US Navy in the Medical Corps. He joined Drs. Caldwell and Kjeldgaard in the Division of Pulmonary Medicine. Responsibilities for patient care and teaching were now shared among the five physicians.

From 1975 to 1980, the pulmonary fellowship expanded to two years and by the end of the decade four pulmonary fellows had completed or were completing their training. They include Dr. John Tooker, Dr. Irving Paradis, Dr. Earl Robinson and Dr. Steven Zimmerman. Of these, Dr. Zimmerman would join Dr. Tooker as being the first MMC trained pulmonary fellows to become attending physicians in the Division of Pulmonary Medicine.

These years also featured new programs at the MMC with exercise testing as part of pulmonary rehabilitation in patients with chronic lung disease, the first sleep testing for sleep apnea in Maine, inhalation challenge testing for the diagnosis of asthma, and transthoracic fine needle biopsy of lung masses and nodules using bi-plane fluoroscopy in the cardiac catheterization laboratory. Other programs were superseded by better methods such as venous ultrasound replacing impedance plethysmography in the diagnosis of deep venous thrombosis. In the SCU, intracranial monitoring techniques enabled critical care medicine physicians to participate in management of intracranial hypertension in a variety of clinical situations through protocols involving positioning, sedation, hypothermia, hyperventilation, control of glucose, and use of osmotic agents in support of neurosurgical patients giving a foretaste of neurocritical care in years to come.

Outpatient Pulmonary Medicine opportunities increased in several areas including occupational lung disease as the effects of asbestos exposure in the workplace brought requests for lung function testing, image interpretation, and patient consultation from retired shipyard workers as well as firefighters exposed to asbestos during the course of their employment. As these forms of pneumoconioses became less frequent through control of exposure measures more challenging illnesses replaced them in the form of hypersensitivity lung disease. The epidemic of lung cancer secondary to tobacco use and radiation exposure in the environment increased demand for diagnosis through bronchoscopy and the application of new diagnostic technologies in imaging. Collaboration with colleagues in thoracic surgery, pathology, radiation oncology, and medical oncology increased during these years along with efforts to decrease, or better end, smoking in Maine and making MMC a smoke-free environment. The efforts to actually eliminate smoking at MMC took far longer.

1980 to 1985 represented the beginning of new challenges on a global scale as well as in Maine and at the MMC in which the Division of Pulmonary Medicine and the Department of Critical Care Medicine rose to the challenges with the arrival of additional physicians with expanded areas of expertise. Dr. Francis Altman and Dr. Steven Zimmerman joined the Department of Critical Care Medicine. Dr. Altman joined after completing pulmonary medicine fellowship at the University of Florida under Dr. Jay Block. Dr. Zimmerman joined after his fellowship in pulmonary medicine at the Maine Medical Center. Dr. Zimmerman expressed an interest in working half-time. When this proposal was accepted he shared a single full time clinical position with Dr. Tooker. As a result Dr. Tooker had additional time to devote to administrative and program development projects. These projects included an intensive care medicine course in SCU for residents, physicians from around the state and fellows. Dr. Zimmerman believes this was possibly the first physician job-sharing arrangement at the MMC. Dr. Cox agreed knowing that he would get in return more than from a single full-time equivalent (FTE) clinician.

Dr. Cox and Dr. Gus Lambrew from cardiology supported the Outreach Council for Critical Care in assessing the needs of 15 critical access hospitals in Maine for a shared educational program by profiling services performed at the hospitals. A proposal for programs, on-site teaching with modules in a variety of services including neurosurgery, heart failure, ventilator support was created to name but a few. The program expanded over the years as part of wider collaboration among hospitals in Maine.

Dr. Altman had been additionally trained as a microbiologist and was Board Certified in Infectious Diseases, having previously completed an infectious diseases fellowship at the University of Pittsburgh Medical Center. His duties included developing a teaching program in critical care medicine for medical students and residents from all disciplines rotating through the units. Rotations on the pulmonary medicine consultation service for a week each month and an afternoon in the outpatient pulmonary clinic balanced out the working responsibilities.

Within a year of their arrival the first cases of acquired immunodeficiency syndrome (AIDS) began to appear at the MMC. Many presented with fever, wasting, and acute respiratory failure with diffuse pulmonary infiltrates due to *pneumocystis carinii* pneumonia. The same illnesses were being seen throughout the nation, especially in urban areas. The underlying disease was poorly treatable at the time, a problem coupled with concerns about risks of transmission during casual contact and routine care. Diagnosis generally required invasive measures including bronchoscopy, biopsy, and lung lavage before induced sputum methods were perfected. Support often required intubation and ventilator management until treatment with steroids and antibiotics could have an effect. All these measures required some level of personal exposure which was mitigated though precautions available at the time. Dr. Altman, in collaboration with infectious disease consultants, helped to develop protocols for diagnosis and treatment with the assistance of the other members of the Division of Pulmonary Medicine and Department of Critical Care Medicine. These protocols were used until better means of earlier diagnosis, multi drug antiviral therapy and primary prevention reduced the number of cases presenting with the late effects of severe immunosuppression.

During these years the educational programs in critical care medicine continued to evolve through efforts of Drs. Zimmerman and Altman. These included daily teaching rounds, radiology conferences in the SCU reading room attended by radiology staff, and the establishment of a current reference library for critical care medicine. Quality improvement measures developed through the efforts of Dr. Cox included nutritional support services, hemodynamic monitoring services, efforts to reduce nosocomial infections especially venous line infections and ventilator associated pneumonia. Measurable data was collected so the results at the MMC could be compared with like institutions throughout the nation. Another innovation was the assignment of an on-site dedicated social work staff to the SCU which facilitated open lines of communication between the families of patients and the care providers from all disciplines.

Growth continued in the Division of Pulmonary Medicine with increasing referrals for sleep apnea diagnosis and treatment leading to the establishment of a dedicated sleep laboratory with two technicians (Ms. Marge Montejo and Ms. Donna French) working under the direction of Dr. George Bokinsky. Initially the sleep laboratory shared space in the EEG Laboratory by using the facility at night when it was not otherwise in use. Two rooms were available and all data recorded on strip chart paper recorders for data reduction by hand prior to interpretation. Effective treatments other than tonsillectomy or tracheostomy were becoming available in the form of continuous positive airway pressure (CPAP). The demand for consultation, diagnostic testing, treatment using these new methods and monitoring of responses led to expansion of the outpatient pulmonary medicine clinic. The laboratory received its first accreditation for sleep disordered breathing diagnosis and treatment by the American Sleep Disorders Association. The development of the Maine Sleep Institute would follow from these early beginnings.

1982 represented a moment of transition in the leadership of the Division of Pulmonary Medicine with Dr. Caldwell passing the leadership baton to Dr. J. Mark Kjeldgaard after serving 11 years in the role of Division Director. This did not mark a transition into retirement for Dr. Caldwell but an opportunity for him to make two more lasting contributions to the Division. At age 59 he undertook an extended sabbatical in Texas. He returned with expertise in both the diagnosis and management of pulmonary hypertension and adult cystic fibrosis starting programs in both of these areas at the MMC that would eventually grow under the guidance of Dr. Joel Wirth in pulmonary hypertension and Dr. Jonathan Zuckerman for adult cystic fibrosis.

Advances in the management of pulmonary hypertension initiated by Dr. Caldwell soon followed. Using the computer-based exercise system developed at the MMC Dr. Caldwell measured cardiac output by Fick calculation, pulmonary artery pressures, and pulmonary vascular resistance under conditions of rest and controlled exercise. The measurement of cardiac output by Fick equation (which required measuring oxygen consumption and the arterial to mixed venous oxygen content difference) provided a more accurate measure of cardiac output in patients with pulmonary hypertension in whom low cardiac output states were poorly measured by thermodilution techniques. The hemodynamic response to intravenous prostacyclin (Epoprostenol) was measured to determine the efficacy of this form of therapy. Treatment was invasive with central lines and continuous infusion of vasodilators. MMC was one of four institutions in a collaborative clinical trial in 1990 to first report the results of this type of vasodilator therapy administered as a continuous infusion via a central venous catheter in the treatment of primary pulmonary hypertension. Drs. Caldwell and Williams were part of the Pulmonary Hypertension Study Group involving a larger number of institutions in a seminal article to appear later in the February 1996 volume of the New England Journal of Medicine. This form of therapy continues to be used in severe pulmonary hypertension.

Care of adults with cystic fibrosis follows from the survival of children with cystic fibrosis into adulthood. This necessitated an organized approach to this complex disease. Dr. Caldwell led the effort recruiting dedicated nursing and physical therapy support. Therapy focused on clearance of secretions from the airways, suppression of chronic infection using inhaled antibiotics and mucolytic agents, monitoring change in lung function over time with pulmonary function testing, and maintaining optimal nutritional state. The program grew over time as survival of adult patients increased. The current Adult Cystic Fibrosis Clinic at the MMC continues this tradition. Thus Dr. Caldwell made major contributions over extended points in time that determined the future of Pulmonary Medicine at the MMC through his insight and leadership.

The 1980's also saw the start of therapeutic bronchology at the MMC both in the Special Care Unit and in pulmonary medicine inpatient and outpatient settings. A Special Care Unit patient with pulmonary alveolar proteinosis was treated in the operating room under general anesthesia using the technique of whole lung lavage via a double lumen endotracheal tube by Dr. Altman using skills that he had acquired as a fellow at the University of Florida. He passed this skill to Dr. Bokinsky with its continuance in other patients over the years. It was informative to witness the gradual clearance on the sediment from the lungs as up to 20 liters were instilled and drained from a lung. Over time, experience and anesthesia techniques allowed this technique to become an outpatient procedure.

Additional therapeutic techniques were applied to non-resectable lung neoplasms obstructing central airways not amenable to radiation therapy often using a combination of laser photo resection and expandable airway stent placement. Dr. Bokinsky returned to the University of California, San Diego to acquire these skills from Dr. James Harrell. The procedure was used in palliation of symptomatic patients with non-resectable central airway malignant lesions but also benign lesions in non-surgical candidates due to co-morbidities. Stents were also used in the absence of prior laser therapy for obstruction resulting from compressing lesions not involving the mucosa and obstruction resulting from tracheomalacia or bronchomalacia. The need for these procedures was relatively infrequent.

Procedures in the Special Care Unit were more common including percutaneous tracheostomies, central venous line placement for monitoring of volume status for administration of vasoactive drugs or parenteral nutrition. Pleural catheters were placed to drain air or fluid from patients compromised by either pneumothorax or effusions. These became the practice of both the Critical Care Department as well as surgeons.

By the start of 1985 nine pulmonary medicine fellows had completed the program or were in the final year of training. They included Phillip Slocum, DO (1980-1982), Peter Bates MD (1981-1983), Lewis Golden MD (1982-1983), Peter Corrigan MD (1983-1985), and Rick Lambert MD (1984-1986).

Dr. Mark Kjeldgaard died suddenly from an acute illness on 25 October 1986. He had served four years as Division Director of Pulmonary Medicine. Dr. Bokinsky was appointed to replace him, supported at that time of crisis by his colleagues, members of the Departments of Respiratory Therapy and Nursing, and by the institution through hospital administration. Senior fellows shared in pulmonary attending responsibilities having completed this portion of their training and becoming eligible for board examinations. Services were continued and expanded with continued growth in sleep medicine, outpatient referrals, and ongoing development of new programs. The Department set about finding a replacement for Mark and was pleased when Dr. Bates agreed to return from Olympia, Washington the next year.

Dr. Bates returned to the MMC in 1987 joining the Pulmonary Medicine Division and Department of Critical Care Medicine and beginning a distinguished career at this institution. He established a multi-specialty conference with participation from pathology, thoracic surgery, radiation oncology, medical oncology, diagnostic radiology and pulmonary medicine. Patients would be presented, the details of clinical history and examination, radiographs, lung function status, and pathology discussed to determine stage of disease and best treatment options for the patient. This multidisciplinary effort evolved over time to become the Thoracic Oncology Center and continues to the present as a successful innovation.

Pulmonary fellows at that time included William B. Williams MD (1985-1988), Sandra Bagwell MD (1985-1988), and Scott Puringer MD (1986-1988). Drs. Williams and Bagwell were the first to complete a third year of fellowship training focused on critical care medicine as the third year of training had been recently approved. They would also go on to join the Department of Critical Care Medicine and Division of Pulmonary Medicine upon completion of their training.

Dr. Sandra Bagwell attended the University of Miami School of Medicine before coming to the Maine Medical Center for internship and residency in internal medicine which she completed in 1985. She was in the first group of graduates to have the third year in critical care medicine as an option. She recalls having a conversation with Dr. Cox before beginning the fellowship regarding the opportunity to develop specific skills that could be used at the MMC in the Special Care Unit. Pediatric critical care medicine, then under the direction of Dr. Cox, was viewed as most important. After agreement was achieved Dr. Cox arranged for the two of them to travel to Boston Children's Hospital to meet with the staff and visit the facility. Dr. Cox and the MMC provided salary and insurance support for Dr. Bagwell to spend six months training as a pediatric critical care fellow at Children's Hospital. Sandy recalls being given three pagers and a booklet of pediatric dosing information before taking all the call responsibilities of a pediatric critical care fellow.

Upon her return to the Maine Medical Center Dr. Bagwell became Chief of Pediatric Critical Care and sole member of the Section of Pediatric Critical Care. The pediatric

ICU was consolidated in SCU2 along with skilled nurses and respiratory therapists. Dr. Bagwell was supported by Dr. Al Dibbins serving as a mentor with whom to discuss difficult cases and from whom to learn skills necessary to meet the challenges she would face. Call support also came from pediatric neurology and nephrology until a second pediatric critical care attending was recruited in the early 1990's. Pediatric cardiac surgery provided additional admissions to the pediatric ICU as steady referrals from hospitals in the region demonstrated the need for a specialized pediatric transport system and team that Dr. Bagwell helped to organize and train. She also travelled with Dr. Tooker as part of the Critical Care Outreach Education Program. When Dr. Tooker ended his time as Assistant Chief of Critical Care Medicine, Dr. Bagwell took over that role eventually succeeding Dr. Cox as Chief of Critical Care Medicine.

Dr. Mark Kjeldgaard had become Division Director in 1982 and advanced many causes until his untimely death in 1986. Mark was deeply respected as a teacher, clinician, researcher, and for his dedication to the cause of preventing nuclear war as an early member of Physicians for Social Responsibility. In his memory the annual Mark Kjeldgaard Chest Conference was established and continues uninterrupted. He was a capable cabinet maker and builder of furniture. I fondly recall our long conversations and afternoons of skiing at Winter Park in Colorado following a long night of call during our residency.

These stories describe some of the major developments in Critical Care Medicine through the foresight and under the steady direction of its Chief, Dr. Cox and supported by his colleagues.

Dr. Tooker followed his interests in internal medicine joining Dr. Hillman as Assistant Chief of the Department of Medicine and as program Director of the internal medicine residency. He was active in the American College of Physicians serving as the Maine chapter Governor from 2000-2004. He was instrumental in the creation of the Maine Rural Health Network. His career took him to Philadelphia becoming the Executive Vice President and CEO of the ACP and President of AOA before retirement.

By the end of this story, 19 fellows had completed or were in the process of completing their Pulmonary and Critical Care training at the MMC. Along with those mentioned earlier, they included Paul La Prad MD (1987-1990), Frank DiTirro PhD MD (1988-1990), Richard Riker MD (1988-1991), Gary Schafer MD (1989-1992), Barry

Coalson MD (1990-1992), Kevin Brown MD (1990-1992), and Timothy Wells MD (1990-1993). Dr. Riker returned to MMC to continue his career in critical care medicine and make contributions in the areas of critical care research and critical care sedation. All have gone on to their careers well prepared for the challenges ahead.

The author thanks those contributing to this chapter for their recollections, insights, and editing skills. Susan Kjeldgaard Stiker, John Tooker MD, Frank Altman MD, Sandy Zimmerman MD, Sandra Bagwell MD, William B. Williams MD, Clifford Hoover RPT, and John Dzio for bringing to mind events from the early years and for reviewing this document.

RADIATION ONCOLOGY

By Stuart G. Gilbert MD

The last 60 years have witnessed a radical transformation in radiation oncology, largely due to the dramatic developments in computers, technology and advances in medical sciences.

During the 1950's and early 60's radiotherapy at Maine Medical Center (MMC) was supervised by three general radiologists, John Gibbons, Ernie Selvage and Charles Capron. They provided limited radiotherapy services using an Orthovoltage 250 KV machine which is a diagnostic x-ray machine "on steroids". This delivered good treatment for superficial tumors but did not effectively penetrate deep into the body. Attempts to give significant deep doses of irradiation often produced burning of the overlying skin.

In 1962 the first full time radiotherapy physician, Robert Bearor, came to Portland. Dr. Bearor was born in Madawaska and was a family doctor before he trained as a general radiologist with an interest in radiotherapy. Shortly after his arrival a cobalt machine was added to the Department's armamentarium. Unlike the orthovoltage machine, which works off of electricity, the beam from the cobalt 60 machine was

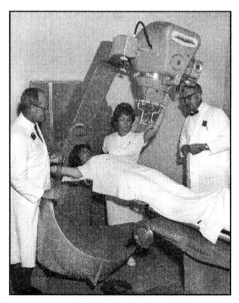

The new Cobalt machine with Dr. Charles Capron on left and Dr. Bob Bearor.

generated by a decaying radioactive source producing a 1.25 Mev beam. This beam was strong enough to penetrate through the skin and deposit its maximum dose more than one centimeter below the surface. This was state of the art therapy until the late 1960's when linear accelerators (linacs) were developed. These machines accelerated electrons and released a homogenous, well defined radiation dose. They were expensive to purchase and to operate, requiring radiation physicists, dosimetrists and highly trained service personnel to maintain and repair the equipment.

At this time a few hospitals in southern Maine had orthovoltage machines. As a result many Mainers went to Boston for up-to-date linac treatments. John Gibbons, the Chief of Radiology at MMC, realized that in order to justify and build a modern radiotherapy facility MMC needed a significant population base since it would require a multi-million-dollar investment that included purchasing a linac, constructing an enlarged facility and hiring additional specialized staff. He contacted all 17 hospitals in southern Maine, from York and Sanford in the south, to Bridgton to the west, and to Camden downeast. He convinced all of them that in order to provide state of the art radiotherapy services one central facility was needed that would service the area, not three or four hospitals that provided cobalt therapy. In 1970 all of the hospitals agreed and the Southern Maine Radiation Therapy Institute was created. Over the next few years the New Diagnostic Facility (NDF) Building was built at MMC housing a beautiful, large radiation therapy department with a 4 Mev linear accelerator and a simulator which was used to plan treatments. It opened in 1974.

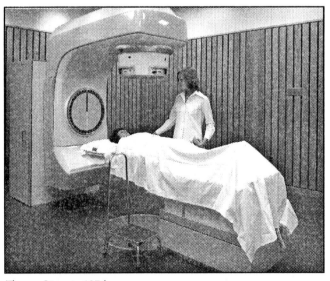

The new Linac in 1974

Dr. Bearor passed away from gastric cancer in 1970 and never saw the new Department. After his passing the general radiologists provided radiotherapy services for a brief time until Sidney Lowery, Maine's first fully trained radiation oncologist, was recruited from the staff at Tufts Medical Center. He was joined by Jake Hannemann in 1971 and by Hugh Phelps in 1973, both from Presbyterian Medical Center in Denver. In 1975 Dr. Lowery decided to return to his native Northern Ireland where he became Chief of Queen's University Radiation Oncology Department in Belfast. Stu Gilbert arrived in January 1976 from the Massachusetts General Hospital (MGH) followed by Chris Seitz in July 1977 from the University of Utah.

Another critical development occurred in 1974-5 when the state formed a committee to establish the guidelines for the future of radiotherapy in Maine. This committee was chaired by Jake Hannemann. It determined that Maine can best be served by having five centers, one each located in Portland, Lewiston, Augusta-Waterville, Bangor and Presque Isle. This would result in radiotherapy facilities located within a one-hour drive for 90% of the state's population. All of these centers except Presque Isle had

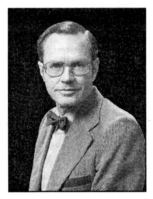

Dr. Jake Hannemann

a sufficient population base to justify a fully staffed and equipped modern center. Although Presque Isle did not have a sufficient population base, its remoteness justified part time coverage to provide the needed tertiary care to the local patients. These guidelines have served Maine well and continue unchanged to this day. The part time coverage for Presque Isle was provided by the Portland radiation oncologists for several decades.

A second linear accelerator was added in 1979 to replace the cobalt machine. The Siemens dual energy machine had 6 Mev & 18 Mev beams which allowed for better treatment for deep tumors and also provided electron beam therapy to treat superficial targets. We publically fundraised to purchase this new machine, emphasizing the major improvements it offered over previous available technology. Several patients delayed their treatment to be on the new machine. Unfortunately, we experienced a 50% down time for the first few months after installation of the unit. Siemens was able to get it running after each breakdown, but the problem was not solved for long. MMC threatened a lawsuit and finally Siemens sent an engineer from the factory in California. In three days he diagnosed the defect and finally fixed it. These are the issues one often faces with new technology.

The 1980's produced a dramatic increase in patients receiving radiotherapy. We attributed this to three causes; the acceptance of lumpectomy and radiotherapy as being equal to mastectomy in the treatment for breast cancer, the introduction of the prostate specific antigen (PSA) test to detect prostate cancer and the development of organ sparing surgical treatment with adjuvant radiotherapy for several tumors. In addition, our radiotherapy physicians actively "spread the word" by attending tumor conferences in our referring hospitals and speaking to community groups. Jake Hannemann, Stu Gilbert, Chris Seitz and Jeff Young all served as president of the local cancer society. Jake Hannemann and Stu Gilbert also served as President of the New England Society for Radiation Oncology. We all took John Gibbons' advice to heart, "you will remain a monopoly as long as you don't act like one".

In 1987 we realized that our two linacs were not enough to serve our patients and there was no easy way to build a third treatment room at MMC. We discussed among ourselves the possibility of building a satellite office and treatment facility that would be more convenient for our patients. Our physicians realized that this would be less efficient for us but better for the patients. We thought that the facility should be located in the mid-coast area since our patients from the Rockland region had to travel one and a half hours each way for their daily treatments. Before we approached MMC's administration we discussed it with the medical oncologists and surgeons in the six hospitals from Brunswick to Rockland. They were very excited about this concept and promised to strongly encourage their administrators and Boards to be supportive of the proposal. We then went to John Gibbons and then to Don McDowell, the President of MMC. Both were supportive of the plan and Don McDowell arranged for Stu Gilbert and him to meet with the Presidents of the other six hospitals. They met monthly but made little progress at first since the hospitals did not want to give a competitive advantage to each other. They also questioned MMC's motives of possible "invasion" into the mid-coast. Bill Caron, then a consultant for Ernest & Whinney, saved the day. He interviewed all six of the hospital CEO's and the chiefs of the medical staffs in their offices. They all agreed that there should be a free-standing facility containing only radiotherapy and it should be located in the Bath-Woolwich area.

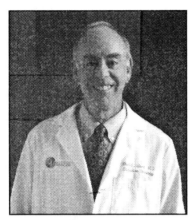

Dr. Stuart Gilbert

The Coastal Cancer Treatment Center opened in February 1993 in a beautiful new building in Bath with easy access to Route One. From the patient waiting room one can only see a pond and trees through the large windows. This satellite was truly a win-win situation. We increased our treatments in the mid-coast area and in the first 15 years of its existence the medical oncologists in the area went from two part-timers to six and a half full-time equivalents, four at Mid Coast Hospital in Brunswick, two at Pen Bay Medical Center and a part time oncologist at Parkview Hospital.

However, the demand for radiotherapy services continued to grow rapidly and the added capacity with a third linac in Bath did not approach satisfying the need. For this an additional facility was required. Please go to the chapter on Maine Med's Scarborough Campus for that story. See pages 336-343.

Further staffing additions to Radiation Oncology included Jeff Young in 1989 from the Mass General, Rodger Pryzant in 1992 and John Mullen in 1994, both from the MD Anderson Cancer Center in Houston. After eighteen years as Chief, Jake Hannemann stepped down and Stu Gilbert took over in 1992.

In the early 1990's radiation therapy was still a division of the Department of Radiology as were general radiography, nuclear medicine, angiography, CT, MRI and ultrasound. Our biggest problem was that our budget for new equipment competed with very expensive CT and MRI equipment which were evolving in dramatic fashion. The hospital agreed to purchase a new CT, MRI or linac each year and asked the Radiology Budget Committee to decide which one. With only one vote, radiation therapy was passed over for several years since our aging machines were still functional.

A major breakthrough for our Department, after several attempts, was the separation from Diagnostic Radiology. It was reconstituted as a distinct Department of Radiation Oncology. One of our first tasks was to get a full time Radiation Oncology Administrator. After several monthly meetings the hospital hired Terry Pickett, who was previously the administrator of a large radiotherapy center in Austin, Texas. One of Terry's first tasks was to review our billing codes and he identified several codes that were not being used for portal films and various physics chargers. The upgraded codes generated an additional $700,000 in billing for the hospital on an annual basis.

Over the following years we went on a buying spree bringing our Department up to date. This was greatly facilitated by Jake Hannemann. He had a close working relationship with the administration since he was very active on several MMC committees and eventually on the Hospital Board. He was able to convince the hospital to modernize our equipment. Stu Gilbert was the Chief from 1992 to 1998 followed by Jeff Young. We replaced our aging linacs and added the Scarborough Campus as well as a new third linac in the Portland area. We also purchased an Impac computer system that is designed for radiation therapy departments and this greatly reduced the risk of human error. This system combined the doctor's radiotherapy prescription with the instructions for treatment set up and the calculations of the dose. The computer was able to communicate directly with the linac so if there was any disagreement with what had been planned, such as the field size, the number of treatments or the blocking system that shaped the portal, then the linac would not be able to give the treatment unless the radiotherapist overrode the warning. All of the typed notes were on the computer and available to anybody in the department, no matter which office they were in.

Other new programs included:

1. Prostate implants: Chris Seitz had a special interest in interstitial (needle & seed) radioactive implants. Aided by his surgical training he developed a regional reputation and had appropriate cases referred to him from throughout Maine. In the mid 90's he went to Seattle for a week and took a course with Dr. John Blasko who had an international reputation since he pioneered many of the techniques for radioactive seed implants for prostate cancer. Interestingly, Dr. Blasko and Chris were first year residents in radiology at MMC when they both decided to go into radiation oncology, to the dismay of John Gibbons. Following his training with Dr. Blasko, Chris started a prostate seed implant program which was very successful. Rodger Pryzant also participated in the program and was able to continue the service after Chris' untimely death in 2002 in an avalanche while helicopter skiing in British Columbia.

2. High Dose Rate (HDR): In 2005 a HDR apparatus using an I-92 iridium source was obtained. This achieved better dose optimization and increased dose homogeneity. There was better patient safety with no further staff exposure to radiation and the treatment was faster and often given without hospitalization. Dr. Pryzant has had excellent results with the HDR prostate implants.

3. Intra-Operative Radiotherapy: In the 1980's Stu Gilbert started an intra-operative radiotherapy program for unresectable pancreatic cancer. This technique was introduced since this tumor needed a high dose of irradiation and was surrounded by several vital structures that were radiosensitive. The procedure started in the operating room, and if the tumor was truly localized, then the abdomen was temporally closed and the patient was transported down to radiotherapy while under anesthesia. On the linac table the abdomen was re-opened and a sterile cone was placed over the tumor and the local irradiation was delivered. We did eighteen successful cases over a two-year period, controlling local pain but we were unable to improve survival with this technique.

4. Pediatric Radiation Oncology: Before Jeff Young joined our Department in 1989 each of us covered the pediatric patients with challenging cases referred to Boston. Dr. Young had a special interest and training in pediatric radiotherapy and took over this section. He had a close working relationship with the pediatric oncologists at the Maine Children's Cancer Program (MCCP) and with the pediatric radiation oncologists at Boston Children's Hospital and at the MGH. He participated in several national pediatric oncology clinical trials.

5. Intravascular Coronary Radiotherapy: Dr. John Mullen performed this technique along with the cardiologists to reduce recurrent blockage of coronary arteries. This technique delivered a concentrated dose of irradiation via a catheter in the coronary artery to the area that was narrowed.

6. Mammosite high dose rate (HDR) radioactive implants: Dr. Celine Godin, who joined our Department in 2000 following her residency at Tufts Medical Center, used our HDR apparatus to give accelerated partial breast irradiation beginning in 2005. This technique spared much of the breast from irradiation and allowed for shorter treatment time, within one week, that was especially beneficial for our patients who lived a distance from our center.

7. GYN HDR Implants: Dr. Phil Villiotte, who trained at Duke University, came to MMC in 2009. He started the HDR implant program for cervical cancer in 2010. Previously these implants were performed with a two-day hospital stay and the irradiation delivered was from a Cesium-137 source. With HDR the patient could be treated as an outpatient with no irradiation exposure to the hospital staff.

8. Cranial Stereotactic Radiosurgery: In the 90's, Rodger Pryzant introduced this novel procedure to our Department. Rather than give a series of treatments to a brain lesion, this technique gave the tumor a lethal dose in one treatment with extraordinary accuracy. The neurosurgeons attached a metallic frame to the patient's skull in the OR and then the dosimetrists, physicists and Dr. Pryzant planned a single radiotherapeutic treatment to the tumor with very close margins using the landmarks of the metallic frame. Later that day the patient was treated. This treatment was well tolerated and had good success rates. Dr. Ian Bristol, who joined our practice in 2007 from his residency at MD Anderson Cancer Center, updated this technique in 2013 with a frameless system that made it much easier and more comfortable for the patient. This has allowed the treatment of multiple brain metastases with radiosurgical techniques, thus shortening the time for treatments.

9. Stereotactic Body Radiotherapy (SBR): Dr. Bristol and Dr. Neil McGinn, who joined our Department in 2003 after a residency at the University of Wisconsin and a staff position at the University of Michigan, introduced our department to this technique. SBR delivers intense targeted treatments using precise localization techniques and treatment planning. This technique has been used very successfully for patients with early lung cancer who are medically inoperable. This program has rapidly evolved to other indications, such as liver, spine and other solitary metastatic disease sites.

The transformation of radiation therapy can best be demonstrated by reviewing the evolution over the past 40 years in simulation of treatment fields, dose calculation and treatment planning and how we delivered those treatments.

1. Simulation: When I was first introduced to radiotherapy during my general radiology residency, I planned the treatments using a diagnostic x-ray machine with metal markers placed on the patient's body. We occasionally used a fluoroscope to assist in tumor localization. At the MGH and at MMC, we had a simulator that could fluoroscope and take radiographs. We could project a lighted field and adjust the size from the control booth.

The major subsequent advance was a simulator with fluoroscopy and CT capability. We took a series of CT scans through the area of interest and then were able to visualize the tumor on a computer monitor and with a mouse draw the tumor's outline on the computer. We were also able to outline structures that we wanted to protect, such as the spinal cord or the eyes. This gave us a three-dimensional target to plan our treatments.

2. Calculation and Treatment Planning: Early in my training we calculated our treatment dose using a slide rule and a depth dose chart and equivalent square calculation. As we progressed and the treatment machines became more sophisticated the treatment planning process became more complex, dosimetrists and radiation physicists became involved. With the information we obtained from CT images, we were able to plan treatments that treated the tumor in multiple directions. The advent of advanced radiotherapeutic computer programs and modern linacs has allowed us to deliver higher doses to the tumor and protect the surrounding, uninvolved tissue.

3. Treatment machines: I have treated skin lesions with an orthovoltage apparatus and had at least a cobalt machine to treat tumors. At the MGH we had a 2Mev Vander Graff accelerator that was two stories tall. The evolution of the linear accelerators over the past 45 years has been truly amazing. Our first linac at MMC was a 4 Mev unit that produced a well-focused beam through a variable rectangular field. We were able to shape the beam using lead blocks that were placed on a table over the patient or screwed to a holder in a lateral position. The blocks were replaced by an in-house manufactured block that was poured to order, using a dense metal compound, Cerrobend, which had the density of lead but the melting point of wax. This was replaced by a mechanical block on the linac that had a series of 1 cm wide "fingers" made of lead that moved in and out of the field from opposing sides to shape the treatment portal.

Under Neil McGinn's leadership as Chief, we have updated our linacs so that our patients can benefit from the latest technical advances. Our linacs used 3-D treatment planning and delivered the treatment via intensity modulated radiation therapy (IMRT) which treated with multiple, shaped beams on a 'stop and shoot' basis. This treatment usually took forty minutes to deliver. Our new linacs can treat with volumetric modulated arc therapy (VMAT), which allows us to treat with a continuous gantry motion and the size of the field and the blocking varies with the angle of the gantry. This sophisticated treatment can be given in five minutes. In addition, we can now treat in 4D mode as the treatment can be synchronized with respiratory motion. Previously, when treating a small lung cancer you had to treat an area to cover the tumor throughout the respiratory cycle, but with gating, you can use a smaller field and cover the tumor with less lung tissue damage.

Our treatment accuracy has benefited from using patient restraints which more securely hold the patient in a comfortable position that can be reproduced on a daily basis. Tumor localization has also improved from using implanted metallic fiducial markers and daily cone beam computer tomography that is attached to the new linacs.

In this era of Google, medical information is readily available and the change is remarkable. I had a patient with breast cancer who I saw in the 80's. Mastectomy was the standard treatment at that time but she had read about lumpectomy and radiation therapy and wanted that treatment. She quoted several research papers and I asked her how she obtained all that information. She told me that she went to the library, looked up the topic in the Index Medicus and then called around for a medical library that had those cited articles and then went to the library and made copies. Today any patient can get that information on their home computer.

Another change is the ability to transmit medical information. I was at our Bath facility when a patient from Boothbay Harbor with metastatic lung cancer called to tell me that he was having significant back pain and trouble walking. I called for a CT scan to be done in the local hospital. Five minutes later the radiologist called and suggested a plain x-ray to start. Thirty minutes later he called and asked me to look at the x-ray on my computer with him. We discussed the findings and agreed to hold off on the CT scan. The patient was in Boothbay Harbor, I was in Bath and the radiologist was in Scarborough. That amazed me.

The technical skills of our radiotherapists (the technologists who deliver the treatments) were greatly enhanced by creating our own school in conjunction with Southern Maine Community College in the early 80's. Scott Soehl was recruited and started the school and he was ably followed a few years later by Dennis Leaver. Our first class was predominately from our own staff who were initially trained as Diagnostic Radiology Technologists and not Radiation Therapy Technologists (RTT). Our first graduating class had the highest average of any school in the country on the national certifying examination and our Vicki Frost had the highest individual grade on the exam. Over the years our school supplied RTT's to the other Maine and New Hampshire hospitals and several of our graduates distinguished themselves nationally. Our school provided an education that helped many young Mainers to acquire a well-paying job and a fulfilling career. In the 1990's the chief radiotherapists at both the MGH and the Harvard Joint Center for Radiation Therapy were women from Maine.

An important measure of how well our Department did its job is how satisfied our patients and their families were with the care they received. In the late 1980's, Bettsanne Holmes was the Chair of the MMC Board of Trustees. Her pet project was doing patient satisfaction surveys and using them to improve patient care. During this time we had medical staff dinners and a lecture on the second Thursday of each month at which over one hundred and fifty physicians attended. One month Mrs. Holmes presented the results of the patient survey with no identification of individual departments, inpatient floors or individual personnel. She reported that 91% of patients were pleased, while a few percent complained about the food, parking and noise in the hospital. At the end of her presentation, one of the surgeons said that he thought this survey was not that useful since if a patient just delivered a baby then she would be thrilled with the experience and everything would be wonderful. However, the feedback wouldn't be as positive if a patient had a serious medical issue. Mrs. Holmes answered that she too was concerned about how the reason for the admission could affect the patient's response but was pleased to note that the Department that had the highest patient satisfaction in the entire medical center was radiotherapy. She added that these patients, with cancer, would have every right to be displeased.

Another experience occurred at Pen Bay Medical Center. At that time, I arranged to see a few follow-up patients from that area in the clinic after attending the monthly tumor conference. As I was examining a patient, she turned to a Pen Bay nurse in the room and told her that "the Radiation Therapy Department in Portland is such a busy place but I always felt as if I was their only patient".

Patient satisfaction and good patient care and caring require staff that is there for the right reason; to treat patients with respect, kindness and concern for their well-being. We were truly fortunate to have such a staff, from the receptionists, transcribers, radiotherapists, nurses and physics personnel. We worked as a team and helped each other and I am sure the patients and their families were reassured by that relationship.

Radiation Oncology

I am proud to say that the Department continues to be in excellent hands. It has been accredited by the American College of Radiology since 2006 and is headed by Dr. Neil McGinn. We have continued to recruit outstanding radiation oncologists, Dr. Matt Cheney in 2015 from the Harvard program and Dr. Jullian Johnson in 2016 from University of California at San Francisco.

I would like to acknowledge the contribution of Dr. Rodger Pryzant who provided valuable information about the Department's accomplishments over the last decade.

Radiology

By Roger T. Pezzuti MD

History Of Radiology at the Maine Medical Center

The Beginnings:

The modern era of Radiology in Portland began with the arrival of John Gibbons MD as the new Chief of Radiology in 1955. However there were antecedents that came before Dr. Gibbons which are worth reviewing. These antecedents set the stage for what would develop once a staff of formally trained Radiologists arrived in Portland in the mid 1950's.

Radiology services in Portland were available soon after the discovery of "x-rays" by Wilhelm Conrad Roentgen in 1895. Maine Medical Center Archives first mention x-ray examinations as early as 1906. The Maine General Hospital Annual Report of 1908 reported that a Dr. Smith requested x-ray equipment adaptable to the demands of surgical work. Was Dr. Smith's request a precursor to portable and intra-operative radiography? The 1908 report also noted that a Dr. Bradford and others had contributed monies to be used to purchase "proper" x-ray equipment to be used in the basement of the Maine General Hospital building.

In the early 1900's the hospital's x-ray equipment was reportedly owned by a non-physician named E. Paul Getchell. He was identified as the "operator" of the x-ray unit or units at the hospital.

In a Maine General Hospital report from 1915-16 it was mentioned that x-ray equipment that would "meet all requirements" would cost in the range of $1200.00. This was likely a substantial sum and percentage of the institution's capital budget at that time.

The first mention of a "Radiology Department" in the archival record is dated 1917. In the 1922 Maine General Hospital Annual Report the increasing use of X-ray services was noted. The report stated that the Department was "one of the most important in the hospital". E.P. Getchell was identified as the department "roentgenologist", with no mention of any physician "roentgenologists".

In 1928 after a reported 50% increase in the number of x-ray exams from the previous year it was recognized that larger space and physician leadership were needed for the

Department. That year Langdon Thaxter, an orthopedic surgeon, was appointed as roentgenologist. Though he was not identified as "chief" until 1941, he served as the leader of the Department until 1948. In 1928, a nurse, Bertha Bernard, was listed as the x-ray technician.

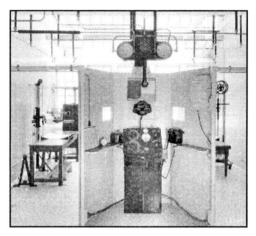

New Victor X-ray machine 1932

By 1940, the physician staff in the Department of Radiology included Dr. Thaxter, along with Associate Roentgenologist Jack Spencer MD and Frank Lamb MD as "consultant". William Holt MD was Director of Radium Therapy, representing the first known archival reference to the use of radiation for therapeutic purposes at Maine General Hospital. The Radiology Department exam volume in 1940 was reported to be 11,726 total x-ray exams.

Dr. Spencer succeeded Dr. Thaxter as Chief of Radiology in 1949 and remained in that position until the arrival of John Gibbons in 1955. There is no archival information as to Dr. Spencer's education or training as a radiologist (roentgenologist). Drs. Thaxter and Spencer were, however, members of the Radiological Society of North America. Together they published an article discussing the radiographic evaluation of acute small bowel obstruction in the Society's journal, Radiology, in November of 1947. In 1938 Dr. Spencer and Dr. Thaxter were permitted by the hospital to open a private x-ray office away from the hospital. This suggests that they were a "private practice" and not hospital employed, which was the practice configuration that was in place when Dr. John Gibbons was recruited to take over the Department in 1955.

The decision to recruit Dr. John Gibbons coincided with the merger of the Maine General Hospital, the Children's Hospital, and the Maine Eye and Ear Infirmary to form the Maine Medical Center (MMC), a process which began in the early 1950's and took several years to complete. This is well described in The History of Maine Medical Center written by Martha Fenton and published in 2012. As the merger was reaching its final stages, the 1956 Pavilion - a major 2 year long building project - was being completed. This new wing included the Radiology Department on the basement level. As Dr. Spencer stepped down as chief in December of 1954 the MMC Board sought new leadership for the department. Dr. Gibbons, whose radiology training was at the University of Pennsylvania under the legendary radiologist Eugene Pendergrass, was recruited from one of the leading medical institutions in the nation, Massachusetts General Hospital (MGH) in Boston, where he was a young attending.

The John Gibbons Era, The Early Years: 1955 – 1970:

The first staffing additions made by Dr. Gibbons as he built the Department were Irving (Ernie) Selvage MD and Charles (Cape) Capron MD who were hired by 1956. Both were strong clinicians and teachers and together with Dr. Gibbons formed a solid staffing core for the Department.

Dr. Selvage did his residency in radiology at the University of Pennsylvania as had Dr. Gibbons. Dr. Selvage was recruited from his initial practice in Presque Isle, Maine. He had an excellent understanding of the physics and the engineering of radiologic equipment. He used this knowledge for teaching technology students and residents for decades until his retirement in the mid 1980's. Dr. Selvage was the radiologist responsible for bringing diagnostic ultrasound to the Department in the early 1970's.

Dr. Capron was a Board Certified radiologist particularly known for his teaching abilities. He became the physician director of the radiologic technologist program that he created in the later 1950's, in conjunction with long time department employee and Chief Technologist Catherine O'Connor. Dr. Capron introduced mammography

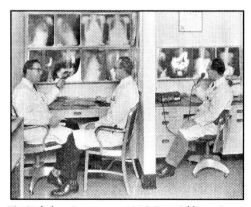

The Radiology Department 1956, Drs. Gibbons, Capron and Selvage

to Maine Medical Center. For several years he was the sole radiologist who interpreted these studies which were at that time performed using a xerographic technique.

In the late 1950's and 1960's the Department had six or seven diagnostic rooms. These included rooms for standard radiography, a linear tomography unit, and fluoroscopy that required special glasses and a period of dark adaption before the radiologist could perceive the fluoroscopic images. One room had a "Franklin Head Unit" that was used for neurologic studies, including pneumoencephalography. This was a painful procedure for the patient no longer necessary due to the subsequent development of computerized axial tomography (CT) and magnetic resonance imaging (MRI) scanning. The Department of the 1960's offered limited angiography, including carotid arterial injections performed by neurosurgeons and peripheral arterial injections mostly performed by surgeons. This preceded the introduction of arterial and venous catheters and dedicated angiographic x-ray equipment in the late 1960's and 1970's.

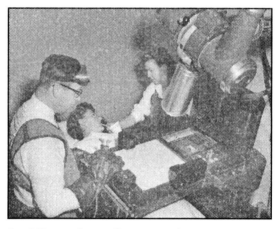

Dr. Gibbons performing floroscopy 1956

In order to support and expand the Department's commitment to education, a formal radiology residency program leading to eligibility for board certification was created around 1960. This was a key factor in the development of the modern Department. Starting a residency program required a major commitment of time and energy on the part of the radiologists. Prior to 1960, individual physicians had apprenticed at the MMC Radiology Department, learning how to perform and interpret radiology exams. Participants were mostly general physicians from around the state who wanted enough training to allow them to serve as the local "radiologist", without formal certification. One individual, Dr. Al Poulin trained in radiology for three years in the early 1950's and later practiced in Waterville. There is no record of any other radiology residents at MMC for the remainder of the 1950's.

Dr. Dick Taylor, the first official radiology resident under John Gibbons' leadership started the three year program in 1960 after a one year internship at MMC. Dr. Taylor went on to practice radiology in Lewiston at St. Mary's Hospital. He was followed in 1961 by Linwood Rowe, a general practice physician from Rumford, Maine. Dr. Rowe became the radiologist for the new Rumford Community Hospital. Others that followed in the mid 1960's included Robert "Pat" Andrews, who practiced in Bangor, Al Swett, who became a radiologist at the Mercy Hospital in Portland, and Jim Binnette, whose practice was in Biddeford. Dr. Bob Milsovic, who was in the program in the late 1960's, was the first resident hired by the practice group upon completion of his residency to fill an acute need for staffing in radiation therapy. He eventually moved on to a career as a diagnostic radiologist in Bennington Vermont. Dr. Andrew Packard, who started his residency in 1968, was the second resident hired back by the group after completing a fellowship in angiography at Tufts in 1972. Nearly all of the early residents, ten of the first 12, practiced radiology in Maine.

In 1962 Bob Bearor was added as the fourth radiologist. He was the first specialist in the Department. He was hired to operate the new Cobalt 60 therapy unit and to develop a Radiation Therapy Division. In the early 1960's the separation of therapeutic and diagnostic radiology was not yet complete. General radiologists were still expected to cover both the diagnostic and therapy divisions of the Department. This would continue through the 1960's, and become an issue following Dr. Bearor's untimely death from stomach cancer in 1970. For about one year after his death, the Division was covered mostly by former MMC resident Bob Milsovic, until a permanent replacement was found in the person of Dr. Sidney Lowery. The subsequent development in the 1970's of the Radiation Therapy Division is fully described in a separate chapter.

Other staff additions in the 60's included H. Randall Deming, in 1966, who came to MMC following his radiology residency at the University of Vermont. By preference he became the Department's designated neuroradiology expert, and later the Chief when Dr. Gibbons stepped down in 1984.

In 1968 Drs. Roland Ware and Russell Briggs, the first two diagnostic subspecialists, were added.

Dr. Ware was the first formally trained angiographer at MMC. He arrived with knowledge of catheter technology learned at the MGH and at the Hammersmith Hospital in London, England. Dr. Ware established a robust angiography division particularly admired by the resident staff.

Dr. Briggs came to MMC in 1968 following his fellowship in nuclear medicine at the University of Wisconsin in Madison. He brought knowledge and experience with the newer nuclear medicine cameras, known as gamma cameras, which were first developed for routine clinical use in the early 1960's. Nuclear medicine had previously been practiced outside of the Department under the direction of an internist, Dr. Stan Herrick. Upon Dr. Briggs' arrival, the Division was moved into the basement space adjacent to diagnostic radiology where it still resides. Dr. Briggs was a strong clinician and teacher throughout his career. He served for decades as an American Board of Radiology examiner. The award for teaching excellence in the department was named after Dr. Briggs at the time of his retirement in the early 1990's.

By the end of the 1960's the radiology staff that began the decade as three had more than doubled to seven, including three subspecialists. A respected teaching program for radiologic technology and a diagnostic radiology residency program leading to board eligibility were in place. This pattern of growth and subspecialization was replicated over the ensuing decades and continues to the present. It is important to note that the successful development of the physician practice group and the Radiology Department were made possible by the cooperative efforts between the hospital and the radiologists. On the surface, this may seem a formula for conflict and gridlock, given the fact that the hospital owns and maintains the physical plant, technical staffing and equipment and the radiologists provide the professional component of the department's work. The arrangement, though not always perfect, thrived through the years. Dr. Gibbons and the early radiologists deserve much credit for creating the excellent working relationship that exists to the present time. Dr. Gibbons and his colleagues from the onset strived to be key players in the hospital and its culture. Whether it was the weekly radiology case teaching conferences referenced by many early MMC residents as the academic highlight of their week, participation in hospital medical staff work, or fund raising, the radiology group has consistently played an important role in the affairs of MMC and its medical staff with obvious benefits to all involved.

Second Half of the Gibbons Era: 1970 – 1984

Additions to radiologist staffing in the 1970's included Andy Packard in 1972, Tony Salvo in 1974, Reed Altemus and Don Bittermann in 1977 and Barbara Luke in 1978. Drs. Packard and Altemus were fellowship trained subspecialists in angiography and neuroradiology respectively. Because there were no retirements during this timeframe this brought the total diagnostic staff by the end of the 1970's to eleven, including four subspecialists. This growth was driven not only by the general increase in the use of radiology as a key diagnostic tool but also by the revolutionary changes in available imaging technology beginning in the 1970's. The first diagnostic ultrasound machine in radiology at MMC was acquired in 1974. In 1976, the first CT scanner was installed. MRI was being developed for clinical imaging in the 1970's, and came to Portland and MMC in the 1980's. Equipment for angiography was evolving rapidly. In the late 1970's two new angiography rooms were installed. One of these was dedicated to peripheral vascular work and the other to neuroangiography. These new or upgraded technologies had significant impact on the development of many clinical departments at MMC including the neurosciences, vascular and oncology services. This positive impact on growth of clinical capabilities at MMC has increased over time as technologies have continued to mature.

In 1974 the "new diagnostic facility" was completed with movement of the pharmacy and lab out of the basement shared with radiology. Expanded space for radiology was used for upgraded multidirectional tomography, dedicated mammography, two new modern fluoroscopy rooms and ultrasound. A radiology conference room was created along with space for the radiology teaching file, an educational office, and new physician and administrative offices. Two radiography rooms were established in the Richards Wing basement to serve the needs of inpatients as well as Emergency Department patients. This represented the first "decentralization" of radiology services. Later in the 1990's decentralization would become a key feature of the Department.

The residency program in the 1970's was becoming better established with its six total slots (two per year for three years) filled by 1980, largely spurred by the expanding and more subspecialized radiologist staff. The addition of the six-week Armed Forces Institute of Pathology course in Washington and the three month Children's Hospital of Boston rotation significantly augmented the educational experience. Although this away time for the residents created staffing challenges the educational value of these rotations was judged to be worth the extra work.

In 1979 the radiology group practice, at that time a partnership of eleven diagnostic radiologists plus four radiation oncologists known as Radiology Associates, was incorporated into a professional association. The new corporation, "Gibbons, Deming and Radiologists, PA", was deemed desirable, even necessary, to allow the group to take advantage of tax, pension and liability benefits afforded by a corporate structure. This also was a highly equitable arrangement for the physician owners/shareholders, all of whom had an equal share in corporation governance. It fostered a culture of shared ownership and responsibility on the part of the shareholder physicians. In the mid 1990's, the successor PA, "Radiology Associates of Maine" was a founding member of the multispecialty group, Spectrum Medical Group, whose formation and history are detailed in a separate chapter.

The last five years of Dr. Gibbons' tenure as Chief, from 1980 – 1984, saw the addition of three more subspecialists - Bob Isler in 1980, Charles Grimes in 1983 and Roger Pezzuti in 1984 with fellowship training in chest (body imaging), pediatrics, and nuclear medicine respectively. All were destined to play important roles as Departmental and corporation leaders. Dr. Isler was instrumental in the development of capabilities for CT of the chest, abdomen, and pelvis. Bob would later become Managing Partner of the practice group and eventually Board Chairman of Spectrum Medical Group. Drs. Pezzuti and Grimes each became MMC Radiology Department Chairman.

Between 1980 and 1984 Departmental space expanded significantly into previous hospital classrooms A and B which respectively became the new file room and reading room. This was made possible by the creation of the Charles Dana Health Educational Center with its multiple classrooms and meeting spaces. John Gibbons played a key role in the combined building projects that resulted in the creation of the Dana Center and the Bean Wing in the early 1980's. His leadership resulted in the medical staff of MMC raising $3 M for these projects which according to "The History of Maine Medical Center" set a national record for hospital medical staff philanthropy at that time. This serves as an excellent example of the cooperative and mutually beneficial relationship between the radiologists' private practice and MMC.

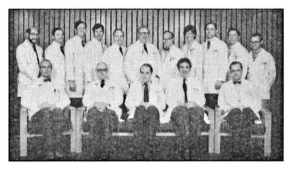

The Radiology Group 1980. Front row Drs. Deming, Capron, Ware, Blinick, Hannemann. Back row Drs. Bittermann, Altemus, Gilbert, Seitz, Briggs, Gibbons, Selvage, Luke, Salvo, Phelps, Packard.

The Initial Years Post Gibbons, 1984 – 1989:

John Gibbons stepped down in 1984 after 29 years as the Radiology Department Chairman. H. Randall Deming, who had been second in command of the Department for many years, became Chairman from 1984 - 1987. He was succeeded by Russell Briggs, the longtime Nuclear Medicine Division Director, whose term as Chief extended to 1989. Despite their relatively short terms, these two leaders were responsible for significant progress between 1984 and 1989. Staff additions included Tod Abrahams (musculoskeletal radiology) in 1986, Steven Amberson (angiography) in 1987, Brett Applebaum (neuroradiology) in 1987, Matt Ralston (neuroradiology) in 1988 and Christopher Pope (musculoskeletal MRI) in 1989. With these additions the diagnostic radiology staff numbered 15 including 11 fellowship trained subspecialists.

The additions of Drs. Applebaum and Ralston were particularly critical as the Department had lost its only fellowship trained neuroradiologist when Dr. Altemus resigned in 1986. They insured the Department had a world class team of neuroradiologists as neurologic imaging exploded with the development of CT and MRI.

Dr. Chris Pope proved to be pivotal to the development of the Department and the practice group. He implemented major improvements in the new MRI division, particularly for musculoskeletal MRI. Dr. Pope significantly stimulated scholarly activity, as well as efforts to measure and improve quality in the Department. He also played key administrative roles as Assistant Chief of the Department in 1994, Managing Partner of the practice a year later and as the key physician leading the effort to form Spectrum Medical Group in the mid 1990's.

During the second half of the 1980's the first MRI was installed in Portland in a private office setting as a partnership of the radiology practices at MMC and Mercy Hospital, along with the neurosurgery and neurology groups and some individual physician investors. Simultaneously, planning for MMC's first hospital-based MRI was underway. This multiyear hospital MRI project, which had to go through the stringent certificate of need process, was completed in late 1989. It required construction of an 8000+ square foot space below ground under the Dana Building and next to radiation therapy. The expense of this project, including equipment purchase and building costs, was in excess of $6 M.

The 1990'S to Y2k:

After developing coronary disease requiring open heart surgery in November 1988, Dr. Russell Briggs stepped down as Radiology Department Chairman in February of 1989. He was succeeded by Dr. Roger Pezzuti, first as interim then as the permanent Chairman in September of 1989. This transition came at a pivotal time for the practice as the group was rapidly expanding and becoming more subspecialized. Radiologists hired in the 1950's and 60's were retired or near retirement. Although MMC pressured the group to bring in an outside radiologist as Chairman Dr. Pezzuti's experience as Medical Staff President at York Hospital in the mid 1970's and leadership in the effort to bring MRI to Portland made him the preferred candidate following a national search. He remained in the position until September of 2004.

Decentralization of the Department accelerated through the 1990's beginning with the establishment of an outpatient imaging facility near the Maine Mall which opened for patient studies in February 1989. This imaging center included plain film radiography, fluoroscopy, ultrasound and mammography. About a year later an imaging facility was established in Falmouth on Bucknam Road. When MMC established its outpatient campus on Route One in Scarborough in the early to mid 1990's a large imaging component was included. The Scarborough imaging center has continued to expand over the years and now includes CT, MRI and positron emission tomography (PET)/CT scanning, along with mammography, ultrasound and standard radiography. The footprint of the Department in the Richards Emergency Department area expanded to include ultrasound and two CT scanners. Movement of imaging resources away from the core space of the department was recognized as important in order to bring imaging to where patients were being seen and treated both at the hospital and away from the congested main MMC campus for outpatients.

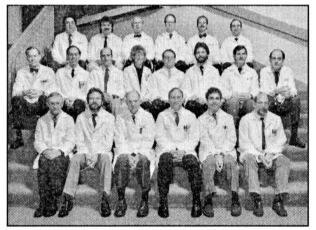

The Radiology Group 1990. Front row Drs. Packard, Abrahams, Briggs, Pezzuti, Applebaum, Bittermann. Middle row Drs. Hannemann, Gilbert, Isler, Luke, Amberson, Young, Seitz, Ware. Back row Drs. Blinick, Pope, Deming, Ralston, Grimes, Salvo.

The residency program, under the dedicated leadership of Dr. Tony Salvo, continued to thrive in the 1990's. The hospital approved a third slot for each of the three years of radiology training. This resulted in an increase in the number of residents in the department from a total of six to nine. By the mid 1990's, related both to the popularity of radiology nationally as a career path and the growing reputation of the Department's training program, the number of applicants to the MMC Radiology Residency grew steadily to as many as 50 or more applicants per available slot. Residents completing the program were finding excellent fellowship opportunities at highly respected university medical centers, followed later by excellent job placements.

Radiologists added in the 1990's included the following physicians:

Barbara Biber, gastrointestinal radiology (1991)
Jennifer Fife, ultrasound (1993)
Jonathan White, nuclear medicine (1994)
James Place, general radiology (1995)
Ken Cicuto, interventional radiology (1995)
Brian Brock, nuclear medicine (1995)
Thomas Dykes, interventional radiology (1995)
Elizabeth Pietras, mammography (1997)
Andrew Landes, pediatric radiology (1997)
Michael Quinn, nuclear medicine (1998)
Andrew Mancall, neuroradiology (1998)
Sharon Siegel, body imaging (1999)
Steven Winn, musculoskeletal radiology (1999)
Eddie Kwan, neurointerventional radiology (1999)
Bernadette Jakomin, body imaging (1999)

These additions brought the number of Diagnostic Radiologists in Spectrum Radiology South (Portland) to 25 by the year 2000. Of these all but three were fellowship subspecialty trained, greatly enhancing the group's expertise and including a fresh generation of individuals who would take on important leadership roles. Examples included Dr. Biber who became Director of the Residency Program after Dr. Tony Salvo held that position for 22 years. Dr. Quinn became Division Director of Nuclear Medicine after Dr. White resigned in 2006 and he also became the group's Managing Partner in 2008, succeeding Dr. Bob Isler. Dr. Mancall provided critical leadership for several of Spectrum Radiology's contracts outside of MMC in the mid 2000's and he went on to become Department Chairman at MMC in 2013, succeeding Dr. Charles Grimes. Drs. Fife, Dykes, Pietras, Winn and Siegel became Division Directors.

The expansion of the Department's space and imaging equipment inventory in the 1990's was considerable. By the beginning of the new millennium the Department had four CT scanners, two MRI's, two new digital angiography suites, five flouroscopy units, along with a range of fixed and portable ultrasound and plain radiography machines. These were distributed over a decentralized Department that included the recently renovated main department, the ED, the Brighton, Falmouth and Scarborough campuses of MMC as well as the MMC operating rooms.

Not surprisingly, given this growth procedure volumes continued to increase steadily through the 1980's and 90's. By the end of FY 2000 total procedure volume was nearly 180,000. This included 90,000 plain film and fluoroscopic studies, 28,000 CT's, 10,500 MRI's, 17,400 US's, 13,300 mammography exams and 4,000 angio-interventional procedures. Comparative Department procedure volumes had been about 65,000 in 1980 and 110,000 procedures in 1990, evidencing the success of the cooperative arrangement between Spectrum Radiology and MMC. Given the critical role radiology services play in the care of most patients treated at MMC, this success supported further development of every hospital service area.

Y2k to the Present:

After 2000, growth of the radiology group and the Department at MMC continued as in previous decades with at least another 18 radiologists added to the Department between 2000 and the writing of this chapter in early 2017. However, counting of "MMC" radiologists has become increasingly complex because the work of the group practice now includes outlying hospitals such as Southern MaineHealth in Biddeford, St. Mary's in Lewiston, Memorial Hospital in North Conway, and Miles Memorial in Damariscotta. Key staffing additions included Drs. Paul Kim, Joe Gerding, Chris Baker, and Derek Mittleider in Angio Interventional, Dr. Steve Farraher in Musculoskeletal and Dr. Scott Fredericks in MRI. These individuals all became clinical and administrative leaders in their areas of interest. Dr. Fredericks succeeded Dr. Biber as Residency Director in 2009. Dr. Kim and later Dr. Mittleider became Division Directors of Angio-Interventional Radiology (IR). Dr. Gerding, together with Dr. Ken Cicuto, were key to the development of interventional oncology. Dr. Baker was instrumental in restarting the neurointerventioal program at MMC after Dr. Kwan resigned in 2008. As of the writing of this chapter, Spectrum Radiology in Portland counts about 38 diagnostic radiologists with a substantial portion of their work done at non-MMC facilities.

Department leadership changed in 2004 with the appointment of Dr. Charles Grimes as Chairman. He provided excellent leadership for nearly a decade. Dr. Andrew Mancall followed him as Chairman in 2013, continuing to serve to the present. Under the guidance of these two individuals the Department has continued to thrive despite the ever increasing challenges and complexity of our nation's medical care system. Interestingly in 2014 when Dr. Mancall and the Department needed a new Residency Program Director, Dr. Grimes, then the Chief Emeritus, volunteered to take on that responsibility. This attests to his outstanding commitment to providing Department leadership.

Nuclear medicine added an important new modality with the addition of mobile PET in 2008 and PET/CT in 2011. These services are provided by a partnership, Maine Molecular Imaging that includes both MMC and Spectrum Radiology. PET and PET/CT play a key role in cancer staging, with important developing applications in neurology and cardiology. MMC plans to create a fixed PET/CT center in Scarborough sometime in the near future.

Residency expansion continued after Y2K increasing the training program to 16 residents by 2006, with four approved slots per year for four years of radiology residency training. Recently, one of these slots has been converted to an AI residency/fellowship track because of the strength of the AI Division and its popularity with the residents at MMC. Interest in the residency program remains remarkably strong with greater than 100 applicants per available slot annually and even stronger interest in the AI fellowship slot.

The Picture Archiving and Communication System (PACS) was implemented in 2001. This was a critical development with profoundly positive effects on all clinical services at MMC. Prior to PACS implementation the Department progressively experienced more and more difficulty handling the increasing volume of studies recorded only on film. There were inevitable problems with lost films resulting in significantly negative effect on the quality and efficiency of medical care at MMC, particularly in the OR where prior imaging is absolutely necessary for good outcomes. Years of attempts to understand and remedy the radiology film library issues during the 1990's had unfortunately failed. It was eventually recognized that a digital solution would be the only means of overcoming the problem. Leadership in moving to a digital, eventually filmless, solution to the film library problem was shared by Spectrum radiologists and administrative staff from the Department, along with the hospital's information services (IS) department. Included were the project's lead physician, Dr. Matt Ralston, Department head administrator Alex Szafran, and Bob Coleman from IS.

The cost for PACS was nearly $6 M. Implementation was challenging. But from the moment it was installed the positive effect of PACS on patient care was obvious. Doctors located nearly anywhere in the region could see patient studies online. Studies were not "lost" because the single film based record had been misplaced or was temporarily in the hands of another physician. Physicians could see imaging studies from the office or from home. This vastly shortened the time needed for them to make a diagnosis and formulate a treatment plan. When seeing patients in their offices physicians could easily display the relevant imaging studies on a desktop computer, greatly enhancing communication regarding diagnoses, treatment options, and response to treatment. Growth in the number of archived images on PACS has been spectacular starting at about 180,000 exams in the first year. By 2014 about 700,000 exams per year were being added to the system. The total number of exams archived in PACS by 2014 was nearly 6,000,000. These studies come from nine hospitals, including MMC, as well as 12 imaging centers. Non-MMC volumes currently accounts for 70% of the archived exams.

Once PACS was in place at MMC efforts began to extend the system to include other MaineHealth affiliated hospitals and other medical facilities. This project became known as Consolidated Imaging (CI)-PACS. Other participants included large radiology departments such as those at Southern Maine in Biddeford and St. Mary's in Lewiston, as well as smaller departments including Stephens Memorial Hospital and Miles Memorial Hospital. Also included were office practices such as Martins Point, Orthopedic Associates and Intermed. CI-PACS became a huge project that over the past 16 years has greatly increased the ability of physicians in our part of Maine to access their patients' images and provide better patient care. CI-PACS, while owned by MMC, is governed by a joint-venture type board comprised of individuals from Spectrum, MMC and MaineHealth. This is another example of excellent cooperation between the hospital and the radiologists from Spectrum. Individuals from Spectrum who played major roles in the development of CI PACS were Drs. Matt Ralston and Steve Winn and the CEO of Spectrum, David Landry.

When considering the development of Spectrum Radiology and the Radiology Department at MMC it is evident that every division of the Department has experienced impressive growth and expanding clinical applications of their imaging technology, increasing the imaging capability available to physicians and their patients. Also important to better patient care has been the participation of radiology in many of the weekly educational and patient care centered conferences at MMC. Examples include Tod Abrahams for rheumatology, Bob Isler and Mike Quinn for thoracic oncology, and Elizabeth Pietras for breast conferences. Another positive institutional effect of improved imaging includes the emergence of CT as the initial imaging technique for most critically ill patients evidenced by two fully utilized CT's in the Emergency Department of MMC. The expansion of mammography services, now including tomosynthesis and stereotactic biopsy, has played a key role in improving the detection

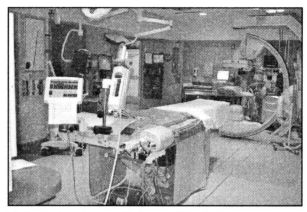

Modern Biplane Angiography Suite used largely for neurointerventional procedures, 2017

and treatment of breast cancer. Similar comments can be made for ultrasound, nuclear medicine, musculoskeletal imaging and MRI.

The Division of Angiography and Interventional Radiology (IR) deserves specific mention for several reasons, including not only the significant expansion of diagnostic and treatment options made available to MMC patients, but also to the particularly important role IR has played for our radiology residents and their careers. The Division was initially developed by Dr. Roland Ware in 1968 and expanded with the hiring of his protégé, Dr. Andrew Packard in 1972. The Division grew steadily through the 1970's and 80's, initially with a focus on diagnostic angiography of the peripheral vascular system. In the late 70's neuroangiography was expanded with the addition of Dr. Altemus. Interventions in urology were developed, along with transhepatic and biliary interventions introduced by Dr. Packard. In the late 80's and early 90's, led by Drs. Packard and Amberson, peripheral vascular interventions were introduced - first angioplasty and then angioplasty with stenting. In the late 1990's, Dr. Eddie Kwan joined the department and began to perform neurointerventional procedures such as aneurysm coilings and carotid stenting. These were totally new procedures to the state of Maine, previously requiring patient transfer to Boston. Although Dr. Kwan left the Department in 2008 the service was restarted several years later with the addition of a neurosurgeon, Dr. Rob Ecker and shortly thereafter Dr. Chris Baker with dual fellowships in IR and neuro IR. Interventional neuroangioraphy remains a critical service offered in the IR Division of Radiology and has expanded significantly in the past five years with the development of intra-arterial acute stroke thrombolysis.

In the mid 1990's Dr. Thomas Dykes joined the IR Division, later to assume its leadership. Together with the Vascular Surgery Division of MMC he developed the highly successful collaborative aortic stent graft program for the treatment of abdominal aortic aneurysms in the late 1990's. This technique was new to the United States at the time, being performed only at a few large regional medical centers. The program in radiology at MMC included approximately 300 aortic stent graft placements over a ten-year period. These were mostly performed in the specifically designed AI suite installed in the Department in early 2000. This program was arguably one of the most successful in the nation at the time, with no fatalities related to these initial 300 procedures. After about a decade, related to competitive issues between the performing services, the program moved primarily to the OR under the Division of Vascular Surgery. However this does not detract from the great success of the Departmental program in introducing this new and highly sophisticated procedure to MMC.

One of the outstanding aspects of the IR Division has been the tremendous career interest it has generated in the radiology residents training at MMC. Perhaps related to the residency program being relatively small and without angiography fellows, MMC's radiology residents have always enjoyed a "hands-on" IR experience perhaps explaining why a large percentage of the residents have become intensely interested in IR. Many have chosen IR for their subspecialty fellowship training, and these residents have often been recognized as "stars" in these fellowship programs. Between 1971 when Dr. Packard chose an IR fellowship at Tufts and 2017, 25 residents of a total of about 125 have made IR their career choice. This is considerably more than any of the other subspecialties.

Looking to the Future:

Certainly no one can confidently predict the future, especially for something as large and dynamic as our medical care system. But no matter what comes to be, the radiology practice group and the Radiology Department at MMC are well positioned to thrive. The level of clinical expertise in the Department is comparable to that present in large university programs around the nation. Administrative support for the radiologists through Spectrum Medical Group is outstanding. The same can be said for the administrative and technical support in the department. IS support through MMC and Spectrum remains strong both for the Department and CI-PACS. The volume of work is remarkable and continues to grow. The radiologists have been able to spread out their base of operations to many facilities outside of Portland. More recently they have established support for off hours work via creative arrangements with radiologists outside the state, some as far away as Hawaii. This allows for true 24 hour "real time" reading of all emergency studies by attending level radiologists, a major improvement in the care of inpatient and Emergency Department patients at MMC. But perhaps as important as anything, the "partnership" mentality between Spectrum Radiology, which is a physician owned private practice, and MMC which is the state's dominant medical center, is as strong as ever and continues to serve both parties well.

Author's Note:

This chapter was a cooperative effort including many colleagues and friends in radiology at MMC. These include but are not limited to Drs. Packard, Isler, Grimes, Salvo, Ralston, Pope, Ware and Dykes. Mary Duffy, Alex Szafran and Bob Coleman of radiology administration, and Jocelyn Leadbetter, the MMC archivist, provided significant factual support. And Dr. Dick Taylor, the first resident in MMC's Radiology Residency Program helped out immensely with the early history of the modern department that otherwise would not have been available. Also, the editing assistance of Drs. Gilbert, Blattner and Weisberg as well as my wife Margaret was critical to the effort. To these and others I consulted during the process, my sincere thanks.

RHEUMATOLOGY

By Larry G. Anderson MD

The field of rheumatology, like so many other areas of medicine, progressed dramatically in the period from 1970 to 2000. Before then, caring physicians provided emotional support and symptomatic relief to Maine patients with diseases like rheumatoid arthritis, which left unbridled, often led to crippling deformities of multiple joints. In this chapter we will explore how the Maine Medical Center (MMC) rheumatology community developed from those early pioneer physicians who entered the field with an extraordinarily limited armamentarium to a robust group practice named Rheumatology Associates that provides patients in our area with cutting-edge therapies to control rheumatic diseases like rheumatoid arthritis.

By 1970 physicians had brought rheumatology experience from Boston to the Portland area. General internist Dr. Philip Thompson spent time with some of the early giants in rheumatology during his training at Massachusetts General Hospital. After working at the Robert Breck Brigham Hospital in Boston, Dr. Melissa Weekly started her rheumatology practice in Portland before relocating to Farmington. After training at the Brigham, Dr. Robert Ritchie, known as the "father" of Maine's biotechnology industry, founded the Foundation for Blood Research (FBR) in the early 1970's. The FBR became one of Maine's first independent, nonprofit medical research and education institutes. The Foundation was dedicated to identifying, managing and preventing human disease through clinical and laboratory investigation. Under Dr. Ritchie's leadership, FBR amassed one of the world's largest clinical databases of serum protein results used for research of a wide range of diseases.

The story of Rheumatology Associates begins with the pivotal decision by Dr. Paulding Phelps to leave academic medicine and enter private practice. He was, indeed, the catalyst that changed rheumatology in the Portland area. Educated and trained in Philadelphia, where he played a major role on the faculty of the University of Pennsylvania Medical School, Paulding had all the triple-threat attributes of clinical skills, natural teaching abilities, and an inquisitive research mind to succeed in academia. His research resume included seminal advances in our understanding of the pathogenesis of crystal-induced joint disease like gout, under the guidance of his mentor Dr. Daniel McCarty, internationally recognized in the field. But, like so many of his future partners at Rheumatology Associates, Paulding realized that what he most enjoyed was taking care of patients. He began searching the country for the best place for a practice, one most in need of rheumatology care and most fitting for raising his family. Portland and the Maine lifestyle, including great opportunities for skiing and sailing, fit the bill. He moved here and started a solo practice in Portland in 1971. The practice grew rapidly and by 1974 he felt the need to expand his practice in terms of space and partners.

Three other private-practice physicians partnered with Paulding to purchase land and build the brick building at 180 Park Avenue in Portland. Each level of the two-story building was divided between two practices: Dr. Bill Leschey in neurology and Paulding in rheumatology on the first floor and Dr. Ron Carroll in oncology and Dr. Jack Davies in internal medicine on the second. Years later the building was expanded to accommodate practices in orthopedic surgery (Drs. Donald Booth and Chip Crothers who went on to help form Orthopaedic Associates) and in ophthalmology (Drs. Bill Holt and Elizabeth Serrage who grew their practice into the Eyecare Medical Group). All of these practices eventually expanded and left the building.

In the summer and fall of 1974 Paulding recruited Drs. George Morton and Larry Anderson to join him, followed by the formation of Rheumatology Associates. While we surrounded ourselves with legal, accounting, and insurance advisers, Paulding was the business mind behind the practice. It took a leap of faith (in Paulding) for us to sign papers to buy into even a small fraction of financing 180 Park Avenue. Words like "accounts receivable" and "depreciation" were not part of our lexicon as we left our fellowship training.

We had monthly evening meetings to resolve issues and fine tune the practice. A turning point was hiring a business manager, Wayne Quimby, whose experience and expertise greatly improved our efficiency and productivity, in areas ranging from human relations to later computerization of the practice. Wayne addressed equitable sharing of overhead expenses, a major challenge in a private practice. He helped design a system of dividing our expenses into fixed (front office salaries, utilities, etc.) which we shared equally and those with uneven use of resources (our individual nurse salaries, proportional use of lab and x-ray, etc.). Wayne was instrumental in guiding our decision to leave 180 Park Avenue and find new space to accommodate the growth of the practice.

Our search for a new practice site led to the discovery of a large empty Sewall Street lot once owned by the railroad. Having experienced the value of having our practices close together at 180 Park Avenue, Rheumatology Associates purchased one sixth of the lot and Orthopaedic Associates (Don Booth, Chip Crothers, and Doug Brown) purchased the adjoining eastern half. We were the first medical group to build on Sewall Street, a building designed by architect Sam van Dam and constructed with oversight provided by Wayne. Our humble wooden office building was eventually dwarfed by ever-expanding brick edifices by Orthopaedic Associates and the Medical Eye Group. The north side of Sewall Street is now lined with medical buildings.

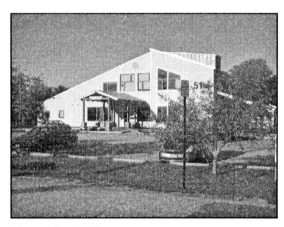

Rheumatology Building

Our initial concerns about having sufficient patients to sustain the practice with three rheumatologists evaporated quickly and at various times as the practice grew the waiting times for new and established patients became unacceptable. In the late 1970's we eventually added Dr. Lewis Cogen to the practice, followed by Dr. Marc Miller in 1981. The good chemistry of our interpersonal relationship was key to the ongoing success of our practice. During the course of our busy workdays, each of us would invite one or more of our group into his office or exam room to share an interesting clinical feature or seek advice about a challenging patient. We also celebrated each other's family events, such as births and adoptions of children and their later weddings. Dr. Lewis Cogen's sudden cardiac death at age 51 in 1991 greatly impacted each of us emotionally. Fortunately the successor partners to the practice assured the continuity of good chemistry, camaraderie, and clinical excellence: Dr. Charles Radis for Lewis, and Dr. Brian Keroack for Paulding and Dr. Brian Daikh for Larry upon their retirements, and others to follow in later years.

Rheumatology Associates was one of the first group practices in Portland to invite a Doctor of Osteopathic Medicine (DO) physician to join the practice. Dr. Charles Radis DO had grown to love Maine during his Public Health Service assignment to serve Peaks Island and other Casco Bay islands. Known to us as a caring and talented physician from sharing patients and consultations at Brighton Medical Center, Chuck had completed strong rheumatology fellowship training in Pittsburgh and was a prime candidate to fill the practice void created by Dr. Lewis Cogen's death. In 1993, the proposal to change the bylaws to include DOs on the MMC Medical Staff was very controversial. We advocated the position that the Medical Staff would be strengthened by inclusion of osteopathic-trained physicians, a position that was confirmed when the bylaws were revised and excellent physicians like Chuck and many other DOs were subsequently embraced by MMC physicians involved in both practice and residency training. Also, in 1998 our practice was among the first in the community to hire a physician assistant, Betsy Evans, who helped increase the breadth and depth of our professional care.

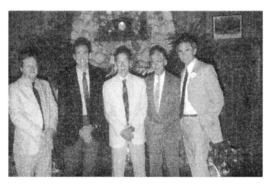

Drs. Lewis Golden, Marc Miller, George Morton, Paulding Phelps and Larry Anderson

The rheumatologic care of our patients also benefitted from the diversity of the training of our partners. We learned from one another about best practices from among the top rheumatology training programs in the country: University of Pennsylvania (Paulding Phelps and George Morton), Robert B. Brigham Hospital (Larry Anderson), University of Michigan (Lewis Cogen and Brian Keroack), Beth Israel Medical Center (Marc Miller), University of Pittsburgh (Charles Radis), and University of Rochester (Brian Daikh).

From the beginning of Rheumatology Associates, the three original partners established systems to assure we stayed current with advances in medicine and rheumatology. We rotated the duty of leading monthly journal clubs to review pertinent articles. We pledged that at least one of us would attend national meetings and report back to those covering the practice back home. Early on we initiated the weekly Rheumatology Conference at MMC. From its inception our conference has started by reviewing x-rays and other imaging studies from our office and MMC with each other and an MMC radiologist, eventually usually with bone and joint specialist Dr. Tod Abrahams. There has always been constructive and informative interaction with our orthopedic colleagues during the first half hour of conference. Only a door at 180 Park Avenue separated our practice from Drs. Don Booth and Chip Crothers who attended our conferences regularly and helped educate us early on about the nuances of carpal tunnel, lumbar spinal stenosis, and total joint replacement. There followed many regular orthopedic conference attendees. Other health professionals like physical and occupational therapists also attended and contributed to the conference sessions. The last hour of conference was devoted to presenting interesting and challenging patients from the office and hospital admissions and consultations, sometimes followed by trips to the floors to interview and examine patients at the bedside. A few years ago we recognized the 40th anniversary of these weekly conferences and noted that the conference was attended most faithfully over the years by Dr. Phil Thompson.

Teaching has always been an important part of our careers. Under the leadership of Chiefs of Medicine Dr. Al Aronson and then Dr. Bob Hillman, MMC residents in internal medicine were assigned monthly rotations with us. Involved in helping care for our admissions and hospital consultations, the residents were expected to present cases at conference, with critique and feedback about their style of presentation. Each resident was expected to present a conference talk after in-depth review of some topic that captured their attention during their rotation. The residents also shadowed us at the office during their rotation. That experience with the residents led to lifelong professional friendships with physicians still active in medicine in Portland and throughout the state. Continuing our group's commitment to teaching and generously sharing his exceptional diagnostic and teaching skills with MMC medical residents, Dr. Brian Keroack in recent years has been the recipient of MMC Teacher of the Year Awards.

One of the MMC medicine residents, Dr. Brian Daikh, perhaps inspired as much by his rheumatologist brother as by his rotation with us, went on to a rheumatology fellowship in Rochester and then accepted an offer to join Rheumatology Associates, where he continues to practice and carry on the tradition.

Our practice also contributed to advances in rheumatology on a national scope. Paulding became active in the American Rheumatism Association (ARA) and in 1987 ascended to the presidency, the 48th ARA president and the first from private practice and not from the academic community. He was instrumental in leading the change in name and structure from the ARA to the American College of Rheumatology. Shortly after his presidency, the ACR created the Paulding Phelps Award, an annual recognition of someone in private practice who has made significant contributions to the ACR and to the field of rheumatology. The annual award continues to this day. Another major contribution from our private practice is that Marc Miller was the original editor of the section on muscle disease of UpToDate.

Success in building a private practice relies heavily on the quality of the supporting staff.

We were very fortunate to carefully to evaluate new hires that were not only conscientious hard workers but also were equally focused on providing excellent medical care. The practice culture included "patient-centered care" and "team approach to care" long before these terms became buzzwords in quality improvement. The majority of our hires stayed with the practice for many years. Two of our original receptionists later became our practice managers. Excellent people ran our laboratory and x-ray and later DEXA and investigational drug studies. Because of the limited mobility of many of our patients, we offered part-time physical therapy to augment our patient education about coping with joint disease. Each of us hired his own nurse, who, along with the front office, PT, lab and x-ray personnel, was as important as the physicians in building patient rapport and trust. The esprit de corps of our office staff remains among our fondest memories of the practice.

It is challenging to find words to articulate the depth of camaraderie and collegiality among the MMC Medical Staff in the 1970's and 1980's. Fostered by monthly staff meetings in the cafeteria, a doctor's dining room at lunchtime, and departmental meetings in small rooms, the staff numbers were few enough that nearly everyone knew one another. The Medical Staff meetings were not to be missed, not only for their informational but also for their entertainment value. Relationships with colleagues were formed and deepened by hospital encounters, such as meeting midway on the flights of stairs between floors in the Richards Wing during late evening admissions or consultations. Conversations there included not only exchanges about mutual patients but also catching up on each other's families and happenings in our practices.

Relationships are important. Many rheumatologists choose their specialty because of the appeal of developing relationships with patients with chronic illness and their families over the years. That expectation was realized by those of us at Rheumatology Associates during our practice careers. Just as important for professional fulfillment are the relationships physicians develop and nurture with colleagues. We valued the professional relationships with each other and our staff at Rheumatology Associates and with our fellow physicians and other health professionals in the Portland community as the practice grew and matured. Changes in the health care delivery system and the significant growth of the MMC Medical Staff may have reduced some of the rewards we experienced during the founding years of our rheumatology practice in Portland. The higher bar for hospitalization has resulted in fewer of our patients being admitted which, along with shorter hospital stays, has resulted in less time for interaction with fellow physicians and other MMC health care professionals. Some of the richness of inter-physician communication by phone or office and hospital records has been eroded by the boilerplate, non-colorful language of the electronic medical records. Increased demands on physicians' time like documentation of quality measures and prior authorization for both imaging studies and medications have encroached upon the time physicians often used to communicate directly with their colleagues and even their patients. We can only hope as these systems mature and improve that we can enrich this much-needed facet of medical practices. The relationships doctors form with their colleagues and patients are the wellsprings that strengthen us to care for the sick and must remain a fundamental component of physicians' lives.

The growth of the MMC and its Medical Staff and advances in rheumatology from 1970 to 2000 were remarkable. In the early days of Rheumatology Associates our waiting room was filled with patients with crutches and hand and other joint deformities. New aggressive approaches to treating rheumatoid arthritis with methotrexate and biologic response modifiers, along with total joint replacement and other reconstructive joint surgery, have greatly improved patient outcomes. We have always been proud of the quality care that MMC and our medical community provide and we greatly admire and respect the primary and specialty expertise of our colleagues. Further, we continue to attract highly qualified and well-trained physicians, insuring that this tradition of excellence continues. However, we cannot forget that the foundation for this success was laid by our physician predecessors. With gratitude we reflect upon our humble beginnings and appreciate what Dr. Paulding Phelps and other key leaders in each of the medical and surgical specialties did to help the Maine Medical Center fulfill its mission as the leading medical care, teaching, and research center in northeastern New England today.

We gratefully acknowledge contributions to this chapter and editing suggestions from Drs. Brian Keroack, George Morton, Marc Miller, Charles Radis, David Giansiracusa, and Ronald Anderson.

Urology

By Samuel B. Broaddus MD

Urology has had a long and distinguished history at Maine Medical Center (MMC). Prior to 1945, either general practitioners or general surgeons with an interest or training in urology during their residency provided most urological services. In the 1950s MMC surgery residents would occasionally rotate on the "urology service". A paper from the 1952 Journal of the Maine Medical Association detailed just such a rotation.

In the middle of the 20th century, there was a shift away from this general approach toward more specialized urological services provided by board-certified independent private practice urologists.

Dr. Donald Marshall has been acknowledged as the first American Board of Urology certified urologist in Maine. Dr. Marshall was born in Portland, grew up on Munjoy Hill, and attended Portland High School. He graduated from the University of Maine in 1931 and then attended Yale University School of Medicine from which he graduated in 1936. He did his residency training in surgery and urology at Strong Memorial Hospital in Rochester, NY. Following his training he and his wife moved to Norfolk, VA, where he practiced urology until the outbreak of WW2. He served with the U.S. Army Eighth Evacuation Hospital from 1941 through 1944. At the conclusion of the war Dr. Marshall returned to Maine and practiced urology in Portland at MMC from 1946 to 1975.

Prior to the initiation of Medicare Dr. Marshall was known to treat his patients without charge if they were unable to pay. In addition he never charged members of the clergy or teachers. He served as Chief of Urology at the Maine Medical Center for most of his career. During the late 1960's he became motivated to "muster the medical and political forces" to start a kidney transplant program in Maine. Dr. Marshall obtained advice from other transplant programs including the Medical College of Virginia, John Hopkins Hospital, and New York Hospital. Maine's U.S. Senator Edmund Muskie lent his support and contributed to the success of the program's development. The first renal dialysis machine was acquired by MMC around 1961 and Maine's first kidney transplant was performed in Portland in 1971. This represented a remarkable collaboration between the divisions of urology, nephrology and vascular surgery. Dr. Marshall, MMC nephrologist Dr. Jan Drewry, and MMC vascular surgeon Dr. Ferris Ray described the program in the October 1973 issue of the "gold journal" of Urology.

Dr. Marshall died in 2001 at the age of 93 at his home in New Harbor, ME. Since the beginning of the transplant program 46 years ago, over 1500 renal transplants have been performed at Maine Medical Center as of 2017. MMC urologists who were involved with the program performed donor nephrectomies and recipient ureteral reimplantations until 2000 when fellowship-trained transplant surgeon Dr. James Whiting assumed surgical leadership of the renal transplant program.

Dr. Frederick Clark, originally from Pittsford, NY, joined Dr. Marshall in 1950. Fred earned his undergraduate degree from the University of Rochester and his medical degree from the New York City College of Medicine. As a veteran of the Korean War, he served abroad at an Army hospital in Seoul. Fred was well known as an affable, knowledgeable and well-respected urologist by his patients and colleagues. Besides his work at Maine Medical Center, he also provided the only urologic care for the Webber Hospital in Biddeford for many years. That hospital predated the newer Southern Maine Medical Center. He retired in 1985 and died in 2005.

Most urologic surgery performed in the 1950's to 1970's involved either open surgery or endoscopic bladder and prostate surgery. The technology for minimally invasive urologic procedures for renal and prostate cancers did not yet exist. Transurethral resection of the prostate and open prostatectomy were the most common prostate procedures at MMC and necessitated dedicated cystoscopy operating room staff and ward nurses who were knowledgeable in catheter care and irrigation. Routine diagnostic cystoscopies were often performed as inpatients until office cystoscopies became routine in the 1970's. Stone surgery was done almost entirely via open approaches. These were usually tedious affairs with extended hospital stays for convalescence. There was some capability of performing retrograde pyelograms in the OR but there was little that could be done to manage upper tract pathology except with open surgery. Percutaneous kidney stone removal, ureteroscopic stone extractions and the placement of ureteral stents would not become available until the 1980's with the development of specialized and miniaturized equipment with improved fiberoptic instruments. The learning curve to perfect these techniques would be steep.

In the mid 1970's, prostate biopsies were only done in the OR under anesthesia using digital guidance of palpable prostatic nodules. Most diagnosed prostate cancers were associated with locally advanced or metastatic disease. Patients with high stage prostate cancer were treated with either palliative orchiectomies or oral diethylstilbesterol. Radiation therapy was beginning to become a common treatment modality for these patients. Transrectal ultrasound of the prostate would not appear in an office setting until the late 1980's. Prostate specific antigen was not discovered until 1979 and didn't become clinically available as a screening test until 10 years later. Screening for prostate cancer with periodic digital rectal examinations and PSA tests would not become routine until the mid 1990's. Following the introduction of these screening tests cancer stages migrated to more treatable and curable prostate cancers.

Besides Dr. Marshall and Dr. Clark, three other urologists played a pivotal role in the development of urology at Maine Medical Center from the late 1950's-1970's.

Dr. Hugh Robinson arrived in Portland to practice urology in 1958. Hugh grew up in Portland under the shadow of Maine General Hospital where his father was the Chief of Surgery and the first Board Certified general surgeon in Maine. When he was just 16 Hugh began his undergraduate studies at Bowdoin College. After 2 years in the Navy working as an operating room technician at St. Albans Hospital in NYC, he attended the University of Rochester School of Medicine then traveled to the Mayo Clinic where he received his urology training under the tutelage of Dr. Ormond Culp, one of the preeminent endoscopists of his time. Upon his return to Portland, Dr. Robinson started a private practice in a back room of surgeon Dr. Isaac Webber's office. He brought the technique of "cold punch" prostatectomy (which he had learned at the Mayo Clinic), and in so doing brought transurethral surgery and the management of obstructive voiding symptoms in Portland to a whole new level. Hugh was also the first urologist to provide services at Stephens Memorial Hospital, a tradition among MMC urologists that continues to this day.

Dr. Robert Timothy completed a urology residency at the Peter Bent Brigham Hospital in Boston and also received training from D. Innes Williams, a renowned pediatric urologist in London. Bob developed a reputation as an astute and talented adult and pediatric urologist, often receiving referrals from other urologists around the state. He was considered the Maine expert in the performance of ureteral reimplantations for pediatric ureteral reflux disease. He also began performing vasectomies in volumes that seem a bit far-fetched today (20+ in a day with technician Jim Cummings setting up 3 procedure rooms at the hospital). Bob retired in 1999.

Dr. Andrew Iverson, a Falmouth native, graduated from Bowdoin and Tufts University School of Medicine. He completed his surgical training at MMC followed by a urology residency at the University of Minnesota under Dr. Elwin Fraley, one of the giants of American urology. Upon his return to Maine, Andy practiced in Portland until 2003.

In 1975, Drs Clark, Robinson, Timothy and Iverson formed Portland Urologic Associates (PUA), which at the time was the largest group of urologists in Maine. Their building sat on Vaughan Street directly across from the then front entrance to the hospital. MMC staff could always depend on the PUA urologists to be "there in a minute." In addition, other independent urologists set up practices in Portland during the 1970's and held privileges at MMC. These included Drs. Bruce Nelson who received his urology training at UCLA, John Dyhrberg (University of Minnesota) and James Pringle (McGill).

In 1984, in anticipation of Dr. Clark's retirement, Dr. Sam Broaddus (a Westbrook native who trained at UVM) was hired by PUA bringing an interest and expertise in minimally invasive urinary stone management. He performed the first percutaneous renal surgery in Maine and was instrumental in bringing the first non-invasive shock wave lithotripsy unit to Maine in 1989.

Dr. Brian Jumper, a Bath native who also trained at UVM was the first fellowship trained pediatric urologist in the state, hired by PUA in 1989. He quickly developed a solid reputation among Maine pediatricians and parents as a technically gifted, passionate and caring pediatric urologist. He was the first urologist in Maine to introduce laparoscopic surgery to the pediatric population.

For over 4 decades, the advances and improvements in urological care and service at MMC would never have been possible without the unwavering support of its dedicated urologic OR nursing staff. These nurses included Annette Dufresne, Lucretia Salvatore, Sue Nelson, Elaine Kerr among many others.

In the early 1990's, the 4 PUA urologists (Timothy, Iverson, Broaddus, and Jumper) took call responsibilities for a week at a time without resident coverage, often receiving referrals from throughout Maine for their specific expertise. Over the next 11 years, 3 other urologists were hired, all with specific sub-specialty expertise: Dr. Thomas Kinkead (UMass, Worcester,1997), Dr. Moritz Hansen (Stanford, 1999), and Dr. Lisa Beaule (Lahey Clinic, 2000).

Collaboration with other specialists at MMC has played an important role in the development of more advanced urologic technologies and services for the last 4 decades. Dr. Marshall's collaboration with nephrologists and vascular surgeons helped create the renal transplant program in 1971. Drs. Andrew Iverson and Broaddus collaborated with MMC radiation oncologists Drs. Rodger Pryzant and the late Christopher Seitz in the early 1990's bringing radiation seed and implant therapy for prostate cancer management to MMC. Collaborations between interventional radiologists and urologists allowed for the development of percutaneous renal access and percutaneous renal stone surgery. Dr. Broaddus worked with gastroenterologist Dr. Douglas Howell on the management of patients with impacted pancreatic stones that were either unreachable or unmanageable with pancreatic ERCP. Together they treated more than 100 patients with shock wave therapy and were among the first to publish their results in the US. Drs. Kinkead and Jumper have had a successful collaboration with MMC pediatricians with the Spina Bifida Clinic. More recently, the creation of the MMC Stone Center and the MMC Pelvic Medicine and Reconstructive Surgery Program have been examples of continuing cross-specialty collaborations.

In order to better serve the regional urologic needs of patients, many local urologists worked at smaller community hospitals on a weekly or monthly rotating basis. These hospitals included the Webber Hospital in Biddeford (Dr. Fred Clark), Stephens Memorial Hospital in Norway (Drs. Hugh Robinson, Sam Broaddus, and Graham VerLee), Memorial Hospital in North Conway (Drs. Robert Timothy and Andrew Iverson), and St. Andrews Hospital in Boothbay Harbor (Dr. Sam Broaddus). In addition, pediatric urology clinics were conducted on a regular basis by Dr. Brian Jumper at a variety of sites.

Visiting Professors of Urology enhanced and showcased the MMC urology program during summer urologic symposia and featured the likes of nationally renowned urologists Drs. David Crawford, Jonathan Epstein, Robert McConnell, and Thomas Stamey, among others.

In 2001, a urologic teaching relationship developed between PUA, MMC and Lahey Clinic. Prior to this, MMC general surgery residents (interns, PGY 2 and 3 level residents) would rotate for several weeks with PUA staff to gain exposure to basic urological diagnoses and procedures. Lahey Clinic chief and senior urology residents rotated on the MMC urology service for several months at a time, augmenting their surgical volume and case complexity, as well as showcasing the MMC program to another highly respected academic program in New England. This relationship ended in 2003.

With the expansion of the Urology Division at MMC, an office move to the present location in South Portland at the "Castle" was completed in February 2006 with Dr. Craig Hawkins joining the staff that year. Craig had completed a fellowship in urologic oncology at the Mayo Clinic. In January 2008 PUA became Maine Medical Partners Urology, a multi-specialty group within MMC. The two main drivers for this merger were to meet the growing demographic demand for urology services by an aging population and to create a urology residency program to help address a urologic manpower shortage in Maine. Close associations existed between the urology service at MMC and affiliated medical schools first with the University of Vermont College of Medicine beginning in 1979 and subsequently with the MMC-Tufts University School of Medicine (Maine Track Program) beginning in 2010. A rotation on the urology service was always a productive hands-on learning experience for students.

Urology

The urology residency at MMC was approved by the Urology Residency Review Committee in 2009 to address critical regional and state manpower shortages. It was the first surgical sub-specialty residency program in Maine. Dr. Moritz Hansen was named the first Program Director and Dr. Otto Sandoval was the first resident. Since then, four residents have graduated from the program and have gone on to either private practice or further sub-specialty training.

Two more urologists were added in 2011 (Dr. Matt Hayn, fellowship trained in robotic surgery and Dr. Graham VerLee with expertise in minimally invasive prostate surgery). Dr. Robert McDonough, a fellowship trained urogynecologist, joined the program in 2013. Dr. David Chalmers, a fellowship trained pediatric urologist, became part of the group in 2014 and two additional urologists were hired in 2016 with fellowship training and sub-specialty expertise (Dr. Jesse Sammon in robotic surgery and Dr. Johann Ingimarsson in endourology).

Clinical research has played an important role in urology at MMC for decades. What may not be known is how urologists in Maine and the MMC played an important role in the health policy debate of the 1980's. Research published in JAMA by Dr. Jack Wennberg and colleagues at the Dartmouth Center for Evaluative Clinical Services in 1988 detailed unwarranted geographic variation in rates of prostatectomy, as well as higher complication rates than expected. The study in Maine was performed with the input of most Maine urologists under the auspices of the Maine Medical Association and was led by Dr. Robert Timothy of Portland Urologic Associates. It showed geographic variation in the rates of prostatectomy and that the rates for death and serious complications such as impotence or incontinence were significantly higher than had been previously believed. It clearly showed that rates of surgery largely depended on where a patient lived and not necessarily on their clinical presentation. The de-identified data was then shared with the participating Maine urologists and within 2 years the rate of prostatectomy among outliers (those with high rates of prostatectomy compared to the group median) dropped significantly.

The urology practiced from 1950 to 1980 at MMC is now a distant echo, as the growth of urology at MMC over the past 7 decades has been truly remarkable. The success of the current program can be traced back to the foundation laid by the many prescient urologists who contributed their vision, courage, professional careers and passion to the effort. They helped to make the MMC urology program into the preeminent Northern New England leader in urologic expertise that it has become today.

How much of a leader?

In 2017 MMC and Maine Medical Partners Urology have the largest team of urologic specialists in northern New England with a breadth of subspecialty care unrivaled in the region. It has the highest urologic volume of any practice or hospital in the area. It has the region's most extensive experience with robotic-assisted laparoscopic urologic surgery, along with a full complement of leading-edge diagnostic and treatment services for adults and children with urologic disease. Its Board Certified physicians include Maine's only fellowship-trained pediatric urologists and its only fellowship-trained urologic cancer and robotic specialists. It has had a consistent ranking of "High Performer" for urology by U.S. News & World Report's Best Hospital rankings. It has a multidisciplinary approach to urologic cancer care, with radiation oncology, surgical oncology, medical oncology, and urology all collaborating on patient care. Its urologic clinical outcomes are consistently rated excellent compared to national benchmarks. The program created Maine's first Genitourinary Cancer Clinical Patient Navigator ensuring that patients receive the education necessary to make an informed decision regarding their treatment and addressed barriers patients faced in receiving timely access to their treatment. It has the distinction of being selected as one of five model prostate cancer programs nationally by the Association of Community Cancer Centers. Its physicians have served in leadership positions for the New England section of the American Urological Association and the Maine Medical Association. Maine Medical Partners Urology also has a full complement of urologic nurse practitioners and physician assistants to facilitate timely patient care. The urology residency at MMC, begun in 2009, has become a highly competitive and sought after residency, providing a wide breath of clinical experience, as well as the next generation of urologic providers.

Landmark urological developments at MMC

- First Board certified urologist in Maine 1945
- Kidney transplant program 1971
- Introduction of percutaneous renal stone surgery for complex and large stones 1984
- Introduction of extracorporeal shock wave lithotripsy SWL 1991
- Collaboration with radiation oncology on the introduction of prostate cancer radiation implant procedures 1990's
- Penile injection therapy for impotence 1990's

- In-office transrectal ultrasound of the prostate with prostate biopsies, evolution of procedure with regional prostate anesthetic pain blocks to minimize patient discomfort during biopsies 1990's

- Introduction of inflatable penile prosthetic surgery 1990's

- Endourology including urologic OR suite with digital X-rays, evolution of techniques including the development of small diameter flexible, directable ureteroscopes utilizing Holmium laser lithotripsy to break and remove small symptomatic renal & ureteral stones 1998

- Introduction of hand-assisted 1994 and pure laparoscopic 1995 renal surgery including radical, simple and partial 2005 nephrectomy & pyeloplasty in adults 2001 and children 2005

- Introduction of diVinci robotic urologic surgery 2003, including radical prostatectomy and continent urinary diversions

- MMC Urology Residency Program begins 2009

- Green light 2006 and Holmium laser prostatectomy 2011

- Microsurgical vasectomy reversal and microsurgical sperm harvesting 2010-2012

- Co-Development of Kidney Stone Center at MMC 2012

- Co-Development Pelvic Medicine and Reconstructive Surgery Program at MMC

My Pathway to the AMA Presidency

By Robert E. McAfee MD

Part One

My first experience at Maine General/Maine Medical Center was waking up in bed with a beautiful woman.

My mother told me I was born on a Sunday. The nurse brought me to her, holding me in one arm while holding a copy of the Sunday paper in the other. My arrival along with the "funny pages" may have been a premonition.

I am pleased to contribute to this book while sharing my journey through the Medical Center as a newborn, surgical patient, medical student, intern, surgical resident, surgical attending, corporator, Commissioner for The Joint Commission, trustee and finally President of the American Medical Association.

The hospital played a major role in my life as my workshop, a comforting refuge for my patients, and an opportunity to work, night and day, with the finest nurses in the world.

Although my career and greatest joy was caring for patients, along the way I felt the need to participate in the greater audience that influenced our health care system. The rest of my story will dwell on that part of my career. I have felt however, that unless one has spent time at the bedside, the operating room, the emergency room, the clinics, one has no idea how the system can meet the needs of our patients. I can only hope more physicians will take leadership roles in the future to meet that goal.

Part Two

I began my surgical practice as a solo surgeon but with a loose coverage agreement and office sharing with my Chief of Surgery, Dr. Emerson Drake and with Dr. George Sager. Dr. Clement Hiebert also shared space and mentored me. I had spent my residency before Medicare, when there were a large number of uninsured patients who relied on our clinics for care. Each resident was assigned to be part of a surgical team composed of junior and senior residents as well as junior and senior attending surgeons. There was a sincere effort to provide equivalent, if not better care, to our "service patients" as that provided to the "private patients".

Medicare and Medicaid, were signed into law by President Johnson in July 1965, the exact month I started practice. Medicare covered all over age 65, regardless of financial need, despite the fact that more than half of those over 65 had their own private health insurance. The American Medical Association had argued for another model, Eldercare, that provided insurance based on ability to pay. To this day, I have a hard time justifying why a 25 yr old father of two in Portland must pay for the health care of millionaires in Portland, just because they are over 65. We continue to struggle with means testing for insurance today.

Don't get me wrong, Medicare was a boon for this young surgeon. I performed an operation, submitted a bill to the fiscal intermediary - Union Mutual Insurance Company - and they apologized if they could not pay it in two weeks! The doctor submitted his usual charge and it was paid in full. Contrast that with today when bills are paid several months later and at an amount that the company deems is allowable.

It only took five years for the cost of the Medicare program to reach three times what was projected. A concentrated effort then began to restrain the growth of the program. State and national planning efforts dominated the news. Comprehensive Health Planning, Certificate of Need, State Health Coordinating Committees, etc., were used to hold down costs. I served on several committees but they didn't work. The advance of technology, an aging population, and the insatiable American desire for the most and best care kept pushing up the cost. How could I help solve this increasing dilemma?

Part Three

Thursday nights were set aside for medical meetings. When I started practice, most physicians used both Portland hospitals based on patient choice and available resources. The first Thursday of the month was for the Mercy Hospital Medical Staff meeting. The Maine Medical Center (MMC) medical staff meeting was the second Thursday and was always well attended. A steak dinner, served by the hospital cafeteria staff, was preceded by a one-hour educational lecture. I can remember the lecture hall filled with tobacco smoke from the more than half of the doctors who smoked cigarettes, pipes or cigars - myself included. A business meeting where the serious business occurred followed dinner. Those who were truly interested in what was happening never missed those meetings. I can recall when the medical staff was asked yearly to approve the hospital budget and could amend it at that meeting.

The third Thursday of the month was for the meeting of the Cumberland County Medical Society. At that time, one joined the Maine Medical Association (MMA) by joining the local county society which had active chapters across the state. These meetings were also well attended by 100-200 doctors, drawing doctors from rural parts of the county that did not have active hospital practices. This particular forum, sometimes abused, provided for a more open exchange of concerns of the practice of medicine than the hospital staffs allowed. The discussions often went on into the night giving rise to the definition of the county meetings as "where everything has been said but not everyone has yet said it!"

The last Thursday was reserved for the meeting of the smaller staff of the Portland City Hospital - a very necessary part, as now, of the Portland health care scene.

All of these meetings were an important part of the practice of medicine during my practice lifetime. Unfortunately, all have since been reduced to either quarterly or annual meetings, that are less well attended. The good news is that medical families can now share Thursday nights!

An interesting situation occurred during my Cumberland County Medical Society Presidency. We always held an annual meeting where spouses were invited. One particular year, the Union Mutual Insurance Company (now UNUM) served as the hosting venue, on suggestion of their Chief Medical Officer, Dr. Stan Sylvester. We wanted to achieve good attendance so I suggested we award the very first Doctor of the Year honor. The other members of the Executive Committee agreed to keep the secret. This allowed us to go to every doctor we met during the month and quietly ask them, no, tell them, that it was important for us to know that they would be there with spouse for this important occasion. Wink, wink. Their faces always brightened and they quickly assured me they would be there. When the after-dinner program began, before the largest turnout ever, I then announced that the Doctor of the Year was every female physician in the county! There were eight of them, all but one was there that night. Each was presented with a plaque and bouquet of flowers and each made brief remarks. While this forever endeared me to the ladies, it may have cut down on my referrals from my male colleagues!

In the mid 1980's, an American Hospital Association initiative asked hospitals to elevate the title of the then Executive Vice President, the CEO of the hospital, to the President of the hospital. Until then the President of the hospital was also the President of the Medical Staff. You can begin to see the evolving struggles of our health system.

Part Four

The leadership of the Maine Medical Association was made up of the President and the Executive Committee. The latter included representatives of each County Society elected by the membership. I was chosen to represent my county in 1970. Also on the Committee was the delegate and alternate to the American Medical Association (AMA). Dr. Dan Hanley, the Executive Director of the Association, was also the Bowdoin College physician as well as editor of our monthly journal. He always encouraged spirited debate on all issues, something I frequently took advantage of. In 1973, the alternate delegate was ill and Dr. Hanley sent me to the meeting of the American Medical Association with specific instructions to "straighten them out!" That was all it took. I was impressed with how democratic an organization it was with any member able to speak and formulate policy. A truly bottom to top organization.

During this same time, I was involved with the American Cancer Society (ACS), as Chairman at both the local and state level before becoming a Delegate Director at the national level. In fact I was asked to chair the Service and Rehab committee, tantamount to ascending to the leadership of the Society. At one meeting, I was able to change policy, I forget the issue, much to the chagrin of the senior staff who didn't care for surprises. At the very next meeting, my policy had been reversed. At this point I had the choice to continue with a top down society, the ACS, or a bottom up organization, the AMA. I chose the latter. I still supported the American Cancer Society, and encouraged others to do so, but with my money not my time. My practice was too busy to do both.

Part Five

Dr. George Wood of Brewer was the Delegate to the AMA when I became the alternate. He was a very busy internist with interest in pulmonary medicine. He also was well known at the AMA and might have been elected to higher office but for a medical problem with his lovely wife. He decided to forego the AMA leadership role and return home, give up his private practice and move to the field of student health at the University of Maine. I always admired him for that dedication to family and profession. Two other bits of info about this mentor of mine - he was a National Delegate to the Republican National Committee for many years, and he was the uncle to Janet Reno, Attorney General who I got to know during my time in Washington. Small world!

I was elected AMA Delegate by the MMA to succeed Dr. Wood in 1975. Dr. Brinton Darlington of Augusta was elected to be my alternate. A lifetime friendship developed with this fine gentleman, even on the golf course!

The House of Delegates of the AMA, the policy setting body, is made up of proportional representation of the states, one delegate for every 1,000 AMA members. Large states - California, New York, Texas, Pennsylvania, etc. - therefore dominated the elections. Because we had four single delegate states in New England, the decision was made to sit in the House not alphabetically, as other sites did, but rather as New England. Combined with Massachusetts (eight delegates) and Connecticut (five delegates) we then constituted one of the larger delegations. This was easily done as the doctors of all New England states had been instrumental in the formation of the Beacon Fund, a retirement fund vehicle that took the place of Social Security until doctors became eligible in 1954. The New England delegation met twice a year about a month before the two AMA meetings - the annual meeting always being in Chicago in June. The interim meeting rotated around the country in late November. I was made Chairman of the Delegation in 1977. I received a call from the then Chairman of the AMA board telling me he had appointed me to the Long-Range Planning Council, a highly sought-after appointment. Most of the other Councils of the House are elected positions, that one has to campaign for, so bypassing that was important to a Delegate from Maine. I became Chair of the Council in 1982.

Part Six

If one wishes to go higher in leadership at AMA, becoming a member of the Board of Trustees is the next step and occasionally the precursor to the Presidency. The Board was composed of twelve Members, each eligible for three 3-year terms, plus a student and resident Member. Since then a young physician and a Public Member have been added. The Speaker and Vice Speaker of the House were ex-officio Members.

After discussion with my family, my surgical partners and the New England delegation, I decided to run for the Board of Trustees of AMA in 1984. There were four slots up for election including two strong incumbents. I quickly found out there were others who had the same thought as I. There were nine candidates for those four slots! I was from the smallest state - second thoughts were overcome.

At that time, one announced his candidacy six months ahead of time. Frank Stred, the Executive Director of the Maine Medical Association, was to manage the campaign. Others from New England would help with the politics of campaigning. Name recognition was the first challenge, especially among new Delegates, despite my having been a Delegate for some time. All candidates have printed campaign literature, small trinkets and some kind of reception. To differentiate us two things allowed us to stand out. This was at a time when hotels did not give free newspapers, so my two sons came out to Chicago, met the Chicago Tribune truck in the early morning applied my sticker on front page, and distributed the newspaper to Delegate rooms first thing in morning. How did we know which rooms? Frank had met and bribed the bell captain as well as the head housekeeper with a six pack of lobsters each a month before. In evening we had prepared a three-pack of chocolates with my face embossed on each. The maid placed one on each Delegate's pillow each night while placing the Marriott chocolates on the other pillow. Next to my chocolates was a new note each night: on the first night it read "We sleep better in Maine knowing Bob McAfee is on the AMA Board" and was signed by Hawkeye Pierce MD, Crabapple Cove, Maine and on the second night it read "McAfee never sleeps!" So, from first thing in morning to last thing at night, "elect McAfee" was on minds of those who were to vote.

During the six-day convention, each Member of the New England delegation was assigned delegations to lobby. I remember meeting the new Delegate from Guam when he got his badge, introducing myself and asking for his vote and welcoming him. With so many candidates running and having to win with a majority, our strategy was to hope that a second and third ballot might elect me.

To make a long and exciting campaign short, I won by one vote on first ballot! An incumbent was displaced, and a second ballot was necessary to elect the four of us. Because the margin was one vote I could go around to all those in the delegation and thank them personally for the fact that their effort had won the election. It had a solidifying effect on the delegation that persists to this day. When anyone who is now running for office calls me for advice, I ask them only one question - "What is the name of the delegate from Guam?" - the margin of victory for me.

Part Seven

Your life suddenly changed when you became a Board member, even as a junior Member. At least twenty days of service (increasing yearly depending on your assignments) were required. There was mandatory media training each year - speech training, podium exercises, personal dress, the hostile interview, radio interviews where you compete with the vacuum cleaner and the screaming kids, etc. The staff carefully graded you so that when a media request came in they would recommend to the Chairman who could handle it best. Each request was grouped into one of four categories: WIN/WIN

- a cub reporter who writes down your every word; WIN /LOSE - a new program of AMA that needs publicity but you haven't the faintest idea what it is; LOSE /WIN - an Oprah or a Donahue show where a contentious topic would be discussed and you could turn a loss into a win because of your knowledge and skills; and finally LOSE/ LOSE - usually a Sixty Minutes session from which your best lines were left on the cutting room floor and which we rarely accepted.

Over the years I appeared on every network morning show - Today, Good Morning America, CBS Morning, etc. as well as every evening news shows, including the PBS MacNeil/Lehrer hour, Nightline with Ted Koppel, etc. The great fun, humor, terror on occasion, and challenges are for another book. I always kept my patients informed. If I had to go to New York with little notice, I would ask my hospital patients if they would allow me to be little late on rounds the next day because of doing the Today or Oprah shows and they never said no but rather organized TV groups to watch! If not for my partners who graciously covered for me on those occasions, I could not have done any of this. More on their importance a little later.

In order to maintain good relations with the nation's media centers, the AMA would send each qualified Trustee and Officer on media visits two to three times a year. These visits would entail about 6-8 contacts in two-day period in the largest media centers of the country. They might include a morning drive time radio appearance, a Rotary club meeting, a Gray Panthers AARP Meeting, a newspaper editorial board, a noon TV news slot, and/or medical staff or county society meetings. They were exhausting but great fun.

Testimony in Washington to either House or Senate would be prefaced by an overnight stay at the AMA guest house in Washington, briefing by Washington AMA staff, a ride to capital and testimony. Staff really grilled you ahead of time to make you as informed about subject as well as politics you might encounter. I always enjoyed the challenge and opportunity to further AMA policy.

I was re-elected for the second three-year term without opposition in 1987 and again for final term in 1990. I truly enjoyed my Board tenure. The twenty days annually steadily expanded to over one hundred fifty days near the end of my term in 1993. I had many requests to represent the Association both within and outside the Federation. I could not fulfill them all and keep my obligation to my partners, my patients and most of all to my family. I was urged to run for AMA President, a long way from the Maine Surgical Care Group and the Maine Medical Center.

During one's time on the Board, each Trustee received a **per diem** plus expenses for each assignment. Over the years, the loss of practice income was balanced by AMA compensation so that one did not lose nor gain income over private practice. As one of the Presidents you received a yearly stipend independent of the number of days spent on AMA business.

Part Eight

As my term on the Board ended, I decided to run for AMA President-elect in 1993. Unbeknownst to me, the then Chairman of the Board also declared to run for the same office. Usually the sitting Chair prevails in such contests, but I had a good feeling that

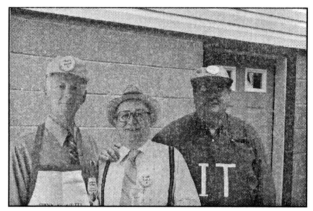

Bob McAfee as IT

the friends that I had met over the years would allow me an even chance. The campaign was intense. My campaign manager was Dr. Mike Collins from Massachusetts, a good politician, then and now. At this writing Mike serves as Chancellor of University of Massachusetts Worcester Health Sciences Center. We felt we were at least thirty votes down as the convention began, so the entire New England delegation went to work. My campaign buttons read "Think About It!" banking on the fact that I might have a more favorable image by comparison of all factors. The night before election, we had our usual New England reception, and I was first in the receiving line wearing a green apron with a large "It" sewed on front - courtesy of Frank Stred. It became hard for voters not to "Think About It"!

The morning of the election, the polls opened early and the credentials of Delegates were carefully scrutinized as only Delegates could vote. About an hour into the House of Delegates deliberations, the tellers handed the results to the EVP on stage and he gave them to the Speaker. He then waited for a comfortable break in debate to announce the results. The minutes can feel like a lifetime as one waits to hear. During this time, my campaign manager, sitting in front of me, turned around and said: "Congratulations

Mr. President." Oh no I said, don't jinx me now! Little did I know he had arranged a secret signal from the stage if I won! The result was announced, there was great cheer among the delegates, especially New England section. Usually candidates, both winners and losers approach one of the six floor microphones to thank their supporters. On this occasion, the Speaker instead invited Doris and me to come to the dais microphone to accept the applause from the house. As I profusely thanked all for their votes and a good campaign from my opponent, I then expressed a feeling of my pride at that moment. "In my wildest dreams, I could not imagine how I would feel at this moment - but then again, in my wildest dreams, I rarely think of the AMA!" It brought down the house and appeared on the front page of newspapers around the country, including the Portland Press Herald.

Part Nine

A fantastic odyssey of three years then began, first as President-elect, then President and finally as Past-President. The travel schedule exceeded 300 days as President and about 220 days for each of the other years. To represent the AMA as well as the profession of medicine in the major cities of the world was indeed the highlight of my medical career. I mention only a few of the hundreds of standout moments as space allows.

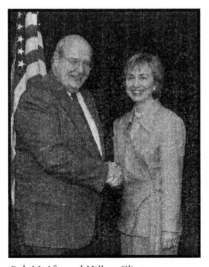

Bob McAfee and Hillary Clinton

Each President is allowed to choose the theme of his or her tenure. Usually some aspect of health system reform or tort reform dominates the agenda. While I would continue those when asked, I became interested in violence in our society as a public health issue - especially violence in the home such as child abuse, domestic violence and elder abuse

295

that I collectively termed Family Violence. The greatest oxymoron I could imagine - two words that should never occur in same sentence.

I was motivated by a study from the Seattle area that simply asked survivors of family violence who came to the emergency room who they would have preferred to have told about the events in their life that led up to this current medical visit. To our surprise the victim's family physician was named 83% of the time - 15% more than those who preferred to tell either priest, pastor or rabbi and 25% more than those who wanted to tell the police.

That motivated me and the AMA to begin a series of initiatives that numbered 15 programs by the time I left the presidency. To mention just a few: the Physicians Coalition Against Family Violence initiative that brought all the major specialty societies together and continued until most had programs of their own; incorporation of family violence into the admitting history taking of all medical encounters (I note that I have since been asked by my primary care physician, my orthopedist, my eye doctor, my cardiologist, etc. on each visit); incorporating family violence related questions into the national boards that all medical students must take thereby elevating the subject of violence into the major public health problem it is; and encouraging violence themed issues of JAMA and state medical journals, priority consideration to manuscripts on violence in the New England Journal among others. We even encouraged the NBA Washington Bullets to change their name to Washington Wizards.

Throughout this journey, I tried to represent my profession and state well. I was able to participate in the appointment of Maine physicians to residency review committees, accreditation activities, and a number of national assignments. I believe there was a significant benefit to Maine, the Maine Medical Association and the Maine Medical Center.

I could not have accomplished any of this without the love and support of my wife, Doris, and my family. My surgical partners provided the coverage that allowed me to continue an active practice. The support that Drs. George Sager, Ferris Ray, Dick Dillihunt, Bill Herbert and later Jens Jorgensen and Bob Hawkins provided made it all happen. I am grateful to my patients who understood my absences and encouraged me to continue. And finally, my gratitude and respect to all the physicians and nurses affiliated with the Maine Medical Center, whose daily commitment to excellence in patient care motivated me every day of my journey.

EARLY HISTORY OF MEDICAL MUTUAL INSURANCE COMPANY OF MAINE

By Jeremy R. Morton MD

The frequency and severity of malpractice claims began to increase dramatically across the United States beginning in about 1970. The reason for this remains unclear, although some believe it represented a cultural trend in which people were becoming less accepting of life's inherent risks and more demanding of accountability on the part of the medical profession. Medicine and surgery were becoming more sophisticated and complex, and the public more conversant with the health care process. Health care became more fragmented with multiple specialists who did not have a long-term relationship with the patient providing care. Suing the doctor for an unsatisfactory treatment outcome, which had been rare in the past, became more common - fueled in part by mounting awards and an enthusiastic plaintiffs bar. The insurance industry began experiencing significant losses from unpredictable malpractice awards which were not covered by existing premiums.

One by one the major companies, including Travelers, Hartford and later St. Paul's pulled out of the medical liability market leaving physicians without available coverage. Physician groups in several states across the country, including Maine, began contemplating the creation of insurance companies of their own to cover their doctors and perhaps reduce their risk of being sued. Convinced that the likelihood of a doctor being sued in Maine was less than in many other states, Drs. William Maxwell, Jeremy Morton and Patrick Dowling came together to explore the feasibility of physician-owned mutual insurance company. With their own company Maine physicians could potentially manage their own liability insurance and pay lower premiums. Before this time, possible cases of medical malpractice were dealt with primarily by the legal profession, with most physicians reluctant to get involved and especially hesitant to testify against a colleague. The concept of a physician owned malpractice insurance company would put the financial and moral responsibility on the medical profession.

In 1973 the Maine Legislature addressed the problem of the diminishing availability of medical liability insurance. It formed the Pomeroy Commission which, in turn, created a state-administered joint underwriting association (JUA) to provide a temporary source of malpractice insurance for Maine's physicians while assuring financial recourse to patients injured through medical negligence. The JUA was intended to be an interim measure. By law it was to expire on July 1, 1979.

The physician initiative moved ahead steadily over the next three years. Working with Dr. Daniel Hanley, then the Executive Director of the Maine Medical Association and with Dr. Douglas Hill, its President, the MMA created an ad hoc Malpractice Insurance Committee. The members included Patrick Dowling (Chairman), William Maxwell, Jeremy Morton and Richard Leck. John McKernan, who later became Governor of Maine, served as counsel. The Committee met with recently formed physician companies from other states and also established a consulting agreement with John Schroeder of Johnson & Higgins, a major insurance broker in Boston, to open discussions with the Insurance Commissioner and with the Maine National Bank.

Additionally meetings with physicians throughout the state were held to introduce them to the idea and to gather their input. The concept gained increasing support among the physicians who, with some encouragement, became intrigued with the idea of having a physician-owned and controlled company representing them and protecting their assets. They were willing to loan the new company an amount equal to one-third of their initial premium to provide start-up capital. In addition, the Company secured a $125,000 loan from the bank underwritten by the initial Board members and a one million dollar letter of credit from the AMA was negotiated by Daniel Hanley. The initial Directors, all physicians, included: Patrick Dowling (Chairman) and William Maxwell, Jeremy Morton from Portland; Richard Leck from Bath; Daniel Hanley and William Medd from Norway; Francis Kittredge, David Sensenig and Philip Hunter from Bangor; John Steeves from Skowhegan; Michael Kellum from Caribou; and Frederick Holler from Lewiston. Dr. Maxwell became the company's first President and ably led the Company for the next twenty years. The first office of the Company was in the same building as Dr. Maxwell's medical office permitting him to look after the day to day activities of the fledgling organization. Dr. Morton (Vice President) was a licensed a pilot. This facilitated his ability to do much of the field work, meeting with physicians around the state.

The Company became Medical Mutual Insurance Company of Maine ("Medical Mutual"). It was the 19th physician-owned company in the country, writing its first policies in the fall of 1978. One-third of Maine's physicians signed up in the first few months of operation, throwing their support behind the new company. The Company soon developed a reputation for integrity and respect and became a leader among the growing number of physician companies nationally. Medical Mutual's initial policy limits were $100,000 per incident and $300,000 in the aggregate. They are now ten times that amount with excess limits available above that. In May 1979, seven months into the Company's first year, Maine Medical Center became the first hospital to purchase its professional liability and general liability insurance from Medical Mutual.

Over time the Company has come to insure 80% of the physicians in Maine. It increased its coverage area to New Hampshire and Vermont in 1992. For a number of years, the Company focused primarily on physician liability and insured only the one hospital, which employed numerous staff physicians and residents. More recently, as more and more physicians have become hospital employees, the Company has come to insure many other hospitals as well.

Early on it became apparent that the mission of the Company should extend beyond legal and financial issues related to professional liability to take on the responsibility for determining the root cause of the medical error or the patient dissatisfaction leading to the claim. It set out to address those issues as well as providing appropriate compensation to patients in the event of concerns about negligent care. Much of the Company's energy and resources now go toward providing risk management services to physicians, physician offices and hospitals, including information and training designed to improve performance and reduce the likelihood of unsatisfactory outcomes and unhappy patients.

All Medical Mutual claims are reviewed and discussed, often several times, by the Claims Committee which meets monthly. It is comprised of 15 physicians from various specialties and the claims adjusters from the Company. As additional data and professional opinions are gathered on a claim, the Claims Committee may decide that a malpractice has likely occurred. In this case it authorizes compensation for the patient and takes actions to prevent that occurrence from happening again. If, on the other hand, the Committee determines that there was no malpractice, the lawyers are told there will be no settlement and the Company will take the case to court if necessary. This has proven to be a powerful deterrent to frivolous malpractice suits which have proven to be highly problematic throughout the nation.

Even when the ultimate findings that confirm the absence of medical error, a malpractice claim represents an attack on a physician's professional integrity. It can be devastating to him or her personally. Medical Mutual has worked diligently to support physicians emotionally through this process and to reduce episodes of malpractice by educating physicians about proper practices, and has had a significant impact on the quality of clinical care.

In 2016, the Company generated $46 M in premiums and had $297 M in assets, including reserves on existing open claims and policyholder surplus. Being a mutual company, Medical Mutual has no stockholders expecting a return on their investment. Any favorable experience by the Company is passed on to the policyholder-owners in the form of dividends. The Company has received several offers in recent years either to merge with or be acquired by other companies. It has maintained its original resolve to remain a Maine company serving northern New England physicians and patients.

InterMed

By Thomas F. Claffey MD

History of InterMed

In the early 1990's changes were occurring in the US medical care delivery system. Health systems were expanding, the market power of insurers was increasing, HMOs and referral restrictions were becoming more common and physicians appeared to be losing influence over important decisions that affected their patients and the quality of physicians' work life. In that environment three internal medicine groups in Portland - Longcreek Center for Internal Medicine, Internal Medicine Associates and Portland Internal Medicine - each recognized the need for physicians to consolidate to be able to play a role in the evolution of medical care delivery.

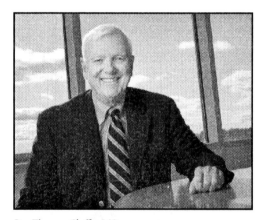

Dr. Thomas Claffey MD

From the outset it took foresight, confidence and determination on the part of the physicians who germinated the idea of a new medical organization to achieve success. Not only were there myriad organizational issues to attend to, but a plan which demonstrated the feasibility of creating a large, self-sustaining medical group was an absolute necessity if we were to get the buy-in of the original 18 physicians to proceed with the endeavor. Tim Carnes, Peter Gordon, Joel Botler, Bill Ervin and I spent countless hours researching the means to accomplish our goal. This included consulting with members of the greater Portland medical community and engaging external consultants to evaluate our plan and assist with the implementation.

At the same time, Maine Medical Center was developing a physician hospital organization (PHO) to address the same issues. Physicians from the three groups considered joining the PHO but were concerned about the possible loss of physician influence over future decisions. The groups wanted to maintain physician control over any new organization, assuming that the future direction of patient care and physician professional satisfaction would be better with that type of model. We also saw that the ability of a physician-led group to deliver a broad range of services to our patients would maintain quality and help keep costs under control. We were joined in the effort by the physicians of Yarmouth Family Medicine and pediatricians including Drs. Talbot, Ritger, and Bennett. Thus in 1993 InterMed was born.

Our early years were spent working out a governance model and a compensation system, both of which had to satisfy diverse constituencies. In fact, many physician organizations flounder on these two important elements. We felt that all our physicians needed to be included and well represented in the governance of the organization and that people needed to feel fairly compensated for their work. Neither task had a simple answer and both took some time and much discussion to work out.

The governance model was perhaps the easier design to accomplish. We established a physician board of directors, initially composed of 9 members which eventually grew to 11. Although we specifically avoided assigning board seats to specific specialties or practice locations, we did recognize the need for broad representation and took those elements into consideration in the nominating process. In the end, we achieved a balance that continues to this day and serves the organization well. It cannot be emphasized enough that having a board of directors (BOD) made up of physicians is critically important for an organization to understand the needs of its patients and providers and to keep the organization focused on patient care efforts and physician satisfaction. Everyone in the organization, from the CEO on down, knows that he or she is ultimately accountable to the physician led BOD. That diverse BOD has proven fully capable to make policy which enhances the quality of care the group delivers.

A compensation system that made everyone comfortable was more challenging to achieve. In fact it took several years and the guidance of skilled professional medical managers to accomplish this. More on management later. The individual groups in the early days of InterMed had diverse compensation systems, practice styles, and levels of productivity. They used ancillary services to varying degrees. The initial InterMed compensation system, established in the late 1990's was entirely work (RVU) based and was importantly payer-neutral. The revenue derived from ancillary services was folded into the calculation of the value of each work unit. That system largely survives today, with additional quality and patient satisfaction metrics also included. As one can imagine, getting the compensation system right - so that all are comfortable with the end result - is critical to group cohesiveness and satisfaction with the professional environment.

Early in the development of InterMed the BOD recognized the need for capital if we were to continue to expand and grow. At the same time several national physician practice management companies emerged and we were in contact with a company called UniPhy. We spent significant time measuring the value of a possible relationship. We concluded that the management expertise UniPhy would bring and the capital they would provide would be worth the cost we would incur. The association did bring us needed expertise in financial management and access to capital. In the end, the cost to our group of continuing the affiliation was too high and we ended the relationship after 3 years.

As one can imagine, severing the relationship with the physician management company created its own set of challenges. The first might have been a lack of confidence in the group leadership. However, the Board developed a plan for continuity of management and access to capital that satisfied the members of the group that we were headed in the right direction.

As a result of the UniPhy experience the belief that strong management expertise was necessary within the group was strengthened. Fortunately among the assets UniPhy brought to us was Robert Wright. Bob had a long track record in managing medical groups and a keen sense of what InterMed needed to move on to the next level. Under his guidance we spent the better part of a year developing and defining the vision, mission, and values of InterMed which remain the bedrock on which the organization is built:

Vision: Care without compromise. Every patient, all the time.

Mission: InterMed is a physician-owned medical group founded on the goals of patient centered primary care that is enhanced by integrated specialty services. Our staff is a team that focuses on putting the patient first to deliver high quality, high value care. We will form partnerships with other organizations to benefit our patients. We will continually innovate and improve how we deliver healthcare towards the goal of healthier patients and better, higher value outcomes.

Values:

- Providing the highest quality care to our patients with a level of service that exceeds their expectations;

- Maintaining a positive attitude and always treating our patients and each other with dignity and respect;

- Insisting on honesty and integrity from each other and our business partners;

- Making teamwork a core component of our relationships between physicians, staff, and patients;

- Embracing change to better serve our patients;

- Using business practices that feature individual accountability and group responsibility to ensure delivery of high value healthcare; and

- Having fun as we carry out our mission to serve.

Bob worked with us for 5 years during which we refined our operational systems, enhanced our management team and refined group cohesion. It is the group's good fortune that Bob was succeeded by Dan McCormack who continues as the CEO of InterMed as of this writing in 2018. Dan's steady management style, his ability to work with people and his vision has continued the growth of InterMed.

That growth has included the addition of Generations OB/GYN group in 1997, adding to the initial specialty division of infectious diseases, the specialties of dermatology, cardiology, ENT, sports medicine, psychiatry and urgent care/emergency medicine. Broadening the number of services InterMed provided increased the convenience for our patients, expanded our ability to monitor the quality of services delivered and improved the value of the services we deliver. It also serves as a tool to provide educational opportunities for our physicians and staff inside the group.

Over the years InterMed has also broadened the range of ancillary services provided by the group. Those services have grown from basic laboratory and plain film x-ray to include a full-service laboratory, CT scanning, a complete range of ultrasound services, nuclear medicine, cardiac stress testing, and MRI services. The practice also has a full service physical therapy department and an outpatient surgery center. These services provide timely and convenient access to most of the services our patients need but also allow us to help control the cost of those services.

The physicians who founded InterMed have always had an abiding commitment to teaching residents and medical students. They have for years served on the faculty of Tufts University Medical School and the University of Vermont College of Medicine and now the Maine Medical Center/Tufts Medical School. That commitment continues today and is a part of the fabric of InterMed. InterMed internists teach inpatient medicine on a dedicated service at Maine Medical Center as well as teaching internal medicine residents in the outpatient setting. The Infectious Diseases Division teaches residents and students in both the inpatient and outpatient settings as well as directing and organizing an Infectious Diseases fellowship program at MMC. InterMed's family physicians, pediatricians and OB/GYN physicians are all also active on their respective teaching services at MMC and in the outpatient setting. The group believes being active in teaching new physicians requires our doctors to be up to date and enhances the quality of care we deliver to our patients.

One of the benefits to the group from retaining an academic focus has been the enhancement of our physician recruiting efforts. Teaching medical students and residents gave our attending physicians first-hand experience with young doctors and allowed us to recruit those that we thought would best fit in our practice. We successfully recruited in each of the primary care departments as well as select specialties. The academic mission also enhanced our efforts to recruit physicians from programs in Massachusetts, Rhode Island, New York, Maryland, Virginia, Illinois, Iowa, and California. Prospective physicians were drawn to a physician-owned practice that would still allow them to contribute to the teaching programs at Maine Medical Center and our local medical schools.

A cornerstone of InterMed's mission has been good relationships with all the members of the healthcare community in Maine. This has included working with statewide organizations such as the Maine Medical Association, the Maine Hospital Association and healthcare policy makers in state government. Locally there have been joint quality of care and access initiatives with oncology, cardiology, orthopedics, radiology and others as well as working closely with hospital partners Maine Medical Center (MMC) and Mercy Hospital. In addition to caring for inpatients at both hospitals, InterMed physicians have served in the outpatient clinics at MMC and have served on multiple hospital committees providing input and expertise across a wide range of disciplines. The Infectious Diseases Division physicians have been especially active in providing services to the hospitals including the hospital Epidemiology and Infectious Diseases Division Directorships at both MMC and Mercy, antibiotic stewardship at MMC and the organizing, staffing and directing the HIV Clinic at MMC. The OB/GYN division supports the inpatient service at MMC with clinical coverage and teaching.

For more than a decade InterMed's physicians and administration have led the way in the areas of quality monitoring and registry development. The clinical team from InterMed was among the founding members of the statewide collaboration - Pathways to Excellence. In that capacity, the team developed quality metrics and registry monitoring systems for the care of patients with diabetes and cardiovascular disease which were incorporated into the care of the group's patients. In addition, tracking systems were put in place at InterMed to monitor patients' needs for preventative care services such as mammography, colonoscopy and cervical cancer screening.

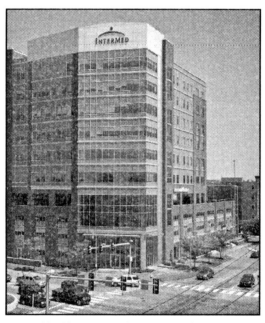

Intermed building, Marginal Way, Portland

Each physician in InterMed receives a quality metrics report on how the management of their patients compares to the established norms in the registries and is provided assistance with practice changes to improve performance. Also, clinical teams devoted specifically to diabetes and cardiovascular disease were established to proactively partner with patients to improve clinical outcomes. Customer service is monitored on an ongoing basis through nationally organized and administered customer satisfaction surveys and the results are published group wide. Finally, physician compensation is tied to performance in care coordination and patient satisfaction.

An interesting and somewhat surprising development as InterMed grew was the evolution of relations with the insurance industry. Historically physician groups and insurance companies have not been the best of friends - and that was the case at least through the first decade of InterMed's existence. In fact the group had several quite contentious negotiations with health plans. There were times when it was likely InterMed would not participate with some major health plans because of these differences.

That situation changed in the early 2000's perhaps for two major reasons. First, InterMed had begun to focus on quality initiatives at the start of the period when the patient centered medical home, disease management, clinical registries and population health management were getting established. Second, InterMed cautiously approached some of the plans with a potentially collaborative approach to our mutual goals of improving care and thereby impacting cost. Some in the insurance industry recognized that more could be gained by constructively partnering with physicians, rather than treating physicians and physician groups as adversaries. As InterMed's care management efforts began to take hold and show results, led by Quality Director Elizabeth Collet, it became clear that supporting those efforts led to higher quality care and lower cost to the entire system as opposed to always negotiating the lowest per encounter price paid to the medical group. Over time the collaboration grew to additional segments of the population, including patients over 65, often with Medicare Advantage plan coverage, in which a substantial decrease in hospital costs was recognized in the care management population. The evolution in the provider-payer relationship continues and has been beneficial in both increased quality of care, lower cost of care and recognition by the payers of the value of such results.

An essential part of success in health care delivery is the patient experience. Every time a patient has contact with a healthcare organization, whether a phone call, electronic communication, or in-person contact, the quality of the interaction registers with the patient and impacts how he or she thinks about the organization and what will be said to others about it. The explicit and implicit culture at InterMed emphasizes that at all levels of the organization all staff are an important part of the team needed to provide a courteous, helpful and knowledgeable experience. InterMed has been fortunate to have management and staff who not only acknowledge the importance of those values but live them. From a patient's first touch of the organization to the conclusion of any encounter, physicians and the full care team work to ensure that the patient is not only satisfied with that individual encounter but also forms a positive opinion of the organization as a whole.

The culture at InterMed stresses patient service while placing equal emphasis on teamwork within the organization. In medical care delivery, all members of the team work closely together. The move to a consolidated building on Marginal Way in Portland had a unifying impact on the entire practice and allowed for further strengthening of the group's culture. Further alignment in the South Portland and Yarmouth offices affirmed the cohesion among the group's physicians. InterMed has been fortunate to have developed a culture of teamwork and of treating all co-workers with friendliness and respect. That attitude is the foundation of the delivery of an excellent patient experience.

Finally, and maybe most significantly, InterMed's evolution and success have been strengthened by its commitment to physician leadership. The physicians on the BOD made an early commitment to the value of dedicated physician leadership. A willingness to pay physicians for this time affirmed that their leadership time was valuable to the practice much like their patient care. For the past decade or more, InterMed has invested in leadership development programs for its physicians. This has allowed for the creation of a pipeline of leaders throughout the organization, many of whom will assume roles on its Board as well as leadership positions in community healthcare organizations. The strong relationship between the physician leaders and management of the practice will continue to be one of the defining elements of the practice's sustainability.

2018 will see the 25th anniversary of the founding of InterMed. The landscape of the medical care delivery system has dramatically changed over that time. There have been tremendous advances in the diagnosis and treatment of illness which have benefitted patients and increased the complexity of medicine. Physicians and all members of the medical community have a vastly increased knowledge base which must be accessed to deliver up-to-date care. The electronic health record has wrought profound changes, both positive and negative, in the way patients and caregivers interact. It has put more information at the fingertips of physicians and has facilitated the transfer of medical records and information within the care team, but it has also significantly increased the workload of some physicians and in some cases decreased job satisfaction. The financing of healthcare has moved from a fee for service delivery model to a more complex interaction of services provided, quality measurement, patient satisfaction metrics, bundled payments and the evolution of large health care delivery systems which now employ, in many markets, more than 50% of the physician delivery force.

In that environment, the continued success of InterMed might seem quite remarkable. InterMed remains an independent, physician led organization which is entirely responsible for its own ongoing management, financing and care delivery model. It is just that independence that has motivated everyone at InterMed to do all that is necessary to ensure continued success. Nothing says it better than the words from our vision that are embedded on the group's logo: Care without compromise.

It was my honor and privilege to serve as InterMed's President for 20 years prior to my retirement in 2014. Over those years the group has navigated through many changes and has become a cornerstone of medical care delivery in Maine. The group is now led and served by a new generation of physician leaders who comprise the BOD and its supporting committees. At this writing the group has the good fortune of the continuing service of President Phyllidia Ku-Ruth, Chief Medical Officer Daniel Loiselle, Treasurer Stephen Dobieski and Secretary Jeff Peterson. They come from diverse backgrounds and medical specialties. Yet they are all united in a shared commitment to provide the best possible care to our patients.

Spectrum Medical Group

By Christopher F. Pope MD

"Even fools are sometimes right."
"No one is smart enough to be wrong all the time."
"Genius is 1% inspiration, 99% perspiration."

Winston Churchill, Ken Wilber, Thomas Edison

Introduction

Most of the chapters in this book focus on the excellent medical care provided at Maine Medical Center (MMC) and on contributions made by individual physician leaders and clinically skilled medical staff. This chapter describes how Spectrum Medical Group (Spectrum) formed and worked with MMC's leaders to improve the quality of the medical care delivered.

Although the difficulty in coordinating physicians is often described as 'herding cats', the medical staff will well remember the challenges of the 1990s and early 2000s trying to focus the hospital on providing quality clinical care rather than on 'profits' as the major management goal. Administrators were guiding the hospital using primarily two financial metrics: cost and revenue. These financial metrics rather than clinical quality measures were directly linked to senior administrators' annual job performance. Those incentives were not tightly aligned with investing resources in clinical care outcomes or patient safety let alone metrics related to satisfaction of patients, nurses, physicians and other clinical staff. Most hospitals at the time did not focus on clinical quality. MMC was not unusual in not having begun to develop quality metrics linked to administrator compensation. Medical quality improvement in healthcare was a relatively new concept - quality was either assumed or left to professional peer review processes distinct from administrators.

Lacking properly aligned incentives, hospital administrators can perhaps be forgiven for holding the following perspective:

"If it wasn't for all these difficult doctors, nurses and patients,
MMC would be running quite smoothly"

This view might be less surprising if the reader realizes: (1) it is truly difficult to coordinate physicians to gain cost efficiencies[1]; (2) MMC had recently faced a vote by the nursing staff to form a union; and (3) caring for sick patients is not a part of the skill set of most senior administrators. Since physicians, nurses and other clinicians actually provide the medical care, it would seem optimal for the views of innovative clinicians and business leaders to be blended. Unfortunately, prioritizing resource expenditures can often pit the views of physicians against those of hospital administrators.

When Spectrum was formed in 1996, the Chairs of those MMC Departments that became members of Spectrum continued their important hospital roles while becoming a vital part of the effort to operationalize Spectrum's early vision:

> *Dedicated to excellence in the diagnosis, prevention and*
> *treatment of illness and the primary importance*
> *of the caring patient relationship.*

Spectrum's initial clinical specialties (radiology, anesthesiology and pathology) provided almost all of their clinical services in or linked to the hospital. Therefore optimizing MMC's clinical infrastructure and focusing on hospital clinical quality were essential steps to achieving the vision.

Most physicians were busy providing clinical services and caring for patients. All were engaged in continuing medical education (CME) but CBE (continuing business education) was not a routine part of their learning goals. Acquiring the knowledge necessary to form a new medical organization as well as the systems[2] and the skills to implement necessary changes that would enhance the quality of practice were new challenges for physicians. Although the performance improvement and clinical quality literature was rapidly evolving[1,3], few physicians had much experience with these new ideas. Complexity[4,5] and systems[2] literature were also making significant contributions to the delivery of cost-effective medical care.

Performance improvement is usually seen as vital and necessary except when it applies to one personally. Resistance to imposed behavior change is felt by most people, even when aware that:

> *"Not all change leads to improvement,*
> *but all improvement requires some change"*

Institute for Healthcare Improvement

Today it is well accepted that organizations in the medical and healthcare business sectors should be guided by metrics that reflect both the quality of clinical services and the financial results.

The Spectrum story is comprised of two tightly interwoven threads:

First, the members of the three independent Portland physician groups that eventually formed Spectrum had to recognize that organizational change was necessary. They also needed to acquire the non-clinical business and leadership skills to create a more effective medical business organization. Some inspiration and a whole lot of perspiration was necessary to accomplish this.

Second, because Spectrum physicians would be working primarily inside MMC it was always clear that Spectrum's success would hinge on redirecting how MMC administration funded clinical infrastructure and measured clinical quality. If a critical objective was to have all MMC patients receive high quality treatment, medical care needed to be both optimized and standardized.

This chapter begins with a summary of the challenging three specialty group merger process that was required to form Spectrum, documenting some key early lessons. When the merger was completed Spectrum became the largest RAP group (radiology, anesthesiology, and pathology) in the USA.

Two anecdotes illustrate the multifaceted approach used to enlarge MMC's focus on clinical quality performance metrics and improving clinical systems. 'Nudging' MMC to become a high performance medical organization required a broad effort from all the medical staff, nursing staff, and other clinicians, and also its business and community leaders. If one could answer 'yes' to both of the following questions, the critical goal of having all patients receive excellent medical care routinely, would be accomplished:

"Will you allow your family member to be treated at MMC or
any Spectrum service site without personally 'guiding' him or her
through the medical system to ensure optimized care?

Do all patients at our service sites get the same optimized care we
want for our families?"

The Spectrum story includes similar efforts in the Bangor, Maine region. This chapter focuses on efforts at MMC only, summarizing Spectrum's formation and the initial 5 years. Many people have made large contributions and served Spectrum in pivotal roles in subsequent years through until the present (2017) making it impossible to tell the full history of Spectrum in one short chapter.

The Spectrum Story Part I:
Why, How & Now: Operationalizing our Shared Vision

WHY: Reasons Spectrum was formed

In the mid 1990's, healthcare was moving away from a physician-patient orientation of care to one that was also greatly influenced by non-clinicians. Health systems, hospitals, managed-care companies, employers, and purchasers of health insurance were taking lead roles in shaping and influencing care delivery and financing. This market evolution threatened autonomy and clinical practice styles for all physicians.

Managed care changes in the healthcare market were most noticeable in California but also in other parts of the USA such as Minneapolis. MMC's reaction, as described in detail in another chapter, was to form a Physician Hospital Organization (PHO). Many questions about PHOs were raised such as how to equitably obtain and share reimbursement. The hospital's share appeared to be non-negotiable with physicians being left to squabble about how to divide the leftovers. MMC's medical staff was beginning the change from being largely independent to being employed in hospital-owned practice plans in which administrators had pivotal roles setting physician salaries, financial metrics and efficiency targets.

Spectrum's founding physicians strongly favored being part of an independent physician-directed organization. This allowed them to avoid the conflicts experienced when they were 'controlled by administrators' and to remain relevant in developing healthcare policy, financing and delivery systems in Maine. Direct contracting outside MMC's PHO necessitated developing new business skills and information systems, as the value of medical care was being measured in the new reimbursement models. Consolidation had the potential for making these infrastructure investments more affordable and permitted the engagement of consultants and creation of a highly skilled, professional, and shared administrative team.

New computerized information systems allowed faster clinical data collection. How to use information to modify and improve physician work patterns[1] was becoming better understood. The value of high performance teamwork[2] was also becoming clearer and the availability of evidence-based decision-making with computer-enabled analysis almost a reality. In the early 1990s, communication networks using email and electronic image distribution were not yet available in Maine. A 'balanced scorecard' business system[6] was increasingly being used in other industries to measure the quality of their delivered products, customer and employee satisfaction and other important variables. These 'quality' indicators tended to be leading indicators in predicting business outcomes in contrast to the lagging indicators of expense and revenue.

The founding members realized that a more cohesive and forward thinking strategic approach was needed to cope with the changing Maine environment. This sparked discussions that eventually resulted in the formation of Spectrum.

HOW: Legacy group mergers

On September 30, 1996 Spectrum Medical Group was 'born' after many months of dedicated effort. It initially consisted of three divisions: Radiology, Anesthesiology and Pathology (the three specialty physician groups decided to complete the Spectrum merger before attempting to include other specialty physician groups). MMC and Brighton Medical Center had merged in 1995, allowing the Brighton radiologists and anesthesiologists to join the radiology and anesthesiology groups working at MMC.

The initial Spectrum merger resulted from a series of interim steps:

- In April 1996 the Portland radiology group (30 members, which included 5 radiation oncologists) merged with the Bangor radiology group (16 members)

- In June 1996 the Portland anesthesiology group (20 members) merged with the Bangor anesthesiology group (18 members)

- In September 1996 the full Spectrum merger was completed as pathology was added to the two prior single specialty mergers (radiology and anesthesiology)

The initial Divisions of Radiology and Anesthesiology included the legacy independent medical groups from Bangor and Portland (in addition the Radiology Division also incorporated a 5-member group from Brunswick) while the Pathology Division was comprised of the 6 Portland based pathologists.

At that point in time Spectrum included 90 physicians: 38 anesthesiologists, 6 pathologists, 41 radiologists and 5 radiation oncologists. By early 1998, Spectrum had grown to 114 physicians: 54 anesthesiologists 11 pathologists, 43 radiologists and 6 radiation oncologists.

HOW: Spectrum's Vision, People and Principles

Vision: The goal of becoming a single fully integrated physician-directed organization was accepted by the leaders of the founding groups in the summer of 1996. Existing concepts from the founding corporations were integrated to create Spectrum's vision, operating principles and guiding documents (See Fig. 1). Workgroups did the countless hours of important work to establish the founding legal documents. These included the new shareholder agreement, the retirement and benefit policies, and the additional legal steps to avoid anti-trust obstacles forming a professional association (PA). Important legal advice was obtained and discussions with the state's assistant attorney general occurred prior to finalizing the Spectrum merger.

Figure 1: Vision, Operating Principles and Decentralized Teams
The existing documents of the founding corporations were integrated,
creating Spectrum's Vision and Operating Principles.

VISION
We are dedicated to excellence in the diagnosis, prevention and treatment of illness, to life long learning, to commitment to our communities, and the primary importance of the caring patient relationship.

OPERATING PRINCIPLES
Integrity & Openness
Respectful Truthtelling
Teamwork & Localness
Accountability & Equitability
Enjoyment & Celebration

TEAMWORK
Participative high performance teams, loosely coordinated with robust communication networks and hardwired feedback loops

Formed as a professional association (PA), Spectrum could function as a fully integrated entity, allowing all business initiatives to be shared without legal concerns. An analysis of the billing practices (anesthesiology had billing employees while radiology and pathology contracted with outside agencies) was completed to enable billing to operate smoothly after the merger.

Administrative leaders: Mary Pinto (anesthesiology), Peter McKenney (radiology), Dick McArdle (pathology) and legal consultants (each practice's attorney, an antitrust attorney and a merger specialist) prepared options for the physician leaders to consider. Many late night meetings after long clinical days, hours of travel to enable face-to-face meetings and meticulous document reviews were needed. The total physician after-hour contribution was never inventoried, but the legal fees alone totaled about $70,000. This included expenses for the two initial mergers of northern (Bangor) and southern (Portland) anesthesiology and radiology. Howard Yates, who joined Spectrum as its first chief executive, provided a crucial corporate-wide perspective.

Governance: The initial Spectrum Board of Directors (BOD) consisted of 12 members elected by the shareholders with the BOD electing its own officers. Each of five subdivisions (anesthesia north/south, radiology north/south, and pathology) elected two members from within their subdivisions (a total of 10 BOD members) with an additional two 'at large' members being elected by the entire group of shareholders. Seven of the elected BOD members were members of the MMC Medical Staff. As operational processes were refined the BOD focused on the corporate-wide view, including both internal and external perspectives. A Divisional Advisory Committee (DAC) governed the corporate-wide operations of each of the 3 specialty divisions. The three elected vice presidents (each previously the President of one of the legacy practices) provided specialty leadership. In Portland, the three MMC Department Chairs continued to manage their MMC clinical departments while communicating Spectrum's views to the MMC administration.

The BOD members (* denotes BOD members who were also MMC Department Chairs): Michael Jones*(VP) & Tim Hayes (Pathology Division); Katherine Pope (VP) & Ken Raessler* (Anesthesiology South Subdivision); Chris Pope & Roger Pezzuti* (Radiology South Subdivision); John Frankland & Gregg Farrell (Anesthesiology North Subdivision); John Long (VP) & Michael Pancoe (Radiology North Subdivision); Doug Cowan (North) & John Darby (South) at-large members. Chris Pope was elected as the inaugural Spectrum President and John Frankland the Executive Vice President. The Divisional VPs were as noted above.

HOW: Spectrum's Early Focus

In the early phases following the merger, Spectrum focused on six key areas guided in part by studies identifying important predictors of corporate longevity[7] (See Fig. 2).

Figure 2: Predictors of Corporate Longevity
Note alignment of predictors with the key areas

Predictors of Corporate Longevity	Key Focus Areas
#1) Cohesion and identity: aspects of a company's innate ability to build a community and a persona for itself	(i), (iii), (iv), (v)
#2) Sensitivity to the environment: a company's ability to learn and adapt to changing market place demands	(i), (ii), (iii), (iv), (v), (vi)
#3) Tolerance and decentralization: Tolerance to new ideas, the ability to build constructive relationships with other entities & within itself, valuing people not assets and a loosening of steering & control	(i), (ii), (iii), (iv), (v), (vi)
#4) Conservatism in financing: defines the ability to govern its own growth and evolution effectively, which is a critical corporate attribute	(ii), (iv), (v), (vi)

These six key focus areas are:

i. **Build good business relationships with other physicians, hospitals and between physicians within Spectrum** *(Aligned with Predictors #1- #3 in Fig. 2)* Spectrum contacted and made presentations to all interested physician groups to explain the vision and guiding principles and to alleviate fears that a monopolistic or market power corporate behavior was planned *(See Fig. 3)*. Spectrum focused on treating each member fairly, aligning incentives to accomplish the vision and preserving advantages of local decision-making as much as possible.

Figure 3: Introducing Spectrum

*An extract from information provided to local medical groups, hospitals
and other interested parties after Spectrum formed in September 1996*

SPECTRUM MEDICAL GROUP

The evolving Maine healthcare market provides an excellent opportunity for a well organized integrated physician-led organization to provide comprehensive medical services that best meet the needs of its customers: patients, employers, insurers, other physicians, managed care organizations and health systems. Spectrum Medical Group will be a multi-disciplinary physician group, representing all specialties (including primary care) and can form the backbone of the emerging integrated delivery systems. To date, many physicians have been drawn into hospital created and controlled organizations mainly due to the lack of a reasonable physician-driven alternative.

Spectrum will develop a corporate infrastructure designed to handle the clinical, business and operational functions that can be consolidated efficiently. Divisional members of Spectrum will enjoy the best of both worlds – the ability to benefit from the economies of scale inherent in a larger, more centralized organization, while maintaining divisional autonomy as appropriate to address the specific needs of each division. Each specialty group will retain its identity as a division of Spectrum. Divisional representation on the Corporate Board of Directors of Spectrum will ensure that divisional issues and needs will be well represented.

Spectrum will provide comprehensive services to customers within its market, including:

- Direct, risk-based contracting with insurers and managed care organizations
- A range of high quality, reasonably priced medical services to patients
- Comprehensive clinical support services to patients and institutions:
  (Quality Management, Outcomes Measurement, Utilization Review, Practice Guidelines, and Credentialing)
- Practice Management services to both divisional members and prospective member practices include:
  (Corporate Planning and Development, Contracting, Finance, Marketing, Corporate operations, Information Systems Management, Human Resources Management, Insured and Uninsured Benefits Administration, Billing and Accounts Receivable Management, Practice Management Consulting)

---

ii. **Strengthen Spectrum's contracting abilities**
(Aligned with Predictors #2 - #4 in Fig. 2)

At the time, capitated contracting and the resources and knowledge to implement such contracts were in the early stages of development in Maine. Spectrum worked closely with insurance plans to develop a unified Spectrum option. This allowed the group to benefit from its broad market presence, and receive fair compensation for the high quality clinical services it continued to improve. Insurance companies recognized the advantages of having Spectrum in an advisory capacity while they developed their own capability to manage both the quality and service utilization of other similar specialty physician groups in Maine.

iii. **Expand Spectrum by mergers with other groups**
(Aligned with Predictors #1 - #3 in Fig. 2)
Although there were many discussions with other physician groups after the
September merger, none joined Spectrum in the first 5 years. Many leading
physician practices (including orthopedic, surgical, emergency medicine, medical
oncology) in Portland and Bangor were approached. The expected managed
care and capitated market evolution did not materialize immediately in Maine
so other groups were reluctant to form a fully integrated multi-specialty group.
Therefore Spectrum initially functioned as a RAP group which resulted in an easier
integration process since the three founding specialties had similar characteristics:

> a.) Primarily hospital-based, had largely solved internal compensation
> conflicts, had similar governance structures and benefit plans;
> b.) Primarily procedure-based, their billing practices were well understood;
> and
> c.) A strong desire to remain a physician-directed organization.

iv. **Actualize the benefits of the initial Spectrum merger**
(Aligned with Predictors #1 - #4 in Fig. 2)
Many of the anticipated cost efficiencies and 'economies of scale' were realized.
Sharing strategic market information as well as extending and sharing existing
infrastructure (such as business and email systems, contracting information and
clinical quality support processes) enabled the 'economies of scale' cost-reduction.
The radiology email system, already integrated into the MMC system, was extended
to all of Spectrum to allow essential information to be shared with reduced cost.
Relationships with MMC were on a different footing due to coordinated contract
conversations. Spectrum clinicians and leaders acted as liaisons with other
hospitals for MaineHealth (MMC's 'parent') services and leveraged the existing
relationships in all the divisions. As MaineHealth continued to grow, Spectrum
benefitted from MaineHealth's outreach gaining some contracting opportunities.

v. **Build infrastructure together while optimizing the hospital systems and
performance improvement efforts** (Aligned with Predictors #1 - #4 in Fig. 2)
Shared process and clinical information systems included the email system
mentioned above. The following are other examples of shared improvements: the
governance decision structure, strategic planning, contracting analysis, clinical
quality information analysis, compliance programs, HR policies (including a
conduct policy), pension investment oversight, analysis of shareholder benefits
such as health insurance options, and purchasing discounts (e.g. computers,
equipment, etc.). The new, fabulous administrative team supported all the

Spectrum members. Improving hospital infrastructure and clinical performance is discussed later in this chapter and also detailed in the other clinical department chapters of this book.

vi. **Develop a new value-added strategy**
Aligned with Predictors #2 - #4 in Fig. 2)
Key goals were to be market leaders for the three clinical services while providing uniformly high quality clinical services at all Spectrum sites. Spectrum members were already involved in many quality initiatives in hospitals and other organizations in Maine. Spectrum's view of quality could be expressed as:

"Walk the talk. Quality is verb not an adjective or noun"

New approaches included the collection of clinical data to profile clinical service utilization. Spectrum contracted with an insurance company to collect and analyze data to optimize image-ordering behavior in its physician panel. Clinical quality anesthesiology systems were used to detect outlier clinical processes and modify clinician performance. Physicians who played key roles in these efforts included several Spectrum BOD members in addition to Craig Curry (Anesthesia Division) and Tim Hayes (Pathology Division) who also played pivotal roles. From the start, Rebecca Murray was a vital member of Spectrum's quality improvement efforts. Spectrum's quality data often allowed MMC to satisfy their hospital certification expectations.

The data driven anesthesiology quality management system called FIDES was further marketed and became an independent product with national clients. Many Spectrum members became part owners of an imaging company (Insight Premier Health) that delivered outpatient MRI imaging at a reduced cost. The mobile PET-CT business was started as a joint venture with MaineHealth. The two companies now provide PET-CT, MRI and CT services at imaging centers and with its mobile scanners.

HOW: Early Lessons Spectrum Learned

In the initial years following the merger, a number of key lessons were learned:

1. **Physicians feared the potential loss of autonomy from joining into a larger group**

   Governance and decision-making processes consume a vast amount of energy and can create many conflicts. Physicians are trained to form opinions and are often accustomed to being the 'expert' in the room. Successful groups work to overcome these hurdles and become high performance teams working towards common goals. Redirecting attention and energy away from physician compensation and benefits toward a focus on developing measurable quality and value-based clinical services is sometimes necessary. Limiting 'negative' energy and avoiding cannibalizing the organization from within are key milestones on a path to success, which of course is always 'under construction'.

2. **Shareholders expected Spectrum to achieve the merger benefits quickly**

   It was necessary to explain that the tangible returns predicted to result from the merger would take some time. For instance, some shareholders anticipated that other single specialty groups would soon join Spectrum. The failure to rapidly meet this and other expectations prompted many shareholder discussions and questions about whether the Spectrum merger could indeed be considered a success. Although some efforts took longer than anticipated, most of the benefits expected from the initial merger were eventually realized. It had been predicted that the organizational changes resulting from the rapid sequence of mergers would cause difficulties. Many shareholders, even some of the leadership group, showed an initial reluctance to accept electronic forms of communication, new clinical systems and business practices. The following statement was often heard at meetings:

   'Everyone wants the benefits of Spectrum, but no one wants to change"

   Group leaders explained the new value-added initiatives Spectrum was pursuing and shared the metrics quantifying the benefits at group meetings (Fig. 4).

Figure 4: Group Performance and Value Measures
Metrics were developed to measure Spectrum's performance.
This is a sample from Spectrum's Balanced Scorecard strategic initiative.

Spectrum Performance and Value Measures

Product Quality: *radiology and pathology interpretation errors, content and format of radiology reports, post anesthesia vomiting, IV contrast complications*

Service Delivery Quality: *reporting delays in radiology & pathology, patient study scheduling wait times, patient satisfaction surveys*

Corporate Strategic Efforts: *achieving the established milestones and timely completion of annual strategic initiatives in all 3 divisions and the overall corporate goals*

Shareholder Surveys: *shareholder satisfaction surveys, inter-shareholder feedback surveys (4As & 1T: Perception of an individual's Availability, Affability, Ability, Afficiency and Team player characteristics).*

Financial: **77%** *to physicians for clinical work (weekday & on-call clinical work)*
8% *for physician administrative and management work*
15% *were general operating expenses including physician extenders, billing and non-physician administrators.*

Charitable Work: *Uncompensated patient care, charitable giving and charity organizational support work hours performed by Spectrum members*

---

3. Balancing the clinical and 'non-clinical' work was challenging

The difficult work of creating Spectrum, including the establishment of new agreements and operating principles, were only the beginning of the effort needed to achieve benefits from the merger. While many after-hours of 'perspiration' were needed in the creation phase, physician leaders also needed time for 'non-clinical' work during usual business hours. Experienced and committed physician leadership is essential to the survival of a physician-directed corporation. Workload adjustments to reduce stress and provide time to gain these new skills were needed. Accepting that 'business work' had a similar value to revenue from clinical work was a big cultural change. Sometimes clinical physicians also thought group leadership had lost touch with the demands of patient care. Acceptance that all team members have important contributions is a characteristic of successful high-performance teams.

Leaders were required to develop familiarity with thinking tools[8], project management skills[2], conflict resolution techniques, high performance team principles[2] and particularly quality improvement processes[1,2] all part of any CBE program. Personal development in ego management and the fundamentals of skillful dialogue[2] (including the primary importance of deep listening) were crucial. Adding CBE needs necessary for leadership development to CME requirements (to retain clinical competency) can often exhaust physicians. It is little wonder that many physicians often trade away autonomy for personal lifestyle.

NOW: Spectrum's Growth and Longevity

Spectrum continued to grow from its start in 1996 with 90 physicians, through 1998 with 114 physicians (Fig. 5) and in 2015, the total number of board certified physicians was 222, with 64 advanced practice providers, making a total of more than 600 physicians and staff working across Maine and Northern New England. Spectrum served 556,927 patients and 1,501,120 services were provided in 2015.

Figure 5: Spectrum Growth in 20 years
The clinicians and specialties 1996-2015

	1996	1998	2015
Total Physicians	90	114	222
Anesthesiology	38	54	80
Pathology	6	11	23
Radiology	41	43	80
Radiation oncology	5	6	6
Orthopedics			33
Advanced Practice Providers			64

Core strategies currently guiding Spectrum are:
- Provide quality;
- Provide for our people;
- Facilitate integration;
- Expand clinical reach; and
- Continue to add specialties.

Today the principles of Spectrum's 'Triple Aim' are: optimize the experience of care, improve the health of populations and reduce the per-capita costs of healthcare.

Having celebrated its 20th birthday in 2016, Spectrum continues to meet the current challenging healthcare environment with 'eyes wide open', remaining cognizant of these predictors of corporate longevity: conservative financing, sensitivity to the local market changes and providing value-based care.

The Spectrum Story Part II:
'Nudging' MMC: Improving Clinical Performance

This section describes two efforts to 'nudge' MMC into becoming a more patient-centered organization: (1) Redirecting MMC to include clinical quality metrics rather than using only financial goals to align administrator incentives with the core purpose of the hospital; and (2) Directing the broad coordinated effort to fund critical clinical infrastructure (for example, modernizing the radiology film library by investing in a computerized image archival and distribution information system).

1.　**'Nudging' MMC: To include Quality of Care Metrics:**

A primary strategic goal for Spectrum was to optimize MMC clinical processes, thereby improving MMC's focus on clinical quality. As was common in hospitals during the early 1990s, MMC leadership focused on expense and revenue indicators of care, which meant that effective work systems designed to collect and measure patient care expenses were well established. Systems to provide easy clinician access to clinical information such as patient allergies, measures of clinical workflow processes, medical treatment errors (e.g. medication Rx errors, surgical complications and patient safety concerns), also became a priority in the late 1990s and early 2000s.

Although MMC administrators were interested in quality, they were uncertain how to address it. Broad support existed amongst MMC clinicians (physicians, nurses and others) for clinical improvement efforts and for developing a more robust clinical infrastructure. The following anecdote illustrates one small effort to shift MMC's Trustees and senior management team's focus from two financial metrics to a balanced set of clinical quality and financial indicators.

In presentations to MMC's Trustees, the following question was asked: *"Who would fly in a jumbo jet that has only 2 dials informing the crew whether all systems are functioning optimally?"*

This visual (Fig. 6) had a powerful effect. All were well aware that MMC was the equivalent to 4 'jumbo' jets and thus the implications and risks of the current focus became evident. By the end of that financial year, the CEO's bonus included the provision that about 25% would be awarded contingent on his successfully implementing a balanced scorecard system[6] that included many pertinent quality-of-care focused metrics.

Figure 6: Introducing Balanced Scorecard Quality Metrics
Who would fly in a jumbo jet that has only 2 dials informing the crew whether all systems are functioning optimally?

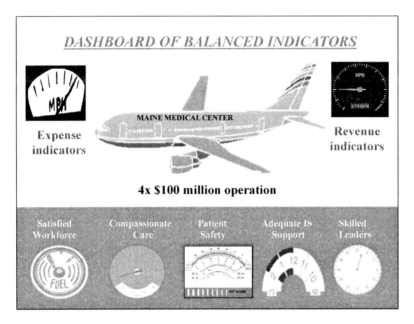

The reader should understand that this example was only one of countless efforts to redirect MMC to adopt a more patient-centered approach. Each MMC clinical department and many Spectrum clinicians worked collaboratively with MMC to accomplish this goal over many years. Their contributions are detailed in the other clinical department and medical group chapters of this book.

2. 'Nudging' MMC: To fund critical Clinical Infrastructure

2(a). Image Storage and Distribution

Details of the radiology image storage and distribution process failures during the 1990s in MMC's radiology file room are already described in the chapter on MMC's Radiology Department. That state of affairs resulted in suboptimal patient care. The following email (Fig. 7: left side) was sent from the Chief of the Radiology

Extract from an email from Chief of Radiology to MMC CEO	Radiology Department Unreported studies (3-month update)
"As you are aware from many prior discussions and presentations dating back at least 3 years, we have had a severe problem with our file room for years. Efforts to fix this have included countless hours of time on the part of departmental personnel, along with others inside MMC, and the services of two outside expert consultants. It is fair to say we have analyzed this problem thoroughly and I doubt there is much detail left that we don't understand. We have suspected but been unable to get a firm handle on the scope of the issue of 'unreported activity', meaning studies performed but not dictated (reported) by the Radiologists. Last week we finally got that firm understanding, and it is horrifying. There are approximately 2000 studies in our system dating back to May 2000 that are still unreported! It is probably quite evident what the implications of this are, but I will enumerate them anyway: poor patient care and possible missed diagnoses, medical legal risk to the institution and to the physicians involved, both Radiologists and non-Radiologists, compliance issues in that these have been billed by MMC but not formally interpreted (completed as a clinical service), as well as economic losses related to the work to clean up the backlog."	**2001** 70 from April 15 from March 19 from February 15 from January **2000** 19 from December 6 from November 9 from October 8 from September 10 from August 2 from July 3 from June 1 from May Oldest May 17th 2000

Figure 7: Radiology Department Film Reporting Improvements

Department to MMC's CEO. The consequences of radiology report delays and lost films due to file room issues are clearly outlined. Follow up about 3 months after this email (Fig. 7: right side) showed that 177 patient films were still without radiologist readings to complete the clinical service. A different solution was clearly needed and required MMC to invest in an expensive computerized system.

"The definition of insanity is doing the same thing over and over again, but expecting different results."

Albert Einstein

2(b). Using "Fake News" to redirect Budget Priorities & improve Quality at MMC

MMC's senior management team met regularly in the early morning. At one particular meeting, a 'fake news' report (Fig. 8) was given to each attendee. It was ostensibly a photocopy of a news clipping summarizing the impact a 'lost' radiology study had on the care of a recent MMC patient:

MEDICAL ERRORS THREATEN PATIENT SAFETY AT MAINE MEDICAL CENTER

Mr. Hammond of Portland recently experienced acute pain in his abdomen while a patient at Maine Medical Center. His physician ordered an X-ray and a CAT scan procedure after surgical consultation. Mr. Hammond has previously been diagnosed with a cancer of the blood called lymphoma.

The Portland Press Herald has learned that the Radiology department lost Mr. Hammond's X-ray films for 2 days and the radiologist doctors (who read these films) did not get to see the old films until 72 hours after he had the procedure. Because all Mr. Hammond's previous X-rays and CAT scans that had been obtained over the past 3 years could not be found until 3 days after the new CAT scan, the doctors thought that some thickening of his bowel on the new CAT scan was a new development. When Mr. Hammond's pain increased, the surgeons recommended that he have surgery because of this "new" bowel mass. When they operated, a mass associated with the bowel was found but the surgeons were unable to remove it.

The family and Mr. Hammond were very disappointed when they were later told that the mass had been present on the prior CAT scan which had been "lost" for 3 days. Had the surgeons known this, they would not have operated. The family members feel that their father has had an unnecessary operation. They indicated that they have already received some bills from the hospital including some for the radiology studies.

Asked to comment on the issue, Mrs. Hammond said, "I am surprised to receive a bill for the radiology work. As they could only read these films properly after my husband already had his surgery, and he would not have had the surgery if they were read completely, I would think that they should not be able to charge anything for this work. My husband had an unnecessary operation and might have lost his life. We pay our insurance and will speak to our insurance company"

Figure 8: Fake News used to improve Clinical and Patient Safety

As anticipated, all were quite disturbed by the news report. After the potential consequences were fully digested and remedial steps to ameliorate the damage to MMC's public image were being discussed, it was revealed to be a 'fake'. The implications were clear to all: given the state of affairs prevailing in the radiology filing system, at any time this news clipping could become 'true news'. The result was renewed interest prioritizing resources to improve clinical workflow and the radiology information systems

Conclusion

Writing this chapter prompted the obvious question: would anyone want to read a story about five private medical groups overcoming the challenges to form a single corporation, acquiring skills to react to rapidly changing market conditions and then work together with MMC to improve the quality of care delivered even as the cost of healthcare was under attack? The answer remains uncertain, but if you are reading this sentence, you will know it's too late to decide.

By avoiding a purely chronologic account this summary has attempted to outline why Spectrum was formed, to clarify the goals and the vision of the founding members, and to provide a description of some key concepts learned during the process. Clinicians have a unique view of patient care and see the purpose of a hospital differently from non-physician administrators. However, the best results are achieved when both perspectives are blended, always recognizing that the hospital is a community-owned resource which need not control all facets of the health delivery market. When all participants in hospital decisions strive to listen carefully and to improve collaboration, meeting patient needs is achievable. Hospitals deliver high quality medical care most effectively when focused on quality indicators of medical care not just on financial metrics.

All those who played instrumental roles in Spectrum's founding, including those providing clinical services in the "trenches" and the physician leaders in Spectrum's beginning, middle and into the present time, deserve to be very proud. Rarely does one have the good fortune to participate in a high performance team that contributes to the needs of human beings seeking help for personal suffering. Are we able to see each radiology image, pathology slide or laboratory test and sedated or clinic patient as the fearful person who is seeking our help? Can we provide the same level of care to all our patients that we want for our own families? Working in modern healthcare and consistently offering the caring relationships our patients need is very difficult. We are privileged to have the resources of Spectrum and MMC to help us in our effort to provide the relief they seek so desperately.

Acknowledgements

I want to thank all those friends, colleagues and family members who spent many hours helping to massage a very rough verbose initial outline into the final more succinct and understandable story. Without their help, this chapter would not have been completed. All the remaining errors, impolitic statements and verbosity are solely my responsibility. Although often it is said that the truth should never spoil a good story, attempting to tell the truth always makes a good story, while remembering all truths are always only partial.

[1] *Enhancing Physician Performance – Advanced Principles of Medical Management* Editors: Scott B. Ranson, William W. Pinsky and John E. Tropman. ACPE 2000

[2] *The Fifth Discipline Fieldbook* – Strategies and Tools for building a Learning Organization by Peter Senge, Charlotte Roberts, Richard Ross, Bryan Smith & Art Kleiner. Doubleday 1995

[3] *Total Quality in Healthcare - From Theory to Practice* by Ellen J. Gaucher & Richard J. Coffey. Jossey-Bass 1993

[4] *Complexity and Emergence in Organizations.* Series Editors: Ralph D. Stacy, Douglas Griffin & Patricia Shaw: The Paradox of Control in Organizations and Measuring Performance by Phillip Streatfield. Routledge 2001.

[5] *The Intelligence Advantage. Organizing for Complexity.* Michael D. McMaster Butterworth-Heineman 1996

[6] *The Balanced Scorecard – Translating Strategy into Action* by Robert S. Kaplan & D.P Norton. Harvard Business School Press 1996

[7] *The Living Company* by Arie de Geus. Harvard Business Review 1997

[8] *Teach yourself to Think* by Edward de Bono. Penguin Books 1995

Maine Medical Partners

By F. Stephen Larned MD and Stephen J. Kasabian

Prior to the 1970's, almost all primary care physicians in the Portland, Maine vicinity practiced alone or possibly with one other physician. Offices were basic, often attached to a physician's home. Managing a medical practice started to become more complicated and costly with the advent of Medicare in 1966 which increased the complexity of billing and the amount of paper work required. One response to these changes was a trend for physicians to merge their practices into four to six physician groups, which became commonplace. This allowed physicians to share overhead and office expertise, and also facilitated the sharing of night and weekend call.

In the 1980's and early 1990's the situation became more complicated and expensive with the advent of the Medicare "Resource Based Relative Value Scale" (RBRVS) and the requirement that all medical claims be coded. The methodology and requirements pioneered by Medicare were quickly adopted by all third-party payers. The cost and complexity of billing accelerated rapidly, requiring more office staff with better training. At the same time the proportion of "straight" fee for service (FFS) reimbursement for most physicians actually decreased. This particularly impacted primary care providers who delivered mostly cognitive (non-procedural) services and thus were already at the low end of the reimbursement spectrum. Other economic pressures presented themselves about the same time, including managed care, which contributed to the need for expensive office business systems and computers for billing and compliance. Although initially elective, these soon became a fundamental requirement for maintaining a practice given ever increasing regulatory requirements, pressures to participate in e-prescribing, and the eventual reality that these would only be possible in the context of maintaining a computerized medical record.

The combination of factors described above raised the cost of running medical practices for all physicians - but resulted in a disproportionate economic squeeze for primary care doctors. They could not simply increase patient or ancillary volumes to compensate for higher fixed expenses – and therefore experienced progressively shrinking practice income. It became increasingly difficult to sustain a private practice, be it solo or small group. The result was the development of large privately owned (e.g. InterMed) or institutionally based (e.g. Maine Medical Center, Martin's Point) primary care group practices. The merger of several primary care groups to form InterMed in the 1990's is chronicled in a separate chapter of this book. The story of the merger of hospital-based specialty practices (anesthesia, radiology, radiation oncology and pathology) in Portland and Bangor into the Spectrum Medical Group in 1996 is also told in a separate chapter. This chapter will focus on the story of the development of the Maine Medical Center (MMC) hospital owned physician practice model (initially Medical Services Corporation) that has grown exponentially over the last few decades and now includes about 500 physicians in a wide range of primary care and specialty practices.

MMC was aware that in order to maintain a first-class medical center, a full complement of primary care physicians as well as specialists and subspecialists to serve the community would be required. Some of the financial problems affecting primary care practices were described above. These problems also affected specialists as well, to varying degrees. However for specialists there was another set of challenges related to the fact that the Portland region lacked a sufficiently large enough population base to support a broad range of subspecialists with enough depth to maintain reasonable coverage and lifestyle. In addition, Portland had a poor payor mix with many patients having no insurance, Medicaid, or forms of underinsurance. This made it difficult for a number of specialties to support enough sub-specialty trained physicians to create a true tertiary care hospital and medical community while preserving financial viability. Ultimately for many specialists the only reasonable solution for these problems was to form a partnership with the hospital.

Maine Medical Partners

In its various forms, Maine Medical Partners (MMP) has been providing care to patients throughout Maine and parts of New Hampshire for approximately 30 years. It is northern New England's largest multi-specialty group practice and serves a direct support role to Maine Medical Center and many other members of the MaineHealth family. The growth and development of MMP can best be described in four significant periods.

Phase 1 – Medical Services Corporation
In the mid to late 1980's, MMC began to explore ownership of medical practices and employment of physicians to support its ambulatory enterprises. Anticipating that such models might grow in the future an entity named Medical Services Corporation (MSC) was formed as the umbrella to house the practices. The earliest of practices included ObGyn Associates, MMC Trauma Surgery, MMC Epilepsy and MMC Pediatric Specialty Group. Seeking to maintain transparency, Maine Medical Center created an MSC Board comprised of physicians from the

community based private practices. The Board reviewed financial MSC performance monthly and was involved in decision making regarding the recruitment needs and ultimate growth of MSC. As additional private practices sought to align with MMC and become employed, MSC was the initial vehicle to accomplish this goal. Subsequent growth included the addition of general pediatric practices, internal medicine practices and several other early entrants.

Phase 2 – Management Service Organization
In 1994 Maine Medical Center, working with private community physicians, developed a business plan to establish a management service organization (MSO). The MSO model was emerging rapidly across the country as a means for hospitals and health systems to best manage their acquired physician practices. By creating a management company uniquely focused on the needs of these practices, hospitals could attract the administrative and technical expertise best suited to provide a strong focus on the unique needs of physicians and their medical practices. The MMC-MSO was activated in May of 1995. Its initial purpose was to provide management, billing, financial and staffing resources to the practices then owned by MMC as well as for several private practices in greater Portland.

Over the following 10 years the MSO continued to grow in its support of new and existing MMC/MSC practices as well as of private practices seeking some or all of these services on a contracted basis. During this period the MMC-MSO changed its name to PracticePartners but continued to provide MSO services as originally designed. The formation of MaineHealth early in this timeframe also contributed to the responsibilities of the MSO which extended its purview to provide physician practice support throughout the expanding MaineHealth system. Initially the MSO provided a wide range of billing and management support activities to the practices at Stephens Memorial Hospital in Norway. That longstanding relationship exists today.

Phase 3– Multi-Specialty Group Formation
After approximately ten years of operation as an MSO the PracticePartners Board of Directors concluded that the opportunity was right to bring Practice Partners, MMC (MSC) owned and MSO managed practices together into a single multi-specialty group practice. The MSO was also included as it was a necessary component to ensure that the new

multi-specialty group had an infrastructure suited for group success. The newly formed multi-specialty group (MSG) was named Maine Medical Partners (MMP) and with that renaming began a decade of significant growth and development. At the outset MMP was comprised of 100 physicians across 11 practice entities. Almost immediately MMP began a prolonged period of significant growth. Initial additions included the MMC Hospitalist group, followed by a host of specialty practices in neurosurgery and spine, pediatric surgery, neurology, ENT, orthopedic trauma, orthopedic joints, cardiology, cardiothoracic surgery, sports medicine, as well as the Portland Urology, Maine Surgical Care and Casco Bay Surgery group practices.

Phase 4 – Integrated Group Practice Formation

During this period of growth through acquisition and integration of practices across the community, MMP and MMC leadership concluded that the time was ideal to fully integrate the cadre of MMC's hospital-based physicians. This included emergency medicine physicians, psychiatrists, and a variety of other physicians previously employed directly by MMC. MMP thus reached a total of just under 500 physicians and nearly 200 advanced practice clinicians (APC). These providers are currently supported by 1200 clinical and administrative support staff located in multiple practice settings but working in coordinated teams to help practices meet the expanding patient access, business, and administrative needs associated with the growth of MMP.

The Future

MMP continues to grow by adding new providers to the existing practice groups while establishing new specialty practices to meet patient demand. An average of over 30 new physicians have joined MMP each year in addition to those who joined as part of new practice acquisitions. The continued reliance on MMC to meet tertiary and community needs will keep MMP focused on growth and services for many years to come.

Two excellent examples of the value added from well managed and highly functional physician-hospital partnerships are the cardiology-cardiac surgery and neurosciences divisions of MMP. Prior to joining MMP, there were two major and competitive cardiology groups in the Portland area - Maine Cardiology Associates (MCA) and Cardiovascular Consultants of Maine (CCM). Early on they realized that each would both benefit from a closer working relationship. This mutually respectful and friendly relationship led to a merger in 2014 as the groups became employed by MMP. The cardiac surgeons had become hospital employees in 2012. With all cardiac physicians under the MMP corporate umbrella, MMC was able to provide a global fee offering for several cardiac procedures thus making MMC price competitive in the national market. A single large and integrated cardiac team was essential to the success of the Acute Myocardial Infarction Response Team. Through this effort, cardiologists and emergency medicine physicians working together with staff were able to achieve a "door to balloon" response time of 90 minutes. Organizing a response team such as this would have been extremely difficult to coordinate with several competing groups, some in private practice and others under hospital employment.

Another great success was the amalgamation of the neurology and neurosurgery physicians into the MMC Division of Neuroscience. Due to changing economic realities in their practice, the neurologists joined Maine Medical Partners in 2010. That group now numbers 22 neurologists - each with some subspecialty training. The neurosurgeons had merged with Maine Medical in 2006. That group has grown to ten neurosurgeons offering, among many services, a robust neuro-endovascular program that treats intracranial aneurysms and vascular malformations. MMC's Neurosciences Center of Excellence is the institution's largest clinical business line. This service line has enabled MMC to provide state-of-the-art neuroscience programs including acute stroke intervention. This program, like that for patients with acute cardiac events is collaborative with the Emergency Department physicians who initiate IV tPA treatment for clot dissolving. More recently intracranial thrombectomy has become a frequent mode of treatment delivered through a collaboration between interventional neurosurgeons and neurointerventional radiologists. The MMC Neuroscience program has reported significant improvement in acute stroke outcomes with these treatment regimens and is a prominent contributor to the medical literature on acute stroke treatment.

As described here and elsewhere in this book, the partnership between MMC and its physicians has had a very positive effect on the success of key service areas. The hospital has been able to recruit outstanding subspecialists by providing modern equipment and technology as well as income and salary support when necessary. This support has allowed physicians in the MMC owned practices to practice high quality medicine while conducting clinical and basic research and delivering excellent teaching programs. The coordination among different divisions under one practice roof - coupled with the added benefit of receiving referrals from throughout the MaineHealth network of hospitals and office practices - has contributed to the growth and quality of the medical care provided and to the satisfaction of physicians and staff. MMC has successfully marketed bundled services with third party payers to provide cost effective, first class medical care.

Although hospital employed physician practices can facilitate coordination of services and reduce the pressures associated with fee for service medicine and other business/economic issues, challenges can arise in this model. Hospitals such as MMC are very large enterprises with huge payrolls and very labor-intensive operations that are required to support 24-hour services over a wide range of disciplines. They have to provide state of the art equipment and facilities as well as competitive compensation to highly trained specialists in order to compete with other practice opportunities both locally and in other parts of the country. By nature and tradition hospitals tend to be top down in management style while also requiring buy-in from a wide range of disciplines in order to reach workable agreements. The influence of physicians in such large and complex institutions can become diluted or marginalized. As a result, the value of the physicians' unique focus on the care and health of the patient can be lost.

Fortunately, MMC was well aware of this potential problem, and made concerted efforts to include strong physician input in the ongoing management of MMP, currently under the direction of Stephen J. Kasabian, its Chief Administrative Officer. This is best exemplified by the Board of Directors of MMP being composed almost exclusively of physicians. In addition, each of the Clinical Service Lines (e.g. Neurosciences, Cardiac and Orthopedics) has significant physician representation in their management structure. Going forward it is critical for physicians to retain a significant voice in management decisions that impact how health care is provided. Since physicians are, in the end, the components of the medical care system most responsible for influencing the quality and cost of patient care, their input should be sought and welcomed.

This book provides many examples of physician-inspired innovations and advances in medical care. It would be unfortunate if going forward the employed doctors are not recognized as critical to the management of the hospital and its medical staff and included routinely in important management decisions.

MMC Scarborough Campus

By Stuart G. Gilbert MD

> *"When you give an order, give it through the Chain of Command. However, if you get your intel through the Chain of Command, you will be dead in the water."*
>
> *Admiral Hyman Rickover, U.S. Navy, Nuclear Sub Command*

Admiral Rickover's comment indicates that subordinates are not likely to tell their superiors that all is not well in their area of responsibility. In the hospital setting the ultimate responsibility for the delivery of quality health care resides with the physician. If the current status affects that quality the physician has an obligation to bring that to the attention of the decision makers. Those decision makers will need data and information to make a decision and to defend it in front of their superiors - often the Board.

Administrators have an awesome responsibility to allocate the hospital's finite resources in the most efficacious manner. They should welcome suggestions and information from all staff on how to improve their institution.

In spite of bringing the Bath radiation therapy (RT) facility on line in February 1993, the two aging linear accelerators at Maine Medical Center were unable to handle a growing demand for services. In August of 1993 I submitted the following unsolicited memorandum to the MMC administration requesting an offsite facility in the Portland area for radiotherapy. That report has been condensed and follows.

Memorandum
To: Paul D. Gray, Vice President of Planning, MMC
From: Stuart Gilbert MD
August 11, 1993

Plan to Fulfill Radiation Oncology Needs at Maine Medical Center
Need for Third Linear Accelerator In Portland

Introduction

In 1970, seventeen hospitals in southern Maine joined to form the Southern Maine Radiation Therapy Institute (SMRTI). They agreed that rather than having several small departments providing cobalt machines, they would cooperate to establish a large modern department to provide state-of-the-art radiation oncology to the residents of southern Maine and eastern New Hampshire. In 1974, that department opened at Maine Medical Center and was staffed by two radiation oncologists. It has now grown so that it evaluates about 1,100 new cancer patients and delivers over 25,000 treatments per year. It is currently staffed by five radiation oncologists.

In 1992, the Board of Trustees of Maine Medical Center has again committed the institution to be a major tertiary oncology center for northern New England and has designated cancer treatment as one of its six primary focuses. Both the cooperative effort by the southern Maine hospitals and the Board of Trustees' commitment obliges us to be able to provide radiation oncology services to the patients of our region. This paper addresses a concern that we will be unable to fulfill our obligations in radiation oncology if current trends continue and the demand is not met with adequate capacity of our Linear Accelerators.

Growth of Patient Demand

In 1987, MMC applied for a Certificate of Need for a third Linear Accelerator. The State approved this request and stated that our patient load justified three accelerators. That third machine began treating patients in Bath on February 1, 1993. Since 1987 the volume of cancer patients treated at MMC and SMRTI has drastically increased, as demonstrated by the following table:

	1987	1992	%
New Patients – MMC Tumor registry	1,360	1,769	30%
New Breast Cancer – MMC	151	195	29%
New Prostate Cancer – MMC	91	198	118%
New Patients – SMRTI	886	1,041	20%
Radiation Treatments – SMRTI	18,942	22,697	20%
Breast Cancer – Lumpectomy & RT	53	96	81%

This dramatic growth in patients with carcinoma over the past five years is related to both the national trend of emphasizing the treatment of cancer with conservative surgery and radiotherapy and with developments in the local oncology community

Current Status

Last year, SMRTI treated 90 to 95 patients per day on their two linear accelerators in Portland. We expected that with the opening of the Bath radiotherapy facility in February 1993, we would off-load 20 to 25 patients per day that lived between Brunswick and Camden and had their daily treatments in Portland. Thus, we anticipated relieving our stressful situation and being able to provide adequate machine capacity to provide for our patients. To our amazement, even though the Coastal Cancer Treatment Center in Bath is treating over 25 patients per day, the department in Portland is inundated with a greater demand for radiation therapy services than we can provide with our two linacs. During the next year, our total treatments will be up 15 to 20% over the past year.

Our Current Status as of August 6, 1993

To illustrate the current status in our department, I obtained the following figures for our two machines in Portland. The 4 MV treated 47 patients on August 6 and has 19 patients who have been seen by a physician and are waiting to start on that machine. The 20 MV Linear Accelerator treated 46 patients on that day and has 23 patients waiting to start. On Monday, August 9, ten new patients were seen by the radiation oncologists in our Portland Department and some of them will not be treated until September. We average four new cancer patients seen each and every day.

Current Options for Dealing with the Crisis Situation

1. *We have been actively off-loading as many patients as we can to our Bath facility. We have treated patients from Biddeford, Westbrook, and Falmouth by providing almost immediate treatment on that accelerator.*

2. *The short-term approach is to increase our staff of radiation therapists and prolong our day. The administration has approved two additional RTT positions, who will replace the two positions lost to our Portland department when we staffed the Bath facility. With these two new positions we will be treating patients for nine and a half hours per day, for a total of two additional machine hours per machine.*

3. *The real solution to our dilemma would be to increase our capacity. Unfortunately, linear accelerators cannot be installed in a few months. If a third linac was available to us in Portland today, the 42 patients waiting for treatment would fill it to capacity. If the current trends continue for another year or two, then three machines in Portland would not be adequate to cope with our patient load. A combination of three linacs and extended hours would probably suffice to address the patient demand. However, realistically, a third machine would not be available to us for at least two years.*

Respectfully submitted,

Stuart Gilbert MD

Seven days later I received the following reply from Paul Gray:

Memorandum

To: Stu Gilbert MD
From: Paul D. Gray, Vice President of Planning, MMC
Date: August 18, 1993
Re: Radiation Therapy Planning

To confirm our telephone conversation of today, at its August 17, 1993 meeting the Management Group endorsed the following approach to the development of MMC's radiation therapy facilities:

Step 1 – Develop offsite facility with two vaults and one low energy machine (replacement of low energy unit currently at MMC)

Step 2 – Do necessary renovations at MMC to install a high/low energy machine (replacement of high energy machine currently at MMC)

Step 3 – Determine need for high/low machine for offsite facility.

We then had several meetings exploring how we were going to proceed. The hospital decided to build a cancer center and house RT and the medical oncology group in the building. A few months later I was informed that MMC had signed a purchase and sale agreement for a lot at the Maine Mall, adjacent to the Hampton Inn. It had approval for an L-shaped footprint that was adequate for our immediate needs but had no space for expansion. Upon hearing the news I immediately went to Bill Caron's office, who was then Executive Vice President at MMC, and told him that that location was a mistake. I said that we did not benefit from the exposure and congestion at the Mall and that we needed room to expand and add services. Bill responded that the site was fully approved and if I "was not a team player, it would delay obtaining an offsite facility by at least one year". I responded that this facility would be used for at least 50 years and we should take the needed time to get it right. MMC was able to get out of the Purchase and Sale agreement since the land was not sturdy enough to support the weight of the linear accelerator vaults.

Shortly thereafter I sent the following Memo to MMC's Long Range Committee in support of establishing an offsite campus rather than an isolated structure for radiation and medical oncology. As I read this memo 23 years after it was written I am impressed that it as relevant today, in the era of Obama Care as it was in the early 90's during Clinton's health initiative. I am also impressed with how close my wish list for an offsite outpatient center has come to fruition through the good work of the MMC administration.

To: MMC Long Range Planning Committee
From: Stuart G. Gilbert MD
Date: April 24, 1994

This is a pivotal time in health care delivery in the United States and it is clear that in the 21ˢᵗ century the way we deliver health care will be dramatically different than it is today. If MMC's primary mission during the next century is to be the best hospital in the area, it will condemn itself to a progressively shrinking role in health care delivery. Its primary goal should be to deliver quality and compassionate care in a convenient, cost effective setting that includes outpatient, home care and when necessary inpatient services.

One does not need an expensive market analysis to determine the following:

• Inpatient care will be avoided and used as a last resort. It is by far the most costly method of providing health care;

• *Location in the downtown of a major city is not a benefit. Consumers have clearly demonstrated their preference for suburban shopping malls that have easy access and parking. Some major medical institutions have moved their entire physical plant from downtown to the suburbs such as the Lahey Clinic's move to Burlington, Massachusetts; and*

• *Some outpatients, especially children, are not comfortable sharing corridors and waiting areas with sick hospitalized patients and would prefer to avoid that experience.*

My recommendation for long range planning would consist of three major areas:

I – To maintain Maine Medical Center as the premier tertiary care facility in the region

  A. *MMC has constructed an excellent state of the art medical center and this should be maintained and enhanced. Some activities that need tertiary care backup such as trauma center, cardiology and so forth should remain at the center.*

II – The development of an offsite outpatient campus that would house non-inpatient services

  A. *It would be located with easy access to the interstate highway system*
  B. *It would provide adequate parking*
  C. *It can be built in stages with a planned interconnecting campus master plan.*
      The campus could include:
      1. *Radiation Oncology Center - 90% of patients treated at MMC are out-patients. It is noteworthy that expansion to an offsite facility is cost effective since the cost of building a third linear accelerator vault at MMC would cost $800,000 while the construction of the Coastal Cancer Treatment Center in Bath with a linear accelerator vault in a 4,800 sq. ft. building cost $600,000 from the ground up;*
      2. *Imaging center with CT scanner and possibly MRI;*
      3. *Phlebotomy and basic lab facility;*
      4   *Pulmonary function test, EKG and other basic testing;*
      5. *Doctors office building;*
      6. *Surgery center and procedure rooms; and*
      7. *Possible hotel.*

This campus would provide easy access for patients in the area but would also attract patients from northern Maine and New Hampshire who need further evaluation. An example would be a patient from Aroostook County with an endocrine problem. That patient could be seen and evaluated as an outpatient in a relatively short period of time with all studies and procedures being provided in a cost effective and convenient manner at the offsite center.

III – To develop a seamless health care delivery system

The most important factor in achieving the goal of delivering cost effective compassionate quality medical care is providing for a continuum of care. An effective health care provider should not concentrate on disposition of the patient to another facility but must be intimately involved in the continuum of health care delivery. In the new era of capitation and cost containment, it is in everybody's interest to adequately care for the chronically ill and dying patient at either their home, or in a hospice or nursing home setting and to avoid inpatient services as much as possible. This seamless health care can be achieved with either close working relationships with other providers or with vertical integration. The former would include working relationships with other hospitals, home health providers and extended care facilities such as nursing homes and rehabilitation facilities.

Thank you for giving me this opportunity to provide input to the committee. If I can be of any further assistance in this most important task, please contact me.

In a meeting with Paul Gray shortly after he received the above memo he smiled when he read about a possible hotel. He said that we can hire a few nurses and make it another hospital. I told him that I was thinking about a facility such as the Children's Inn, built next to the Boston Children's Hospital on Longwood Avenue.

A few months later, Bill Caron arranged a meeting with me and Ron Carroll, the Chief of Medical Oncology and presented seven possible sites for the offsite facility. He said the Real Estate Committee of the Board was undecided between two of them. Ron and I strongly favored the old K-Mart site in Scarborough since it had excellent access to both interstate highways and had room to expand into a full campus. Bill Caron agreed and proceeded to secure and develop the site. To his great credit, the Scarborough campus has developed into a beautiful, accessible campus that includes:

1. A cancer center with:
   a. Radiation Oncology Department with two linacs and a simulator
   b. Medical and gynecologic oncology offices and infusion centers
   c. The Maine Children's Cancer Program, a pediatric oncology center with a play area and colorful decorations
   d. Radiology with full outpatient complement including a CT, MRI, and PET/CT
   e. Cancer clinics and outpatient support facility
   f. Laboratory facilities

2. A doctor's office building housing several specialty groups

3. An outpatient surgical and procedure building

4. An excellent medical research building

They decided we did not need a hotel.

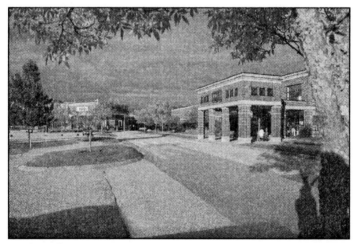

Scarborough Cancer Center

The Foundation for Blood Research

By Robert F. Ritchie MD

Prologue

The story of the birth and development of the Foundation for Blood Research ("FBR" or "Foundation") is largely the story of physician entrepreneurs. The FBR was in existence as a free-standing, not-for-profit medical research and education organization grown from the Portland community from its inception in 1973 until its dissolution in 2017. It was devoted to the conduct and promotion of medical and scientific research and to the provision of community education relating to disease prevention and early detection. For over 40 years it maintained cutting-edge laboratories, clinical, public health, biostatistical and educational facilities, equipment, and both clinical and research scientists.

The Foundation's initial focus on arthritis and allied diseases was the result of interest expressed by Dr. Phil Thompson in having Dr. Robert Ritchie spend a two-year clinical and research fellowship in Boston at the Robert Breck Brigham (RBB) and Peter Bent Brigham Hospitals (PBB) from 1963 to 1965.

Fellowship

At the Robert Brigham Hospital Dr. Ritchie's program was divided between research into antinuclear antibodies (ANA) and clinical practice in rheumatic diseases. The RBB patient population provided a wide scope of different rheumatic diseases while the PBB was involved in the start of a kidney transplant program. Many transplant cases were being identified as suffering from systemic lupus erythematous (SLE) a disease spectrum demonstrating autoantibodies of many types.

During the preparation for the research program it became evident that the study of ANA would require technology to investigate the immunoglobulins which formed autoantibodies. Two techniques were prominent at the time: protein purification and fluorescent labeling of these antibodies. The technique of fluorescent labeling had been initiated by Alfred Coons MD, an immunologist at Harvard Medical School. In the neighboring institution the New England Deaconess Hospital, Wadi Bardawil, a pathologist with a broad interest in immunological testing of the rheumatic diseases provided key samples and advice to Dr. Ritchie.

Early in the program, serum protein electrophoresis in the form of cellulose films was required. This method was not suitable to detailed investigation so other methods were sought. A new electrophoretic medium, acrylamide gel, became available. However the procedure used thin glass tubes that were not suitable for Dr. Ritchie's needs. He felt that a gel in slab form would work better. After extensive development and the manufacture of prototype apparatus in his home shop he put a working unit into operation producing separate protein bands of unparalleled detail in 1966. During the latter portion of this investigation both Dr. Ritchie and his counterpart Dr. Chester Alper, a colleague in Boston, were introduced to each other. Synergy rapidly developed.

When Dr. Alper, a pediatric hematologist with a keen interest in serum proteins, heard about the acrylamide gel system being used by Dr. Ritchie he visited the RBB laboratory. Projects quickly developed. A second plexiglas chamber was built for Dr. Alper at the Blood Grouping Laboratory (BGL) to be used to purify proteins as antigens for immunizing animals. The work at the RBB on acrylamide electrophoresis was also being carried on independently in Philadelphia, without either entity being aware of the other. Publication of these identical processes occurred almost simultaneously in 1969. Fortunately, commercialization was not on Dr. Ritchie's agenda.

Projects to expand knowledge on ANA in human populations and pursued through the two institutions revealed the ubiquity of these antibodies in the general population - beyond patients with rheumatic diseases. This work continued for several years and was published in 1967. Development of the slab acrylamide electrophoresis was brought essentially to completion in 1966.

Upon his completion of the RBB fellowship in 1965 Dr. Ritchie was offered salary support from the Maine Medical Center (MMC) Research Department headed by Dr. Peter Rand. He was the first fellowship-trained arthritis specialist to provide this clinical expertise within Maine as a rheumatology consultant. He subsequently recruited the next generation of rheumatologists when his lab activities became sought by clinicians. Maine's Arthritis Foundation provided funding for the early phase of the Rheumatic Disease Laboratory (RDL) in 1964-1965. A start-up grant of $22,000 was obtained from the Arthritis Foundation from a reserve fund of private donations to support startup funds for the lab including Dr. Ritchie's and Mr. Ronald Brunelle's salaries plus instruments and reagents. (1964-1965) This made it possible to create, in a very modest way, a clinical laboratory service which added tests previously unavailable in Maine.

The newly developed special tests for rheumatic diseases utilizing a fluorescent antibody technique for the demonstration of autoantibodies in the serum of patients with rheumatic diseases as diagnostic tools had initially been offered by the RBB in Boston to the rest of the Harvard hospitals. This service was transferred to the RDL in Portland in 1965 to take advantage of the startup financial support that had become available. Virtually all such testing for the Boston area hospitals was eventually provided by the RDL. After some political effort, the clinical revenues derived from this testing were allocated for the RDL operation by the MMC administration.

Early Research

The roots of what was to become the FBR therefore date to 1965 when Dr. Ritchie and his medical technologist Ronald Brunelle, arrived at the MMC in Portland from the RBB to set up the rheumatology consultation service and the RDL.

At about this time protein electrophoresis was introduced to clinical medicine. However, the support media were of poor quality and were of limited clinical use in the years from 1965-1969. Recognizing this early on, Dr. Ritchie made contact with Marine Colloids, in Rockland, Maine (soon to become FMC Corporation and now a part of DuPont USA). Their research scientists were testing newly developed forms of carrageenan isolated from seaweed believed to have potential use as the medium for serum electrophoresis. Materials were provided to the RDL for trials. One such sample, to be called agarose, proved to be superior. The company further developed this product for the medical laboratory market. After considerable effort it was clear by 1969 that this product was ideally suited to the application and became the basis of today's clinical analysis of serum proteins.

One of the first techniques to be of clinical use was the determination in 1967 that immunoglobulin levels in spinal fluid were an indicator of central nervous system infection and immunological diseases. The basic method employed was simple in the extreme, having been used for other purposes in laboratories around the country, and could be performed in a small test tube with small volumes of cerebrospinal fluid (CSF) and antiserum to immunoglobulins. It had previously never been used for CSF immunochemistry. The combination produced turbidity after incubation for 5-10 minutes which by 1972 proved to be analyzable by turbidimetry (light-scattering analysis). This ultimately replaced the previous, relatively laborious analytic technique of immunodiffusion in gel. The project produced the first publication from the laboratory on the subject of immunologically based serum protein quantitative analysis. It received wide exposure and was responsible for a shift in thinking by RDL staff members to research oriented towards the development of new protein analysis technologies.

By the spring of 1967 Dr. Ritchie had conceived the idea of automating protein analysis. With the investment of a few thousand dollars and some assistance from members of the Technicon Corporation (TC) in New York, it was possible to purchase used equipment. It rapidly became evident that the concept was viable. For the next several months, the subject was carefully investigated and shown to be of great potential interest to laboratorians studying serum proteins. A meeting with scientific members of the TC resulted only in "continued interest" but no substantive financial support. The prevailing thinking by TC administrators at that time was "If this is such a good idea, why hasn't somebody thought of it before?" Dr. Ritchie and his colleagues were urged to return to work and come back with more information.

It became immediately evident from this project that commercial antisera were of very poor quality. Much more monospecific and potent preparations were needed. Thus began an entirely new project that brought the RDL into cooperation with Dr. Alper's BGL and spawned a new entity, Atlantic Antibodies (ATAB). Based on a goat farm in Windham Maine, by the 1980s ATAB was the largest producer of high quality antiserum in the world, holding a nearly exclusive market share as the supplier of high quality antisera nationally and serving as a reference laboratory for clinical serum protein analysis in Maine and New England for over a decade. The antiserum and standards for proteins were the primary resources in use in the Pacific Rim and much of Europe. The prime producer previously had been the Behringwerke in Marburg Germany with whom Dr. Ritchie had also worked extensively.

Light Scattering Analysis

Drs. Ritchie and Alper remained in frequent communication. In 1969 they became intrigued by the challenge of fully automating protein analysis. Dr. Alper favored designing and modifying a new instrument using light transmission (turbidimetry), whereas Dr. Ritchie pursued the idea of redeploying "off-the-shelf" hardware from the Technicon Corporation. As it became evident that there was definite commercial interest in Dr. Ritchie's approach this time around a grant was obtained from TC to support parallel projects by Ritchie (at the RDL in Maine) and Alper (at the Brigham's BGL in Boston). Dr. Louis Diamond, an iconic figure at Harvard University and considered one of the founders of pediatric hematology and then of the BGL at the Brigham Hospital was instrumental in facilitating the project designed to demonstrate the economic feasibility of producing antiserum for the quantitative measurement of human serum proteins in an instrument similar to the one originally assembled by Dr. Ritchie in Maine. The project ran for one year, meeting all goals. At that point, MMC assisted with the creation of a contract for the sale of antiserum to the Technicon Corporation. TC in turn marketed roughly 400 of the Automated ImmunoAnalysis (AIP) instruments in a worldwide distribution effort with a price of $ 24,000 each!

Antibody Production And ATAB

A developmentally critical result of Dr. Ritchie's use of automated nephelometric protein analysis was the increasing need for high quality antiserum to be used for automated protein analysis. Antiserum production was initially carried out in an arm of the RDL which prior to the actual creation of ATAB (see below) rented space on a farm in Windham, Maine supported through the TC grant to RDL and BGL. These antisera rapidly became the most sought-after reagents in the country due to their high quality and potency. This necessitated revision of the RDL's business model.

By 1972 ATAB had become the sole source for high quality antiserum verified by the Protein Division of the Centers for Disease Control headed up by Charles Reimer, PhD. Research on the automated methods for serum proteins mentioned above had progressed with the continuous flow methods marketed by TC. In 1980 Dr. Ritchie was asked to share his work with Beckman Instruments, Inc. of Brea California. Beckman produced a wide variety of superior laboratory instruments for clinical use as well as industrial applications at the time. Within a year this new project grew exponentially as the result of greatly improved precision. With analysis time completely computer-controlled (see section below on Computerization and Analytics), it could be accomplished in seconds leading to a greatly expanded number of analytes. Also of great interest to the FBR was the ability to recover digitized data for computer applications for population-based research applications.

With the availability of high-grade antibodies produced by ATAB, the project, named the Automated ImmunoChemistry System (Auto ICS) became the primary means of measuring human serum proteins in the clinical laboratory worldwide.

FBR is Formed

The Foundation for Blood Research ("FBR" or "Foundation") was chartered as distinct from the predecessor Maine Medical Center Rheumatic Disease Laboratory (RDL) in 1973. It had become apparent by late 1972 that antibody production could generate revenue and profit. Dr. Ritchie, believing that the revenue producing activities should be separated from the scientific efforts, proposed the creation of two separate corporations. The Foundation would be a 501(c)3 nonprofit organization furthering a scientific and educational mission while Atlantic Antibodies (ATAB) would be formed as a traditional for-profit corporation to produce high quality antisera. RDL and BGL principals and MMC leadership agreed to this approach. MMC transferred equipment from the RDL to the newly formed FBR while Atlantic Antibodies was formed as a 50:50 equity partnership between RDL and BGL which, at about this time, evolved to become the Harvard Center for Blood Research (CBR). While the RDL provided the initial scientific and administrative groundwork for FBR, both the FBR and ATAB eventually grew to prominence that was both unimaginable and unpredictable at that early stage.

From 1975 to 1992, Drs. Ritchie and Alper, as a result of the FBR and BGL serum protein research and development, were named to the Food and Drug Administration's Immunology Panel overseeing approval of immunological Testing and Devices. In 1978 as the result of recognition of the need for standardization of serum protein testing ATAB began to offer the first Reference Standard for Human Serum Proteins, worldwide. The International Federation for Clinical Chemistry (IFCC) and later the American National Committee for Clinical Laboratory Standardization (NCCLS) embraced the ATAB Serum Protein Standard which ultimately became the Clinical Reference Material for Serum Proteins (CRM470) available from the World Health Organization and distributed in the US by the American College of Pathologists. This reference material is still available today. The FDA Immunology Devices Panel, including FBR consultants, approved AFP tests for neural tube defects (1990-1997) under the Chairmanship of Dr. Ritchie.

Immunoelectrophoresis

During early work Dr. Alper had demonstrated a new approach to better separation of human serum proteins, primarily the immunoglobulins. It was called *immunoelectrophoresis,* largely developed in Europe. Dr. Alper had used a more precise method involving coating or exposing the gel to a liquid antiserum to a single serum protein with genetic polymorphisms. All these gel-based methods were time consuming with diffusion times ranging from one to two days. Dr. Ritchie realized the potential in the demonstration of monoclonal immunoglobulins which would have immediate clinical application with minimal investigative effort, except for clear demonstration of practicality. This proved to be the case and with the application of specific antisera to the agarose surface by a moistened strip of cellulose acetate. The name *immunofixation* was coined and within a short time was being introduced to laboratories worldwide and remains in use until the present. However it was not quantitative and therefore did not meet the needs of expanded protein automation.

Dr. Alper gave the FBR 100 ml of a crude antiserum to alpha-fetoprotein (AFP) which at that early time had no obvious use. This antiserum was purified by Dr. George Knight at FBR which provided the wherewithal for the AFP assays. Several years later this was to be pivotal in the development of the FBR AFP program.

Computerization and Analytics

Dr. Ritchie's concept of transforming crude protein electrophoresis measurements into quantitative, specific protein measurements had represented an advance, even without automation. Transforming manual turbidimetric measurements to automated nephelometric measurements was another advance. Immunoanalaysis with instruments, however, was not yet on the horizon. The earlier immunoanalytic methods were only qualitatively judged visually. Light scattering analysis had been described many decades ago but had been abandoned because technology and reagents were not of sufficient quality. During an invited lecture at The Catholic University of Leuven, Belgium arranged by a close friend, Dr. Pierre Masson, whose department head was Prof. Joseph Hermans - a renowned immunologist responsible for many original concepts in that science - a discussion of antiserum production developed in which Dr. Ritchie was told of Dr. Masson's work on improving antiserum potency and monospecificity. Instead of massive doses of antigen injected intramuscularly, used widely in the immunization of rabbits, they used microgram quantities injected intradermally with adjuvant into many sites. The results revealed dramatic increases in both potency and specificity. ATAB resolved the issue of potency and specificity with this single event, applied to goats. The method is "standard operating procedure" today.

Dr. Ritchie combined an extensive medical knowledge base in a specialty (arthritis) with a pre-existing experience in electronics (gained in the Navy) and laboratory skills to learn and apply computer programming. Between 1972-1974 Dr. Ritchie started to automate and computerize nephelometric determinations of serum proteins, initially using the TI Automated ImmunoPrecipitin System (AIP). He worked with Beckman Instruments' Auto ICS device which ultimately became the primary protein analysis system in the US, Europe and the Far East. Computerization improved efficiency and reduced potential human error during the analyses. Analytical time was reduced from 1-2 days with previous methods to less than 10 minutes at first and ultimately to a few seconds with refined and computerized instruments. He and the computer staff had been able to develop software to:

1. Accept computerized antigen-antibody reaction signals and identify and quantify fourteen different serum protein fractions;

2. Assist clinicians in interpreting results and significance of serum protein patterns; and

3. Store data with patient demographic information for population-based research.

The concept of unifying interpretation of the serum protein panel in 1974 was a unique advance "before its time". Dr. Ritchie had initially interpreted protein analysis data manually, as an aid to clinicians. When he learned how to write computer programs he rapidly discovered a way to enhance the process. His computer-generated protein analysis report stands as an early effort in merging quantitative analytics with clinical data to yield diagnostic assistance to clinicians. The standard lab report at the time had been a number, attached to a normative range, but without expert interpretation. Dr. Ritchie's groundbreaking software innovation provided an explanation of protein patterns, advising on how the multiple component measurements fit together to tell a meaningful clinical story.

Ultimately over 1.3 million anonymized records were preserved online for research purposes.

Although this is incidental, MMC was heavily influenced by Dr. Ritchie's computer knowledge and experience to select and install an early version of what was to evolve to the electronic medical record. In the late 1970s he was asked by MMC administration to take the lead in determining the most appropriate company for a hospital-wide system for clinical data retrieval, physician ordering (now CPOE), and a wide range of patient management capabilities. He also took responsibility for answering questions from physicians during the introductory period of the Technicon Medical Information Systems (MIS) product. MMC was one of the first hospitals worldwide to undertake a project on this scale. Many clinicians would call to scream into the telephone, especially when he might gently ask a high-tech question like, "have you tried turning it off and on again?".

People, Growth, And Expansion After 1974

By 1974 it became possible to take a major growth step. Dr. Ritchie recruited James E. Haddow MD, to be Associate Director of the Foundation. Dr. Haddow, who had been Director of the Pediatric Metabolism and Endocrinology Unit at Boston City Hospital prior to his appointment at the FBR, introduced a prenatal diagnosis effort at FBR which was to become a crucial focus to its ongoing programmatic and scientific development. Among other accomplishments, Dr. Haddow and his colleagues published seminal articles in the New England Journal of Medicine on the benefits of enhanced alpha-fetoprotein (AFP) screening for the prenatal detection of Down Syndrome (1992) and the impact of subtle maternal thyroid deficiency on postnatal development which contributed to widespread thyroid screening during pregnancy (1999). Dr. Haddow fostered a major ongoing collaboration with Dr. Nicholas Wald, one of the world's leading epidemiologists and neonatal health experts at the Wolfson Institute of Preventive Medicine, Barts and The London School of Medicine.

By the end of 1977, Ritchie, Haddow and 15 other staff members moved from MMC into their own 15,000 square feet, building on a 15-acre campus in Scarborough. The purchase was successful because the loan was secured by the personal assets of the two principals and their spouses. This marked the beginning of autonomous life of the FBR as an institution distinct from MMC.

In 1978 George J. Knight Ph.D. joined the FBR as Director of its Radioimmunoassay (RIA) Laboratory. His expertise in the development of immunodiagnostic tests and reagents substantially strengthened the institution. The serendipitous availability of an antiserum to alpha-fetoprotein, given several years earlier by Dr. Alper (see above) spawned work on the detection of AFP in maternal serum. Considered, but postponed for the time being, was the introduction of tests to diagnose carriers of genetic disorders such as cystic fibrosis. However the FBR became the nationwide External Quality Control Agent for AFP testing for prenatal diagnosis.

In 1979 new regulations governing organ transplant programs required that tissue typing be performed under the direction of a certified Ph.D. with considerable training and experience in that specialty. Therefore in 1981 the FBR recruited Richard J. Mahoney Ph.D. and became home to the FBR Histocompatibility and Immunogenetics Laboratory which served both FBR and MMC. Dr. Mahoney had been a research fellow in immunogenetics at the Dana Farber Cancer Institute and in pathology at the Harvard Medical School. Over the next few years, the Foundation also developed innovative programs in the emerging technology of flow cytometry by sponsoring Drs. Kenneth Ault and E.J. Lovett. The flow cytometry program eventually found a permanent home at MMC

In 1984, Barbara A. Chilmonczyk MD, a pediatric allergist-immunologist, joined the FBR to head the Clinical Immunology program. Dr. Chilmonczyk had completed a three-year fellowship in immunology/allergy at what is presently the National Jewish Center for Immunology and Respiratory Medicine, Denver, Colorado.

In 1986, A. Myron Johnson M. D., Clinical Professor of Pediatrics at Tufts University School of Medicine and Medical Director of the CBR in Boston, came to the FBR to head the Rheumatic Disease Laboratory, and what was to become the Center for Cardiovascular, Liver, and Lung Disorders. He was an expert in plasma proteins, plasma lipids and related laboratory technologies.

In 1987, the FBR started a new program in Reproductive Immunology. It evolved from the University of Southern Maine's (USM) Graduate Program in Applied Immunology. Neal S. Rote, Jr., Ph.D., came to USM and FBR to head both programs from the Department of Obstetrics and Gynecology at the University of Utah Medical School. where he had been an Associate Professor. His main research interest lies in the immunologic causes of recurrent pregnancy loss.

In the 1990's the FBR faculty included an impressive staff of scientists, physicians, analysts, and educators from the Portland community as well as regional and international institutions. These included senior systems analyst and biostatistician Glenn Palomaki, B.A., B.S., education expert Paula K. Haddow M.A.T., collaborating scientists Chester A. Alper MD, Dennis Barrantes M.S., Laurent Beauregard Ph.D., Harry W. Bennert, Jr. MD, Jacob Canick Ph.D., Marshall Carpenter MD, J. Chipman Ph.D., Frank Lawrence MD, Donald J. McCrann, Jr. MD, Wayne A. Miller MD, Alistair Philip MD, Nadir Rifai Ph.D., Donna Thompson MD, Olga Navrotolskaia MD, and Nicholas J. Wald M.R.C.P. (London) and Research Associates Wendy Craig Ph.D. and Christina Goldfine Ph.D. Tom Ledue MA, and Andrea Pulkkinen provided many years of technical support to these laboratories.

The Foundation also enjoyed major collaborative relationships with organizations that included MMC, USM locally, the Centers for Disease Control (CDC), the National Institutes of Health (NIH) including the National Institute for Child Health and Human Development: NICHD), the New England Regional Genetics Group (NERGG) nationally, the Department of Environmental and Preventive Medicine at the University of London internationally, and The Bigelow Laboratory for Ocean Sciences.

Investigative pursuits at the FBR spanned three research centers by the early 1990's: 1) the Center for Perinatal and Child Health; 2) the Center for Cardiovascular, Kidney and Liver Disorders; and 3) the Center for Arthritis, Immunological Disorders and

Cancer. Each Center also provided laboratory and clinical services and graduate education. By the mid 1990's these Centers evolved into three distinct laboratories, the Rheumatic Disease Laboratory which also included a Neuro-Immunology Laboratory created by Walter Allan MD, the Prenatal Screening Laboratory and a new Molecular Genetics Laboratory.

Along with the laboratories, an expanded education program serving physicians, teachers and students was established. FBR created a Clinical Genetics Program and Cleft Palate Clinic to complement prenatal testing for neural tube defects, molecular testing for cystic fibrosis (CF), and the other known genetic disorders at that time. The Genetics Clinic was staffed by a full-time geneticist and genetic counselors. The geneticists included Thomas Brewster MD, Allan Donnenfeld MD, Richard Doherty MD, Rhonda Spiro MD, and Rosemarie Smith MD. Edward Kloza had joined FBR in 1976 as the first genetic counselor in Maine. Later, Dale Lea RN, also a genetic counselor, directed the genetic counseling program. The clinic was funded through the Maine Department of Human Services and closed in 2005 when funding was moved to Maine Medical Center and Eastern Maine Medical Center to provide more statewide coverage for patients and families. FBR continued the Molecular Lab testing and introduced a couples-based carrier test for CF. Research on CF continued along with research on Fragile X Syndrome.

FBR's education program began informally with Dr. Ritchie and Dr. Haddow's contact with interns and residents at Maine Medical Center. When FBR moved to Scarborough, a series of small, invited meetings was convened known as "The Scarborough Conferences" held at the Atlantic House in Scarborough. The first three of these conferences (1977-80) were responsible for launching the new field of prenatal screening in the United States, a process enhanced by links established at these meetings with investigators in Canada, the UK, and elsewhere in Europe. The prototype model, a statewide prenatal screening program in Maine, was established at FBR during that time, building upon an integrated laboratory/programmatic design that had been conceptualized and introduced by Dr. Ritchie during the RDL's formative years.

One of the subsequent major Scarborough Conference topics was the impact of environmental tobacco smoking on non-smokers. Cotinine, a metabolite of nicotine serves as a laboratory marker for smoke exposure. The results of the cotinine conference led to developing a test to measure cotinine in pregnant women, allowing FBR investigators to better understand adverse consequences of "passive smoking" among women in Maine during pregnancy and delivery. FBR's research showed that fetal growth was adversely affected, even when exposure to cigarette smoke was limited to non-smoking women. The ability to measure cotinine in pregnant females was of considerable interest to Maine obstetricians, as it served as a motivating force for encouraging avoidance of both "passive" and active smoking. FBR continued this testing until smoking cessation programs became a part of routine physician visits.

Dr. Haddow and his team, having developed an AFP marker test for prenatal screening, wanted to educate physicians and caregivers locally, nationally, and internationally to the techniques of prenatal screening and started holding annual short courses in Portland. As more knowledge of prenatal testing developed at FBR, including the triple screen (AFP, unconjugated estriol, and human chorionic gonadotrophin) and integrated testing (first and second trimester testing) each year the courses were updated. Haddow's partnerships with Nicholas Wald, (London), and Jack Canick (Women and Infants Hospital, Providence R.I) provided an opportunity to host these courses for more than 20 years. FBR also provided quality control prenatal testing for the American College of Obstetricians and Gynecologists.

At the same time, Dr. Ritchie was traveling to Europe to meetings of the Protides of the Biological Fluids (1975-1985) and making presentations on FBR's work on establishing reference ranges for testing (1998-2007). Dr. Ritchie and his staff did several presentations at conferences related to the development of his Western blot method for Lyme disease testing and immunofixation. Dr. Ritchie published a two-volume syllabus on serum proteins and trademarked his computer generated interpretive program STANDX. This lengthy project was greatly assisted by the support of Olga Navrotolskaia MD, a Russian trained physician with a broad understanding of serum proteins.

Paula Haddow established FBR's *ScienceWorks* program, a multifaceted program to provide summer workshops for Maine's high school science teachers, a used equipment exchange program to equip school laboratories, and an in-house wet lab program for high school student field trips. Along with Edward Kloza (a genetic counselor), she developed and introduced a curriculum unit in human genetics for use in high school biology classes throughout the state. She also provided oversight for FBR's medical library, a vast collection related to all of the research and testing done at FBR. When Paula left FBR, Walter Allan MD took over the leadership and expanded the program to include computer software development programs for Maine's school laptop program.

Jane Sheehan, J.D, former Commissioner of Maine's Department of Health and Human Services, joined FBR as Vice President for Administration in 1996, becoming President after Dr. Ritchie's retirement in 2007. She had followed Sondra Everhart, the prior VP for Administration, who left FBR to pursue other interests. In addition to her administrative duties, Jane became involved in the formation of the Maine

Biomedical Research Coalition, a group of biomedical research institutions including Jackson Laboratory, Maine Medical Center Research Institute, University of New England, and Mt. Desert Biological Research Institute. This group was instrumental in getting Maine Governors and the Legislature to support bond initiatives for biomedical research infrastructure. The bond funds allowed FBR to upgrade its facilities and technologies. Jane also promoted FBR on the national level by leading the Association of Independent Research Associations (made up of 90 nonprofit institutions in the US including Salk, Fred Hutchinson, Cold Spring Harbor and Jackson Lab to name a few). She served on the Maine Technology Institute Board and established an incubator at FBR for startup companies to fill vacant FBR space. FBR already had a rich history of helping local startups with laboratory services, knowledge, skill and experience.

Funding for the FBR was primarily derived from laboratory revenues supplemented by grant funds, contracts, and private foundations. Non-laboratory revenue included grants for hypothyroidism in pregnancy and alpha-fetoprotein screening, FBR funding for Smith Lemli Opitz research, evidence-based medicine, and diagnostic algorithms and tools for arthritis, and genetic disorders. Sources of funding included: National Institutes of Health; National Science Foundation; Howard Hughes Medical Institute; March of Dimes, State of Maine; Maine Technology Institute; The Branta Foundation; The Davis Family Foundation: Technicon Instruments, Inc. and Beckman Instruments, Inc. Changing payment and delivery models for health care services in the 21st century and shrinking federal research grants ultimately worked against small free-standing organizations like FBR. The Foundation ultimately could not maintain solvency in a market requiring competition with consolidated hospital systems with salaried physicians and large-scale laboratory services.

Epilogue After 43 years of serving Maine, the nation and the global community, on June 30, 2016, the Foundation for Blood Research closed its doors. At the time of closing, many colleagues expressed their appreciation for the one on one professional relationships they had built with FBR scientists and personnel. FBR's innovation, science, and culture of collaboration will live on in those who have participated and benefited from the FBRs educational, scientific, and clinical work and in the methods for prenatal screening, quality control, nephelometry and serum protein testing that endure.

Konbit Sante Cap-Haitien Health Partnership

By J. Michael Taylor MD

Konbit Sante was conceived in 2001 by me (Michael Taylor), my wife Wendy and a group of Portland citizens who included physicians, nurses, nurse practitioners, residents, lawyers, businessmen, hospital administrators and community activists. There are too many individuals to count, but many members of the Maine Medical Center (MMC) family including Mike Ryan, Don Nicoll, Don McDowell, Jim Moody (MMC Board member), Sam Broaddus, Steve and Polly Larned, Marc Miller, Eva Lathrop, Anne Lemire, Peter Bates, Ronnie Ervin, Elna Osso, EJ Lovett, and more have been involved. The goal was to use Portland's medical and community resources to improve the well-being and the health of people living in the second largest city in Haiti, Cap-Haitien, and its public hospital, the Justinian University Hospital.

Four of the original Board members were former Peace Corps Volunteers.

The original Board was comprised of twelve members affiliated with MMC. Since its founding, there have been more than 45 volunteers affiliated with MMC. Not only has MMC generously contributed financially, materially with donated equipment and supplies, and with its staff, but it has hosted visiting Haitian professionals including not only physicians but nurses, therapists, administrators, and residents. The Board now includes members from Atlanta, Switzerland, Boston, and Haiti and the volunteers also come from throughout the US as well as from Canada, Europe and Israel.

Konbit Sante is a 501 (c) 3 organization with a four person US staff and more than 40 Haitian employees including physicians, nurses, educators and agents sante (home health workers). Although it is not an emergency relief organization, it played the key role organizing the responses to the earthquake and the cholera epidemic in coordination with Doctors Without Borders and the United Nations. Konbit Sante also initiated a Sister City relationship between Portland and Cap-Haitien which has encouraged the exchange of City Representatives, priests, Roman Catholic and Episcopalian, and artists.

Konbit Sante has an annual budget of $820,000. More information can be obtained by visiting our website: www.konbitsante.org.

SURGICAL MISSIONS IN HAITI AND EAST AFRICA

By Michael R. Curci MD

My interest in international medicine was a chance occurrence that presented itself when I was a 4th year medical student at Columbia. The head of the parasitology department offered a 2-month elective at the Firestone Plantation Hospital in Liberia. I thought this would be a one-time experience. To my surprise, the Yale general surgical residency offered a 3-month rotation in our 3rd year at the Albert Schweitzer Hospital in Haiti, HAS, (created by Larry and Gwen Mellon in 1956). I spent an additional 6 weeks as a Chief Resident to replace a 3rd year resident who couldn't travel to Haiti. This entire time block was almost 5 months during my 5-year residency, which would be completely unacceptable today by the ACGME.

I first arrived at HAS in 1969 and have continued to work there for 2 weeks on an annual basis. Initially my family accompanied me until my children entered college. Beginning in the early 1990s, the 3rd year surgical residents from the Maine Medical Center (MMC) surgical residency program spent 2 weeks at the hospital using their vacation time since they had no elective time block. More than a decade later, this was extended to a 4 week elective when an additional categorical position was added to the general surgical program. I was also the surgical residency Program Director (2000-2008), which permitted me to arrange the rotations in Haiti to provide the experience in international surgery.

I retired at the end of 2008 which allowed me to spend more time working in low and middle-income countries (LMIC) in east central Africa. For the next 3 years, my wife (a PhD social worker) and I worked in Kigoma, Tanzania for 8 months/year. I worked in a regional hospital, 1000 miles from the capital on Lake Tanganyika training non-physician clinicians to improve their surgical and obstetric skills to bring needed services closer to the population in need. My wife taught social work and was the acting head of the local social work school. This project was supported by the Michael Bloomberg philanthropy. I was also able to bring our surgical residents for a 1-month elective each year.

During the year following completion of the Tanzania project in 2011, we spent several months in Malawi working with Physicians for Peace. The present "chapter" began in 2013 in Rwanda. The US government and the Rwandan Ministry of Health launched the largest known bilateral effort to strengthen health care training and expand the work force in LMICs. This is a 7-year, $ 170 M program to populate the district hospitals and provide a self-sustaining teaching faculty since most of their physicians died or left Rwanda during the genocide in 1994. The project's goal was to provide an educational experience for the recently graduated medical students and not just service, which is more characteristic of short-term volunteerism. One surgeon has already completed a 3 year pediatric surgery fellowship in Kenya and a second surgeon will begin his fellowship this July. I have just completed my 5th year, serving 3 months per year, and anticipate returning for my 6th year in January 2018. I have also continued to bring our MMC surgical residents for a 1-month elective.

My wife and I have been fortunate to have these opportunities and provide an educational service in our later professional careers. We have also mentored individuals to work in an international environment after completing their training. This has been a very fulfilling experience and we will continue this work to make the world a better place to live for its marginalized population.

Urological Missions

By Samuel B. Broaddus MD

I first started thinking about international medical volunteer work in 1976, while I was doing a month-long rotation on the urology service at the VA Hospital in Seattle. The war in Southeast Asia was winding down. I had several patients who had been wounded in Vietnam. I also met a woman who worked for the International Rescue Committee who introduced me to a group of Cambodian refugees who had immigrated to Seattle. It piqued my interest in contributing my skills to the urological needs of people engulfed by war, conflict and calamity.

After completing my urology residency at the Medical Center Hospital of Vermont in Burlington in 1982, I spent two years teaching transurethral prostate surgery to general surgeons in mission hospitals in St. Lucia, Egypt, Pakistan, Sri Lanka, and Thailand. After soliciting, collecting, and shipping donated fiberoptic resectoscopes to each hospital ahead of my arrival, I spent two to four months in each locale teaching general surgeons how to perform transurethral resection of the prostate (TURP). This educational exercise ensured that the technique and its benefits would continue after my departure.

After returning to the US in 1984, I was appointed to the International Relations Committee of the American Urological Association (AUA), where I had the opportunity to meet other like-minded volunteer urologists. I represented the AUA at the Pan-African Urologic Surgeons Association congresses in Zimbabwe in 1992 and Kenya in 1995. In 2001, I was invited to be a visiting professor of urology at hospitals in Ho Chi Minh City and Hanoi, Vietnam. Through a chance discussion with pediatric surgeon Dr. Michael Curci at Maine Medical Center (MMC), I then began a series of annual trips with my young family to the Albert Schweitzer Hospital in the Artibonite Valley of central Haiti, working as a volunteer urologist from 1994 to 1997.

In 2002, I learned about MMC dermatologist Michael Taylor's efforts to start a Portland-based medical NGO in Haiti and joined Konbit Sante and its Board of Directors soon thereafter. Since then, I have traveled to Cap Haitian in northern Haiti on 15 medical mission trips to collaborate with Haitian colleagues and help them improve urologic and surgical care for their patients at the Justinien Hospital. In 2008, I helped bring two Haitian chief surgical residents to MMC for six weeks each to make sure they received an adequate experience in U.S. surgical training skills. I co-authored (along with Dr. Brad Cushing, Chief of Surgery at MMC) a surgical needs assessment that became a model for other medical departments at Justinien, helping Haitian health care providers understand what resources they have, what resources they need, and how to get from one to the other. In 2009, I helped facilitate a visit by the Justinien chiefs of surgery and anesthesia to Maine so that they could see first-hand both surgical and hospital efficiencies that they could bring back to their own hospital in Haiti. In 2010, I led a Konbit Sante and MMC surgical response team to Haiti 10 days after the catastrophic M7 earthquake that killed more than 200,000 people, severely injured as many as that, and left the country in the depths of despair. Later that year, I was honored with the American College of Surgeons Surgical Volunteerism Award for International Outreach. To me it was a reflection of the immeasurable work that Konbit Sante has done and continues to do in Haiti.

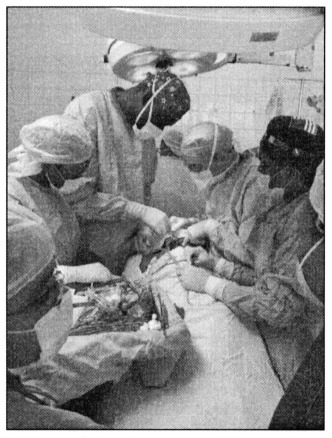

Dr. Sam Broaddus operating with Haitian surgeons at the Justinien Hospital in Cap Haitian after the earthquake in January 2010

RECONSTRUCTIVE SURGICAL MISSIONS

By Therese K. White MD

One of the unique opportunities available to a reconstructive surgeon is the ability to bring our skill set to remote locations and foreign countries. As many of my colleagues have found, volunteering is one of the greatest experiences of our professional careers. Most trips are self funded. Volunteer physicians are expected to cover all of their personal expenses including flights. There is no financial compensation. Personal time, often meaning "vacation" time, is used. Accommodations are often marginal by American standards. Work conditions are often far less modern and far less sophisticated than what we are used to. The work days are long and the cases often challenging. Despite all of these true issues, volunteer surgery is far more rewarding than one can easily explain.

I have personally travelled to numerous Central and South American countries to volunteer. Among them: Columbia, Guatemala, Peru and Brazil. These trips were organized through various medical charity organizations including Healing the Children, Interplast and Operation Smile. My colleagues from Plastic and Hand Surgical Associates have literally spanned the globe performing charity work. Drs. Jean Labelle, Dick Flaherty, David Fitz and Alan Harmatz traveled to Asia, Africa, Central and South America, all performing cleft lip and palate surgery, burn reconstruction, hand surgery and micro surgery. These adventures were numerous and often lasted approximately 2 weeks. The work at the office before and after the trips was often difficult, as preparing and returning was in itself a major effort.

The motivating factors were many: the opportunity to travel and work with peers, the opportunity to see another culture and be immersed in a foreign community and the opportunity to give back to a world in which we are extremely privileged.

For each of us, these experiences had career changing impact. I have found them to be the "purest" medical experiences I have encountered. Mission teams were expected to bring all supplies including medications and any surgical instruments that would be required. We set up in the local hospital facility, some of which were quite modern, others more modest, but all lacked supplies that we take for granted.

I learned that excellent surgery could be accomplished in these settings. It was liberating to do what was medically indicated without insurance approval and reams of paperwork. Medical records were carefully documented but were quite simple. The medical teams were energetic, motivated and selfless.

The missions typically started with days of screening. This involved evaluating patients, assuring their health status was adequate for anesthesia, surgery and recovery. This was a crucial part of the mission as most of the facilities had no intensive care capabilities, no blood banks and in many, the family members provided much of the post op care under the guidance of the mission team.

Next was the planning and performance of the surgical schedule. The routine was typically 4-5 long days of surgery, a day or two of break followed with another 4-5 days of surgery, then departure for home. The "break" days were an opportunity to see the local community and culture. We were often treated to local cuisine and sightseeing by host families.

After completing the operative schedule the surgical team departed. A "follow - up team" was predesignated to stay and assure supervision and assistance for recovery for the patients.

I will never forget the honor I felt when the parents handed me their child. Unable to speak a common language they trusted that I, a complete stranger, would do my best to restore the smile of their child born with a cleft lip. These families often had traveled days to arrive at the surgical sites. I was and remain to this day profoundly humbled. The gratitude in their eyes when their children were back in their arms is unforgettable.

For many of us, surgical volunteer work is a way to contribute. I am proud of the work we have been able to offer. As medical ambassadors we have been able to leave a positive mark around the world as testimony to our genuine concern for the welfare of others. Ironically the rewards have been far greater than any contribution we have made.

GYNECOLOGY FOR IMPROVERISHED WOMEN

By Hector M. Tarraza MD

It began 21 years ago in the remote mountains of northern Peru. A small team of 14 doctors and nurses set out on a surgical mission trip to a region devastated by poverty, terrorism (the Shining Path), and despair. Imagine caring for patients but not having technology (ultrasound, CT scan, a laboratory, a blood bank, or healthcare workers), medicines, or medical supplies. Everything is challenging – electricity and running water is sporadic. One could be in the middle of surgery and the overhead lights would go out. It wasn't uncommon to be operating in a hot, sweltering room. Toward the end of mission trips you could often be running low or completely out of supplies.

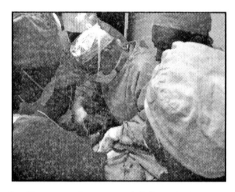

Dr. Tarraza teaching surgical skills to OBGYN surgeons in Africa

Despite the many inconveniences, medical missions became a very important part of the Department of Obstetrics and Gynecology at Maine Medical Center. Many OB/GYN residents and attending physicians began to participate. Chief Residents were offered a rotation where they could attend and participate as part of their training. They were exposed, in a supervised fashion, to an opportunity to operate on very challenging cases in an effort to help patients while improving their skills.

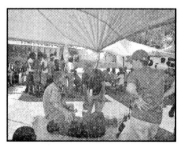

Dr. Tarraza at the massive earthquake in Haiti

Initially trips were confined to the western hemisphere. We would travel to Guatemala, Haiti, Brazil, and Colombia with several NGOs. Most of the trips were two weeks long. We would bring supplies and staff to be able to perform approximately 150-200 major surgeries. All patients throughout this time were offered free care. Priority was given to patients who were suffering or had significant quality of life issues. Beginning in 2004 we expanded our reach to include Africa and Asia. We provided care for people in the grasslands of Ethiopia, the slums of Sierra Leone, and the overcrowded cities of Bangladesh.

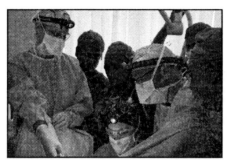

Dr. Tarraza in Bangladesh with MMC Chief Residents
Dr. Caroline Foust Wright (center) and Dr. Kristi Maas (left)

Our goal was always threefold. We would provide direct patient care with surgical interventions. We would teach our in-country colleagues surgical techniques and new innovations. We would also offer our OB/GYN residents the opportunity to learn and care for patients in a resource poor environment.

Everywhere we went we worked hard to care for those who have nothing. Our patients were predominantly uneducated women with no jobs, future, or hope. They often lived in one room shacks and each day struggled to figure out where their next meal was coming from. Being a woman in an undeveloped country is an extreme hardship. It is our goal to provide medical care for them alongside our in-country partners.

We bring kindness, compassion and caring where there is no care.

Project Guatemala

A Story of a Cooperative Medical Enterprise

By Frank W. Read MD and Peter S. Hedstrom MD

In the 1980's and 90's the Portland medical community supported two successful and competitive ophthalmology practices, each having coalesced from largely solo legacy practices. Project Guatemala ("the Project") ultimately evolved into a cooperative effort between these two practices - Maine Eye Center (MEC) and Eye Care Medical Group (ECMG) - to provide basic optical and surgical services to a Mayan region in the highlands of Guatemala.

The Project developed from a small group of enthusiastic ophthalmic technicians. In 1997 Bonnie Tagliatti persuaded her New Hampshire ophthalmologist employer, John Detweiler MD, to come to the Quiché district of Guatemala and perform cataract surgery. She had earlier witnessed a high incidence of blinding cataracts when she and two of her friends - one of whom was Sonja Liaho, who was employed by MEC - joined a mission to provide optical correction for visual impairment near the city of Santa Cruz del Quiché in the western highlands of Guatemala. This nation had the largest indigenous population in Central America.

The Quiche district supports a rural, remote population of Mayan people - the Kíché. Many Kíché, especially the elderly, speak no Spanish and seldom leave their villages. Travel typically is on unpaved serpentine roads traversing hillsides too steep for mechanized farming. Ten miles travel by car can take one or two hours - even on paved roads 60 miles is 4 or more hours. Essential medical services for these mostly subsistence farmers are often not available.

Of note, all of the families in the district suffered grievously from the 36-year civil war that began in 1960 and in which 200,000 indigenous people were killed, primarily by government troops. Any Kíché family member over the age of 40 years personally witnessed the murder of a close family relative. An uneasy peace began in 1996.

Dr. Detweiler died suddenly and unexpectedly in 1998. The core of his mission team, now employed by MEC, urged 2 MEC surgeons, Peter Hedstrom MD and Fred Miller MD, to join the effort in 1999.

The first team organized around those two surgeons included optometrists, technicians, anyone who could speak Spanish, and family members willing to work. Many had no clinical experience whatsoever. Few knew what to anticipate except that a throng of people was likely awaiting their arrival and expecting help to see well again. The team was not disappointed as on arrival they were greeted by a very long line of patients waiting outside the Santa Elena Hospital.

The Santa Elena Hospital was found to be a well-designed, sunlit, airy, one story extended building with a medical clinic, open wards for inpatients, an ER, and multiple operating rooms. It was constructed in the 1970's with USA funding. Equipment, however, was remarkably limited, especially consumables like tubing (often washed and reused), gowns, face masks, gloves, sutures, soap, scrub brushes (also reused) and toilet paper.

A quick pass down the line with a flashlight looking for those people with two white pupils from advanced cataract separated the most urgent surgical cases from those needing optical correction. Screening for glasses and surgical procedures began promptly.

The success of this first team could not have happened without the support of local people with boots on the ground knowledge. For this first team that support was provided by a group of women - Sisters of Charity - from New York City and environs. These women had been involved in the Quiche district through an organization called Caritas for at least 20 years. The leader of that group was a remarkable woman, Sister Barbara Ford. She had good relations with hospital administration smoothing the team's entry to use a large room for screening exams as well as use of an operating room. Caritas had stored critical equipment like the operating microscope, surgical instruments, and slit lamp safely off site from when Dr. Detweiler had last used them more than a year previously. Equipment like that would not have survived in the hospital. We had planned to stay nearby in the city of Santa Cruz and walk the 1/2 mile to the hospital. Barbara Ford worried about our safety and arranged for the entire team to occupy a large room - an unused ICU - within the hospital. Caritas efficiently organized patient visits by assigning a day to surrounding villages in rotation and promoting the team's arrival date. Long lines formed each morning before the clinic opened for the day.

Barbara Ford and Caritas ran nursing homes, alcoholism treatment programs, and programs to empower women within the local society and within families. Barbara Ford was also involved in exhuming bodies from mass graves created during the war and returning these bodies to their villages. Distinctive clothing found with the remains provided village identification. She would hear of fighting during the war years and jump in her Toyota pickup to collect the wounded. We were amazed by her bravery and kindness.

From these humble beginnings grew a much larger organization. Frank Read MD (MEC) and Nancy Read joined the team in 2000 and were largely responsible for expanding fundraising, equipment and supply donations, and promotion. In 2003 Frank invited Bruce Cassidy MD and Bob Daly MD, both partners from ECMG, to create a second surgical team. This proved to be highly successful. A new corps of talented clinic and OR staff accompanied Bruce and Bob as well as the CEO of ECMG, John Wipfler.

Typically the patients requiring surgery were elderly, and some had been blind for years. They may have been led by rope on a several hours walk to a bus line, followed by a 7-hour bus ride to Santa Cruz del Quíché, they were accompanied by several family members. Kíché people are durable, lithe, and reluctant to show any anxiety or emotion. Their very straight backs had no trouble lying flat on a pillow-free OR table. Only a very few flinched even a little as a 3-inch needle passed beneath their eye into the orbit to provide anesthesia. The obvious trust placed with complete strangers, and the faith that the very best would be done to give valuable service was humbling and demanded the highest possible standards of care. Many cases were a formidable challenge to a surgeon's skill, sometimes due to equipment limitations, but more often to the degree of cataract development.

Project Guatemala was entirely independent, self-supporting and all volunteer. Everything needed to screen 150-200 people per day and provide eyeglasses or cataract surgery as required was hand carried to Guatemala by the team. The first airline checked bag was personal, the other checked duffle was loaded with supplies. Each person was instructed to say they had packed both bags. Frank Read's office gradually filled with donated equipment and supplies over the months before a trip at a level only comfortable to a hoarder. The Project raised funds in small generous donations from many, and large generous donations from a few.

The team attracted dedicated and talented people. Among these include the culturally aware, and native Spanish speaker Fernanda Darrow, a language teacher from Cheverus High School who would bring along a personally selected, bright, adaptive student brushing up on Spanish language skills. Rebecca Evarts of Yarmouth, involved with Safe Passage, learned of and joined the group providing high level executive and organizational skills, excellent Spanish and financial support. She and Nancy Read took upon themselves myriad details that allowed confidence that travel would be smooth, a place to stay existed, and food was provided. Tom Dykes MD, a steadfast man, performed his Peace Corps work in the Quiche region years before medical school and volunteered his language and cultural skills, valuable whenever a tight spot developed.

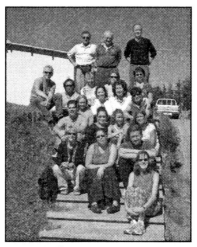

Mission Staff

Any volunteer who could afford it was required to pay his or her own way including airfare, lodging and food. This included all physicians and lay volunteers. But the success of our efforts also entirely depended on technical help both in the clinic and the OR. Remarkable people from both MEC and ECMG volunteered to staff these needs using their own vacation time. The Project covered the expenses of these fine men and women too numerous to name, but all fondly appreciated.

Eventually a team drawn from MEC and ECMG grew to as many as 26 people who learned to cooperate and to support each other. For instance surgeons might alternate cases in one OR, but typically the non-operating surgeon would sit nearby in kinship and in case their input was needed in a difficult case. It was largely that kinship that kept people coming back year after year, beyond the satisfaction of giving service. Similar relations developed in the clinic.

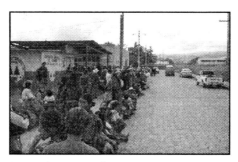

Patients line up outside

In 2001 Barbara Ford was assassinated while in Guatemala City to pick up a water heater. Her assassins staged the event to look like a robbery. Her loss was felt by many. Amnesty International notes that *"a blight of organized crime and corruption....has seeped out of criminal networks formed by veterans of the Guatemalan Army that ravaged the country in its long civil war....creating a Corporate Mafia State."* (Ref: Showdown in Guatemala, Editorial Board, NYT 9/4/17). Project team members could not help but notice that in later years our transportation personnel, hired privately by the Project, carried side arms. For safety reasons Project Guatemala was discontinued after 2011.

The Maya are one of the 5 founding civilizations of the world, prosperous and complex enough long ago to have developed their own script independent of any other civilization. They knew in ancient times that the earth went around the sun. It was news to most of the team to learn that this ancient culture yet exists, and a thrill to hear that old language spoken. Thanks and gratitude to the Kíché people for all that they have revealed to us in our time with them.

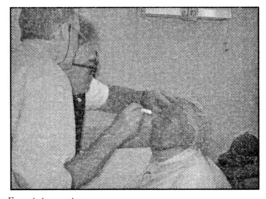

Examining patient

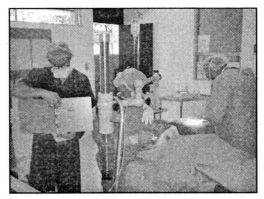

Surgery

Global Health Activities of Maine Medical Center Department of Family Medicine

Alain Montegut MD

"To reap a return in ten years, plant trees.
To reap a return in 100, cultivate the people."
Ho Chi Minh

The Department of Family Medicine of the Maine Medical Center over a journey of almost 30 years has participated in the development of primary care in several regions of the world. It has done so through teaching, advocacy, and mentoring. Just as it has contributed to the growth of family medicine and health care in the United States, it has also embraced its responsibility to improve health globally.

In 1989, the Department of Family Medicine (DFM) began a long journey in global health through its support of the work that the Maine Academy of Family Physicians (MAFP) was doing as a consultant to the Ministry of Health in the USSR. The MAFP and Maine Medical Center (MMC) provided consultations and partners to establish a collaborative team that assisted the USSR and then the Russian Federation to create the specialty of family medicine in 1992. These efforts were led by Drs. John Randall, Alain Montegut and David Massanari. This in turn led to assistance in creating the first family medicine (FM) post-graduate training program at the I. M. Sechenov Moscow Medical Academy the following year. This project was completed in 1995.

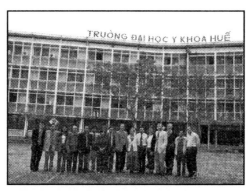

MMC Family Medicine team at Hue University

In 1994 a Division of International Family Medicine Education (DIFME/Division) was established within the Department of Family Medicine by Dr. Robert McArtor. Alain Montegut was named the Director. In 2005, DIFME changed its name to the

Division of International Health Improvement (DIHI). It did so to better reflect its vision and mission and to recognize the designs of the consulting work it was doing.

In 1995, the Division began discussions with the Ministry of Health (MOH), Vietnam to consult about their vision for primary health care reform. This led to a four-year grant from the McKnight Foundation for a needs assessment. This work included multiple visits to both urban and rural areas of Vietnam, discussions and interviews with medical school leaders, practicing physicians and patients. The MMC faculty involved included Drs. Alain Montegut, Steve Cummings and Ann Skelton. As well Julie Schirmer and Cynthia Cartwright made significant contributions. This team engaged in teaching activities, advocacy and regular meetings with the Ministry of Health. The needs assessment was completed in March 2000 with a report to the Ministry of Health. This resulted in the creation of family medicine as a specialty in Vietnam.

The Division was then invited by the MOH, Vietnam to propose a project that would lead to enhancements in primary health care education and delivery. The Vietnam Family Medicine Development Project, was proposed, accepted and then funded in 2001. The grant was awarded from the China Medical Board, Inc. The goal of the project was to develop a network of three medical universities that would develop and implement a training program for the new specialty of family medicine. The duration of the grant was for five years.

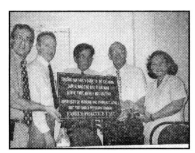

Dr. Le Hoang Ninh (MMC FM Fellow)
opening first Family Medicine clinic in Vietnam-
with Alain Montegut, Steve Cummings and Robert Higgins

The Division provided consulting teams to the Vietnamese network, provided faculty development, assisted in the creation of a new curriculum, supervised implementation of the new training model and assisted graduates with return to practice. It hosted many Vietnamese physicians both in yearlong fellowships at MMC and in short term learning activities. It developed and led a consortium of US residencies to partner with each of the new residency programs in Vietnam including Boston University and

University of Massachusetts. In 2003, a grant from the Unocal Foundation funded the addition of a fourth medical university to join the project and the Maine Dartmouth program was recruited as a consortium partner. This was facilitated by a team from the Maine Dartmouth Residency including Drs. Jim Schneid, Bill Alto and Dan Meyer. A grant from the New York Life Foundation permitted the beginning of evaluation of the project.

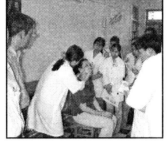

Teaching in outpatient setting in 2000

An expanded primary health care manpower development project was funded for DIHI from the China Medical Board for an additional five years in Vietnam This grant was awarded to assist the Hanoi Medical University to develop a Primary Health Care Faculty Development Training Center. This new model was to train teachers of family medicine to the MSc and eventually PhD level for lifelong careers in academic family medicine departments within medical schools throughout the country. This grant also funded the development of both an urban and a rural training site.

Behavioral medicine became noted as a need in Vietnam. Under the guidance of Julie Schirmer and Dr. George Dreher from MMC, the MOH developed curriculum and training programs for behavioral medicine in primary care. This team continued its collaboration with other ministries in Vietnam to enhance the care of the underserved population of people with mental illness.

In 2005, DIHI was awarded a large grant through the Atlantic Philanthropic Foundation to develop a rural retraining program in Vietnam and integrate the University of Hue into the national training network. This grant also led to the integration of the last three medical universities in Vietnam into the network, such that by 2007, all of the medical universities in Vietnam were engaged in the training of family medicine specialists.

In 2004, the Division performed a needs assessment in Cambodia for primary health care changes and in 2005, did the same in Laos. Consultation was requested and given to the Ministry of Health, People's Republic of China and the Association of Medical Colleges and Universities of China in 2005. This consultation was to assist in the revision of the primary health care education model.

Foreign Medical Missions

The initial needs assessment consultation in Laos led to a five-year grant from the China Medical Board to enhance primary health care training programs in Laos. This effort was led by Dr. Christina Holt. DIHI worked with the Faculty of Medical Sciences in Vientiane to provide faculty development, create curriculum enhancements to train physicians at the central level and in three rural provinces to upgrade their knowledge, skills and attitudes in the newly designed Family Medicine Training Program.

Family Medicine residents joined the MMC faculty teams mentor new residents in Vietnam. These experiences also allowed them to enhance their knowledge and skills in developing cultural competence. These activities blended well with the Department's curriculum in enhancing cultural awareness through its work with medical students and residents in the US.

This 20-year relationship that the faculty of the MMC Department of Family Medicine has had with the universities in Vietnam is the longest sustainable Family Medicine Development Project in the world. Over the last decade, the DFM has remained engaged in the continued development and expansion of the specialty in Vietnam. It has supported curriculum revisions, faculty development and advocacy for enhancing access to primary care for all patients in Vietnam.

Since 1990, the faculty of the Department of Family Medicine has taken a leadership role in the development of primary care in many parts of the world. It has cultivated promising leaders, young physicians and interested organizations to understand the importance of primary care and the need for training of competent primary care physicians and health care teams. It continues to enhance health care for all and cultural competency for our learners through the discipline of Family Medicine.